CHILDREN'S HEALTH, THE NATION'S WEALTH

ASSESSING AND IMPROVING CHILD HEALTH

Committee on Evaluation of Children's Health

Board on Children, Youth, and Families
Division of Behavioral and Social Sciences and Education

NATIONAL RESEARCH COUNCIL *AND*
INSTITUTE OF MEDICINE
OF THE NATIONAL ACADEMIES

THE NATIONAL ACADEMIES PRESS
Washington, D.C.
www.nap.edu

THE NATIONAL ACADEMIES PRESS   500 Fifth Street, N.W.   Washington, DC 20001

NOTICE: The project that is the subject of this report was approved by the Governing Board of the National Research Council, whose members are drawn from the councils of the National Academy of Sciences, the National Academy of Engineering, and the Institute of Medicine. The members of the committee responsible for the report were chosen for their special competences and with regard for appropriate balance.

This study was supported by contract number 282-99-0045, task order number 6 between the National Academy of Sciences and the Department of Health and Human Services. Supplementary funding for a report synthesis and dissemination of the report and report synthesis was supported by contract number N-01-OD-4-2139, task order number 125. Any opinions, findings, conclusions, or recommendations expressed in this publication are those of the author(s) and do not necessarily reflect the views of the organizations or agencies that provided support for the project.

Library of Congress Cataloging-in-Publication Data

Children's health, the nation's wealth : assessing and improving child health / Committee on Evaluation of Children's Health, Board on Children, Youth, and Families, Division of Behavioral and Social Sciences and Education.
  p. ; cm.
 Includes bibliographical references and index.
 ISBN 0-309-09118-7 (hardcover)
 1. Children—Health and hygiene—United States. 2. Child health services—United States.
 [DNLM: 1. Public Health—Child—United States. 2. Child Welfare—United States. 3. Data Collection—methods—United States. 4. Health Policy—Child—United States. 5. Research Design—United States. WA 320 C5379 2004] I. National Research Council (U.S.). Committee on Evaluation of Children's Health.
 RJ102.C4895 2004
 362.198'92'000973—dc22

                    2004016741

Additional copies of this report are available from National Academies Press, 500 Fifth Street, N.W., Lockbox 285, Washington, DC 20055; (800) 624-6242 or (202) 334-3313 (in the Washington metropolitan area); Internet, http://www.nap.edu.

Printed in the United States of America.

Suggested citation: National Research Council and Institute of Medicine. (2004). *Children's Health, the Nation's Wealth: Assessing and Improving Child Health.* Committee on Evaluation of Children's Health. Board on Children, Youth, and Families, Division of Behavioral and Social Sciences and Education. Washington, DC: The National Academies Press.

THE NATIONAL ACADEMIES
Advisers to the Nation on Science, Engineering, and Medicine

The **National Academy of Sciences** is a private, nonprofit, self-perpetuating society of distinguished scholars engaged in scientific and engineering research, dedicated to the furtherance of science and technology and to their use for the general welfare. Upon the authority of the charter granted to it by the Congress in 1863, the Academy has a mandate that requires it to advise the federal government on scientific and technical matters. Dr. Bruce M. Alberts is president of the National Academy of Sciences.

The **National Academy of Engineering** was established in 1964, under the charter of the National Academy of Sciences, as a parallel organization of outstanding engineers. It is autonomous in its administration and in the selection of its members, sharing with the National Academy of Sciences the responsibility for advising the federal government. The National Academy of Engineering also sponsors engineering programs aimed at meeting national needs, encourages education and research, and recognizes the superior achievements of engineers. Dr. Wm. A. Wulf is president of the National Academy of Engineering.

The **Institute of Medicine** was established in 1970 by the National Academy of Sciences to secure the services of eminent members of appropriate professions in the examination of policy matters pertaining to the health of the public. The Institute acts under the responsibility given to the National Academy of Sciences by its congressional charter to be an adviser to the federal government and, upon its own initiative, to identify issues of medical care, research, and education. Dr. Harvey V. Fineberg is president of the Institute of Medicine.

The **National Research Council** was organized by the National Academy of Sciences in 1916 to associate the broad community of science and technology with the Academy's purposes of furthering knowledge and advising the federal government. Functioning in accordance with general policies determined by the Academy, the Council has become the principal operating agency of both the National Academy of Sciences and the National Academy of Engineering in providing services to the government, the public, and the scientific and engineering communities. The Council is administered jointly by both Academies and the Institute of Medicine. Dr. Bruce M. Alberts and Dr. Wm. A. Wulf are chair and vice chair, respectively, of the National Research Council.

www.national-academies.org

Acknowledgments

T his report is the work of the Committee on Evaluation of Children's Health, a project of the National Research Council (NRC) and the Institute of Medicine. The expertise and hard work of the committee was advanced by the help of our sponsor, able consultants and staff, and the input of outside experts. The funding for this project was provided by the Office of Disease Prevention and Health Promotion of the U.S. Department of Health and Human Services. Woodie Kessel served as project officer and provided valuable insights and guidance in framing the project. The National Institute of Child Health and Human Development provided supplementary funding to print and disseminate the report and a report brief summarizing the report's findings.

The committee's early meetings included presentations by experts in a range of disciplines as well as representatives from other federal government offices: Duane Alexander, National Institute of Child Health and Human Development; Brett Brown, Child Trends; Merry Bullock, American Psychological Association; John Cohrssen, Public Health Policy Advisory Board; Jose Cordero, National Center on Birth Defects and Developmental Disabilities, Centers for Disease Control and Prevention; Michael Donnelly, Integrated Health Information Systems, Centers for Disease Control and Prevention; Lauren Fasig, Society for Research in Child Development; Lynn Goldman, Children's Environmental Health Network; Wayne Holden, OCR Macro; Eric Kodish, Rainbow Center for Pediatric Ethics; Kristin A. Moore, Child Trends; Tom Sinks, National Center for Environmental Health, Centers for Disease Control and Prevention; Sandra Tirey, American Chemistry Council; Peter van Dyck, Maternal and Child Health Bureau, Health Resources and Services Administration; Rachael Wallace, Children's National

Medical Center; and Randolph Wykoff, Office of Disease Prevention and Health Promotion, U.S. Department of Health and Human Services.

The committee commissioned papers that provided information incorporated into this report from Eric Kodish and Rachael Wallace; Howard Frumkin, Emory University; and Elizabeth Vandewater, University of Texas. We wish to thank Brett Brown for providing the framework and core information on data sources included in Appendix A and Greg Stevens of the Center for Healthier Children, Families and Communities, University of California at Los Angeles (UCLA), for preparing the analysis of major national surveys included as Appendix B.

In addition, several experts helped prepare background or related materials that were incorporated into this report, and we wish to acknowledge their advice and assistance: Lee Pachter, St. Francis Hospital and Medical Center; Deborah Klein Walker, Abt Associates (formerly Center for Health Information, Statistics, Research and Evaluation, Massachusetts Department of Public Health); and Ellen Wartella, College of Communication, University of Texas, Austin.

Matthew Zerden, a research associate at the UCLA Center for Healthier Children, Families and Communities, provided valuable assistance in confirming references. Camelia Arsene and Jennifer Roberts, National Academies interns, helped manage and identify references and provided valuable research assistance.

This report has been reviewed in draft form by individuals chosen for their diverse perspectives and technical expertise, in accordance with procedures approved by the NRC's Report Review Committee. The purpose of this independent review is to provide candid and critical comments that will assist the institution in making its published report as sound as possible and to ensure that the report meets institutional standards for objectivity, evidence, and responsiveness to the study charge. The review comments and draft manuscript remain confidential to protect the integrity of the deliberative process.

We wish to thank the following individuals for their review of this report: Beverly Bauman, Department of Emergency Medicine and Department of Pediatrics, Oregon Health and Sciences University; Janet Currie, Department of Economics, UCLA; Allen J. Dietrich, Community and Family Medicine, Dartmouth Medical School; Andrew S. Doniger, Monroe County Health Department, Rochester, NY; Lynn R. Goldman, Occupational and Environmental Health, Johns Hopkins Bloomberg School of Public Health; Tamara Halle, Early Childhood Development, Child Trends, Washington, DC; Marie C. McCormick, Department of Society, Human Development and Health, Harvard School of Public Health; Susan Redline, Pediatrics, Medicine, and Epidemiology and Biostatistics, Case Western Reserve University and Rainbow Babies and Children's Hospital, Cleveland, OH; Lynn Singer, Provost's Office and Department of Pediatrics and Psychiatry, Case Western Reserve University and Rainbow Babies and Children's Hospital, Cleveland, OH; Richard D. Todd, Child and Adolescent Psychiatry, Washington University School of Medicine; and Deborah Klein Walker, Abt Associates (formerly Center for Health Information, Statistics, Research and Evaluation, Massachusetts Department of Public Health).

Although the reviewers listed above have provided many constructive comments and suggestions, they were not asked to endorse the conclusions or recommendations nor did they see the final draft of the report before its release. The review of this report was overseen by Aletha C. Huston, Human Development and Family Science, The University of Texas at Austin, and John C. Bailar, III, Department of Health Studies (emeritus), University of Chicago. Appointed by the NRC, they were responsible for making certain that an independent examination of this report was carried out in accordance with institutional procedures and that all review comments were carefully considered. Responsibility for the final content of this report rests entirely with the authoring committee and the institution.

The committee appreciates the support provided by members of the Board on Children, Youth, and Families under the leadership of Michael I. Cohen. We are grateful for the leadership and support of Michael Feuer, executive director of the NRC's Division of Behavioral and Social Sciences and Education; Jane Ross, director of the Center for Economic, Governance, and International Studies; Rosemary Chalk, director of the Board on Children, Youth, and Families and her predecessor, Susan Cummins; and Susanne Stoiber, executive officer of the Institute of Medicine.

Finally, the committee benefited from the support and assistance of several members of the National Academies staff. Bill Selepack (until April 2002 and between October 2002 and April 2003) and Anthony Mann (between April and October 2002 and since April 2003) managed all administrative aspects of the project. The research needs of the project were greatly aided by the able assistance of William McLeod of the Institute of Medicine library. Final preparation of the report, including incorporating edits, helping to respond to review comments, and finalizing references, was handled with grace, competence, and patience by Elizabeth Townsend and Neesha Desai. We are indebted to Christine McShane who provided superb editorial guidance, Yvonne Wise, who helped prepare the report for publication, and Kirsten Sampson Snyder, who guided the report through the review and release process.

Greg Duncan, *Cochair*
Ruth E.K. Stein, *Cochair*
Mary Ellen O'Connell, *Study Director*
Committee on Evaluation of Children's Health

Contents

Executive Summary   1
1   Introduction   13
2   Children's Health: A New Conceptual Framework   28
3   Influences on Children's Health   45
4   Measuring Children's Health   91
5   Measuring Influences on Children's Health   116
6   Developing State and Local Data Systems   164
7   Conclusions and Recommendations   192
References   211

Appendixes
A   Datasets for Measuring Children's Health and
    Influences on Children's Health   253
B   Gaps Analysis of Measures of Children's Health and Influences
    on Children's Health in Select National Surveys   262
C   Selected Indicators from National Children's Data Syntheses   288
D   Glossary   302
E   Acronyms   305
F   Biographical Sketches of Committee Members and Staff   308

Index   315

Executive Summary

Many things we need can wait. The child cannot. Now is the time his bones are being formed, his blood is being made, his mind is being developed. To him we cannot say tomorrow, his name is today.

Gabriela Mistral

Despite substantial progress in improving children's health, communities vary considerably in the ways they address their collective commitment to children and their health. This results in part from a lack of appreciation of the short- and long-term implications of suboptimal health and in part from the fact that the nation's systems for monitoring and optimizing the health of its children are inadequate. This report seeks to address and remedy those issues.

It is in the national interest to have healthy children. Healthy children are more ready and able to learn and, in the longer term, are more likely to become healthy adults who will contribute as a productive citizenry and workforce to the continued vitality of society. Health surveillance and monitoring systems have evolved largely from models of health based on preventing and treating childhood morbidity and mortality that resulted primarily from infectious diseases, as well as monitoring chronic diseases among adults. Future systems need to incorporate a refined conceptualization of children's health that considers prominent developmental characteristics of children as well as positive aspects of health, and they should include new methods for assessing both children's health and its influences. To ensure healthy children and create a healthy nation, meaningful information must be collected to support a broader conceptualization of health; this information must be used by federal, state, and local decision makers to inform interventions, programs, and policies.

In earlier eras, disease and death in children were due largely to infections. Childhood deaths were common. Childhood mortality and infectious disease rates in America have been radically lowered over the past century. These medical

1

triumphs are significant, and the medical and public health systems should take pride in what has been accomplished. Despite these accomplishments, however, there are growing numbers of children in the United States with serious chronic diseases, including many emerging disorders that reflect the interaction of genetics, behavior, and the environment. Childhood obesity, diabetes, and asthma rates are among the highest in the world and are increasing rapidly. Intentional and unintentional injuries, mental health disorders, and attention deficit disorder are highly prevalent. Moreover, many of these conditions are not equally distributed across the population; some groups experience substantially higher rates than others. Finally, the long-term consequences of these disorders are significant, because unhealthy children often become unhealthy adults. Health during childhood must be a major concern both because children are important in their own right and because the nation cannot thrive if it has large numbers of unhealthy adults.

THE COMMITTEE STUDY

In response to a congressional request, the Board on Children, Youth, and Families of the National Research Council and the Institute of Medicine formed the Committee on Evaluation of Children's Health: Measures of Risk, Protective, and Promotional Factors for Assessing Child Health in the Community. The committee was directed to review definitions of children's health, factors that influence it, the data and methods used to monitor children's health and the factors that affect it, and how data can be used to inform policy and practice. The committee used the term "children" to refer to the period between birth and 18 years and focused on population-level issues. Although data to monitor population health are often collected at the level of the individual, the committee's focus is on the health of local, state, and national populations of children.

In beginning our work and reviewing the available literature, the committee agreed on six guiding principles:

- children are vital assets of society;
- critical differences between children and adults warrant special attention to children's health;
- children's health has effects that reach far into adulthood;
- the manifestations of health vary for different communities and different cultures; and
- data on children's health and its influences are needed to maximize the health of children and the health of the adults they will become.

FRAMEWORK FOR A CHILDREN'S HEALTH MEASUREMENT SYSTEM

Over the past century, the United States has instituted important health monitoring and surveillance activities. It also has adopted important research strategies to better understand the influence of various factors on health outcomes. A measurement system for children's health, building on what has already been achieved, should be able to:

- Measure and monitor important trends in health and its influences. These measures would span the developmental stages of childhood and be gathered from important subgroups defined by ethnicity, income, geographic region, and special needs (e.g., children with chronic conditions, in foster care, in special education).
- Provide a surveillance and early warning capacity for the detection of significant changes in health, as well as increase the capacity to forecast the effect of changing influences on children's health and anticipate the need for specific services and interventions.
- Improve understanding of the mechanisms of children's development and determine how changes in behavior, new health practices, and new policy interventions affect children's health.
- Measure the performance of the personal medical care system, relevant community service systems, and the broader public health system and how they affect children's health. Such activities would not only measure the quality of services, but also encourage the improvement of the integration and coordination of personal, community, and public health services.

CONCLUSIONS AND RECOMMENDATIONS

The committee identified five action areas to move toward a comprehensive children's health measurement system:

1. establishing a definition and framework for children's health;
2. establishing children's health as a national priority;
3. improving measurement of children's health;
4. increasing state and local leadership and use of data; and
5. promoting research to better understand children's health and its influences.

This report is intended to provide a foundation and a framework for children's health measurement rather than specific measures to monitor children's health. Appendix B provides a review of the approaches taken by key national surveys, and Appendix C summarizes many of the indicators used in national monitoring efforts.

Definition and Framework

Few existing definitions of health are specific to children, and none accounts fully for issues particularly salient to them: the developmental process; how biological, behavioral, and environmental influences are embedded in developing biological pathways during sensitive and critical periods of development; the vulnerabilities and sources of resilience of growing children; and the implications for health and health influences in one stage for all subsequent life stages, during both childhood and adulthood. Children interact with their environments in ways different from adults; their body size and behaviors make them more susceptible to some environmental influences; and, particularly in their early years, they are more dependent on their families and communities to meet their needs than adults.

The committee developed a definition of health that builds on the definition adopted by the Ottawa Charter in 1986. While this definition emphasizes health as a positive construct and accounts for the positive attributes, capacities, and reserves that determine how well an individual or population is able to respond to the challenges that life presents, it is more appropriate for adults than for children. The committee modified the Ottawa definition in light of research on developmental processes that affect health, especially for children, and to acknowledge that children's health results from a range of influences.

Recommendation 1: Children's health should be defined as the extent to which individual children or groups of children are able or enabled to (a) develop and realize their potential, (b) satisfy their needs, and (c) develop the capacities that allow them to interact successfully with their biological, physical, and social environments.

Based on current thinking, the committee's expertise, and current research on children's health, the committee further defined three distinct but related domains of health: health conditions, which capture disorders or illnesses of body systems; functioning, which focuses on the manifestation of health on an individual's daily life; and health potential, which captures the development of assets and positive aspects of health, such as competence, capacity, and developmental potential.

There are a variety of potential schemes for classifying health influences. It is generally acknowledged that factors in children's social and physical environments, as well as the services and policy contexts in which they live, affect their health. Research demonstrates that these factors interact with children's own biology and behavior to determine health. One visual model that illustrates the interaction of multiple factors on health is that adopted by the *Healthy People 2010* initiative. The committee refined this model of health to illustrate that multiple influences interact over time and that the relative weight of those influences and interactions changes in relationship to a child's developmental stage. At each stage the previous set of influences and health set the stage for the effects of future influences and health (Figure ES-1).

While much has been learned about children's development and how specific factors influence it and are embedded in biopsychosocial pathways, increased

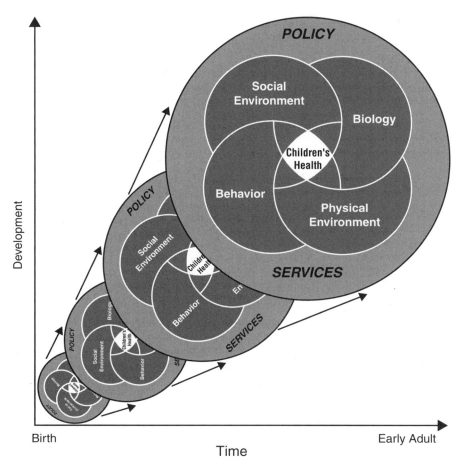

FIGURE ES-1 A new model of children's health and its influences.

understanding is important if cost-effective programs and policy interventions are to be developed, targeted, and implemented to support healthy children.

A National Priority

It is necessary for a single federal-level agency to take lead responsibility for measuring and monitoring children's health and its influences. The majority of relevant data is collected by offices in the Department of Health and Human Services (HHS), the lead federal agency on health issues. This includes the Maternal and Child Health Bureau in the Health Resources and Services Administration, the National Center for Health Statistics and other offices in the Centers for

Disease Control and Prevention, the Agency for Healthcare Research and Quality, the Office of Disease Prevention and Health Promotion and the Office of the Assistant Secretary for Planning and Evaluation in the Office of the Secretary, the National Institute for Child Health and Human Development and other units in the National Institutes of Health, and the Administration for Children and Families. Coordination among these agencies and with the other federal departments who collect data and fund services or research that affect children's health is essential to minimize duplication, increase efficiency, and ensure that data collection focuses on the most important variables.

Recommendation 2: The secretary of the U.S. Department of Health and Human Services (HHS) should designate a specific HHS unit with a focus on children to address development, coordination, standardization, and validation of data across the multiple HHS data collection agencies, to support state-level use of data, and to facilitate coordination across federal departments. The designated agency's long-term mission should be to:

- **monitor each of the domains of children's health (i.e., health conditions, functioning, and health potential) and its influences over time;**
- **develop the means to track children's health and identify patterns (e.g., trajectories) in it over time, both for individual children and for populations and subpopulations of children; and**
- **understand the interaction and relative effects of multiple influences on children's health over time.**

The designated unit should (1) translate recommendations on domains, subdomains, and dimensions of health and its influences into improved data collection strategies; (2) identify duplication and gaps in data collection efforts and develop recommendations to make data collection efforts more economical and standardized; (3) ensure that necessary data validation efforts are carried out; (4) ensure that as many data collection activities as possible are usable at the state and substate levels; (5) ensure that thoroughly documented data are released on as timely a basis as possible; (6) develop a process for assessing the potential effect of key policy changes on children's health; and (7) facilitate continued research, particularly longitudinal research, on children's health and its influences.

Improving Children's Health Measurement

Although numerous national surveys collect relevant data on children's health, serious gaps remain. Health is not measured in sufficient detail to distinguish the special developmental issues of infants and toddlers (ages 0–3 years), preschool children (4–5), school-age children (6–11), early adolescents (12–14), and older adolescents (15–18). Data on children between toddlerhood and adolescence are especially lacking. Surveys usually do not capture information on multiple individual and environmental influences necessary to improve under-standing of the interactive nature of health influences. Data on functioning and health potential, integral to a broader conceptualization of health, are particularly deficient. Biomarkers and environmental samples, important measures of envi-ronmental toxins, are not usually included in survey studies. Oversampling to ensure sufficient numbers of respondents in racial, ethnic, and socioeconomic subgroups is common in many but not all general population surveys, and most instruments and measures are not validated with major population subgroups.

It is unlikely that the nation will scrap its existing system of children's health measurement and design an entirely new system. However, improvements to existing measurement systems, coupled with continued rigorous research, can provide a solid foundation for analysis and action related to children's health. The committee recommends immediate action in several areas:

- Improved data collection in selected national surveys;
- Improved monitoring of the origins and development of health disparities among children and youth;
- Continued collection of local-area data and linking of those data with other data sources;
- Increased inclusion of geographic identifiers in health-related surveys and administrative data;
- Improved access to survey and record-based sources of health informa-tion by the research and planning communities; and
- Increased federal support of state and local monitoring of children's health and its influences.

Longitudinal surveys are needed to determine the relative contribution and roles played by individual and contextual characteristics in overall health. Such surveys should be a priority of federal and foundation funders. Comprehensive data collection projects also should oversample disadvantaged groups; begin to track children early in life; conduct frequent interviews and assessments with these children throughout childhood and into adulthood; measure assets as well as deficits; provide comprehensive measurement of all contexts that affect chil-dren's health; measure gene-behavior-environment and other contextual interac-tions; and chart health and disease trajectories and the relative contribution of various influences on health outcomes.

Data Collection in Select National Surveys

Existing data collection vehicles can be modified to provide more useful data over time (e.g., repeated cross-sectional data) and more comprehensive informa-tion. As a short-term response, this could include follow-back studies and addition of specific comparable health measures to the most comprehensive current surveys.

Recommendation 3: National surveys of health and health influences, such as the National Health Interview Survey, the National Health and Nutrition Examination Survey, the Early Childhood Longitudinal Studies, and the National Children's Study initiative, should address gaps in what is now collected and reported to reflect a more comprehensive, developmentally oriented conceptualization of children's health and its influences. Particular attention should be paid to adding data on functioning and health potential.

Monitoring of the Origins and Development of Health Disparities

Although in the committee's view policy makers should attend to the needs of all children, certain subgroups of children defined by race, ethnicity, immigration status, and socioeconomic status experience poorer health outcomes and receipt of services in ways that affect their future potential for healthy, productive adulthood. The factors leading to the development of health differences at all socioeconomic levels are poorly understood, although many have origins early in life. Better information and more conclusive evidence are needed to target interventions and to design effective policies to ameliorate these disparities. There also are differences in how various cultural and ethnic groups interpret symptoms and signs of disease that, in turn, alter their interpretation of inquiries about health and patterns of services.

Despite a large body of research on health disparities across subgroups defined by socioeconomic status, standards have not been established to characterize socioeconomic status across surveys and administrative records; the same is true for social discrimination and the effects of culture. However, ample methodological research has led to thoughtful recommendations on how surveys and administrative records could gather reliable measures of the education, household income, or occupational dimensions of socioeconomic status.

Recommendation 4: National and state surveys and records-based sources of data on children's health and its influences should gather systematic, standardized data on racial, ethnic, immigration, and socioeconomic classifications in order to measure the origins, distribution, and development of disparities in children's health and facilitate linkage and analysis across multiple datasets.

Collection and Linkage of Local-Level Data

An emerging body of evidence demonstrates a clear association between health and aspects of geographic location, such as neighborhood socioeconomic conditions, crime and cohesion, ambient noise, traffic flow, and air quality. Efforts to monitor and understand environmental influences on children's health have been facilitated by the systematic collection of regional, neighborhood, and community-level information. Demographic and economic data about neighborhoods (e.g., census tracts), communities, cities, and states have been collected and made available to planners and researchers every 10 years as part of the decennial census. The emerging American Community Survey has been proposed as the vehicle for more frequent collection of these detailed local data. Continued collection of these data is vital. Other local and regional environmental data are also necessary for health planners and researchers to specify gradients in the impact of different influences. Improving the availability of data at the neighborhood, community, or regional level can improve the ability of a local community to target its own efforts and institute community-specific interventions. (See recommendations 8, 9, and 10 for additional recommendations affecting state efforts to monitor and improve children's health.)

> **Recommendation 5: Federal agencies and departments, particularly the Environmental Protection Agency and the U.S. Department of Health and Human Services, should promote the systematic collection, dissemination, and linkage of data on children's exposure to toxins, air pollution, and other environmental conditions, as well as data on policies likely to affect children's health. The Census Bureau should continue to collect and distribute local-area data and facilitate efforts to match these data to existing sources of information on children's health and its influences.**

The geographic dimension of health patterns can be exploited only if subjects' locations (e.g., home, school, workplace addresses) have been coded with geographic identifiers and these geocoded data are made available to the planning and research communities.

> **Recommendation 6: Government and private agencies and academic organizations that conduct health-related surveys or compile administrative data should geocode addresses (i.e., provide geographic identifiers) in ways that facilitate linkages to census-based and other neighborhood, community, city, and state data on environmental conditions. With adequate protections to ensure the confidentiality and security of individual data, they should also make geocoded data as accessible as possible to the research and planning communities.**

Access to Data by Research and Planning Communities

The importance of maintaining the confidentiality and privacy of data on specific individuals is clear. In the case of health data, specific rules govern the acquisition and use of data. Data are necessary, however, to inform and guide public decisions and to advance public health knowledge. Administrative data *can* be integrated without identifying specific children, data security protocols *are* in place, and access to individual-level data *is* limited. Many surveys and records systems have been linked using geographic identifiers with mechanisms to both safeguard data and make them available to the research and planning communities. Yet these mechanisms are not as widely used as they could be.

> **Recommendation 7: Administrators of survey and records-based sources of health information should take all necessary legal, ethical, and technical steps to ensure respondent or subject confidentiality while also promoting the availability of needed data to the research and planning communities.**

Federal Support for State and Local Monitoring

Technical, methodological, and measurement challenges common at the state and local levels define a role for the federal government in convening and supporting efforts to reengineer state and local health information systems. This could include providing guidance on standardized data collection; funding demonstration projects that use standardized data collection methods, aggregating data by local geographic units, and providing deidentified data on readily accessible web sites; and providing technical assistance.

> **Recommendation 8: The U.S. Department of Health and Human Services should formulate strategies to improve the capacity of state and local communities to monitor children's health and its influences, including funding state or local demonstration projects, standardization of data elements, and technical assistance.**

State and Local Leadership and Use of Data

At the state and local levels, numerous agencies provide services to children and collect data relevant to children's health or its influences. To maximize use of these data to guide state and local decisions about interventions and policies and to inform communities about the status of children's health, it is necessary to have a single agency at the state and local levels responsible for monitoring children's health and reporting the results to policy makers and the public. This may be the state or local health department, a children's cabinet, or a senior official appointed by the governor or mayor. Most important are the mandates to relevant agencies to provide relevant data, institutionalize responsibility for coordinating data efforts, and use the data to promote and evaluate children's health.

> **Recommendation 9: Governors, mayors, and county executives should designate a central coordinating agency responsible for measurement and monitoring of children's health across agencies, as well as an individual responsible for reporting on progress toward integrating data on children's**

health. The state coordinating agency should facilitate use of standardized data at the local level.

Although there have been increased efforts at the federal, state, and local levels to collect state- or local-level data, comprehensive state- and local-level measurement of children's health is still relatively uncommon. Substantial administrative data are collected and have been used by some states and communities to characterize children's health. Data integration—both aggregation of data from multiple sources and linkage of individual-level data across multiple sources—is an available mechanism to improve children's health in specific communities. Data standardization, provision of data at the smallest feasible geographic level, and targeted surveys to fill gaps in data, ideally drawing on standard models available at the federal level, will be needed as states develop approaches to integrating data sources.

> **Recommendation 10: The designated state and local coordinating agencies should advance strategies for standardizing and integrating records, including available administrative records and survey data, to maximize their potential for monitoring children's health and understanding its influences.**

Promoting Research

Great strides have been made in conceptualizing the dynamic processes by which external influences interact with individuals' biology and behavior over the course of childhood. Still, additional research is needed to refine understanding of specific influences, to take advantage of new technologies for measurement, and to further advance understanding of children's health. There is a particular need for comprehensive, longitudinal surveys. The value of biomarker data is substantial, particularly as their collection and genomic testing become less invasive. More needs to be known about the relative importance of the range of influences, including the exposure of children to the large number of chemicals introduced into their environments. Valid and reliable measures are needed to assess the influence of culture and discrimination on children's health. Efforts should also be made to support application of newly developed statistical strategies using longitudinal data and to train researchers in the use of these methods. Finally, research is needed to translate potentially effective measures used primarily for research purposes into wider application for population health measurement and policy development.

> **Recommendation 11: The U.S. Department of Health and Human Services and the Environmental Protection Agency should prioritize research and training on emerging methods for characterizing children's health and understanding influences on it, including research on:**

- creation of improved measures of functioning and health potential;
- the relative importance of and interactions among the range of influences;
- biopsychosocial pathways of development;
- assessment of children's exposures to environmental toxins and other environmental health hazards;
- reasons and remedies for health disparities;
- longitudinal methods that can identify causal relationships between developmental and functional levels and the health status of children;
- development of profiles and integrative measures of children's health; and
- construction of trajectories for each domain of children's health.

In sum, health extends beyond traditional notions of disease and disability and is influenced by myriad factors external to the individual. Conceptualizations of health have generally not considered development as part of health. The committee has proposed both a definition of health and a framework that portrays these interactions. New measures need to be developed that capture the multidimensional nature of children's health.

Although numerous data collection efforts capture data on children's health and health influences, none has kept pace with the evolving understanding of health, and none provides a complete understanding of the interactions between and across influences. Comprehensive, longitudinal surveys are essential to filling critical gaps in data collection. More immediate, short-term approaches could include modifications to existing surveys and better use of extensive administrative data at the state and local levels. Regardless, efforts to improve collection of data need to be supported by additional research that will address key gaps in knowledge (such as limited understanding of disparities in health) and advancing children's health research by embracing new methodologies (such as use of biomarkers and improved health measures).

Finally, federal, state, and local governments need to establish a shared vision to focus on children, the nation's most valuable resource. It is time to develop comprehensive ways of assessing the health of children that will foster the nation's ability to nurture and develop its children with all their inherent richness and potential.

1

Introduction

C hildren are vital to the nation's present and its future. Parents, grandparents, aunts, and uncles are usually committed to providing every advantage possible to the children in their families, and to ensuring that they are healthy and have the opportunities that they need to fulfill their potential. Yet communities vary considerably in their commitment to the collective health of children and in the resources that they make available to meet children's needs. This is reflected in the ways in which communities address their collective commitment to children, specifically to their health.

In recent years, there has been an increased focus on issues that affect children and on improving their health. Children have begun to be recognized not only for who they are today but for their future roles in creating families, powering the workforce, and making American democracy work. Mounting evidence that health during childhood sets the stage for adult health not only reinforces this perspective, but also creates an important ethical, social, and economic imperative to ensure that all children are as healthy as they can be. Healthy children are more likely to become healthy adults.

Within this context, it is reasonable to ask what it means for children to be healthy and whether the United States is adequately assessing and monitoring the health of its children. Do available surveillance and monitoring approaches provide the information necessary to ensure that common priorities and shared resources are aligned with children's needs and deployed to optimize their health? Are there ways to improve methods to better guide policies and practices designed to make children healthier? This report addresses these questions.

Children are generally viewed as healthy when they are assessed by adult standards, and there has been a great deal of progress in reducing childhood death and diseases. But the country should not be blinded by these facts—several indicators of children's health point to the need for further improvement, children in the United States do not fare as well as their European counterparts on many aspects of health, and there are marked disparities in health among children in the United States. Recent improvements in children's health need to be sustained and further efforts are needed to optimize it. To accomplish this, the nation must have an improved understanding of the factors that affect health and effective strategies for measuring and using information on children's health. This chapter starts with what is known about the health of children. It then moves to a discussion of why measuring children's health is important. The chapter concludes with an examination of why critical differences between children and adults establish the need for children's health to be held to a standard different from that used for adults.

CHILDREN AND THE STATE OF THEIR HEALTH

Dramatic improvements have occurred over the past several decades in such areas as reducing infant mortality, reducing mortality and morbidity from many infectious diseases and accidental causes, increasing access to health care, and reducing environmental contaminants, such as lead (Centers for Disease Control and Prevention, 1999b, 2000a). There have been steady increases in the proportion of immunized children, and both acute mortality and long-term disabilities resulting from certain infectious diseases have been greatly reduced. Learning how environmental exposure to lead adversely affects children's development contributed to great reductions in ambient lead and significantly reduced childhood blood lead levels (Lanphear, Dietrich, and Berger, 2003). Average concentrations of lead in the blood of children younger than 5 years dropped 78 percent between 1976–1980 and 1992–1994 (U.S. Environmental Protection Agency, 2000a). Fewer adolescents are having babies—in 1999, the teenage pregnancy rate reached the lowest recorded rate since 1976 (Child Trends, 2003). Daily cigarette use fell by over 50 percent (from 10 to 5 percent) among 8th grade students between 1996 and 2002, and by over two-fifths (from 18 to 10 percent) among 10th grade students (Child Trends, 2003).

Yet despite these improvements, some national indicators raise questions about the health of the nation's children and point to the need for continued progress. The children behind each of these statistics face serious barriers to healthy childhoods and healthy, productive adult lives. For example, 12–19 percent of children in the United States have chronic health conditions (Newacheck, Hung, and Wright, 2002; Stein and Silver, 2002), an estimated 15 percent of children and adolescents ages 6–19 years are overweight (National Center for Health Statistics, 2002b), and 1 in 10 children have significant mental health conditions that cause some form of impairment (Satcher, 2001). Despite the country's great wealth, some children are not surviving past childhood. Even with recent improvements in child mortality, approximately 7 out of 1,000 children die before the age of 1 (Federal Interagency Forum on Child and Family Statistics, 2003), and 44 percent of deaths of children between the ages of 1 and 19 are caused by unintentional injuries (Anderson and Smith, 2003).

Children, particularly poor and minority children, are not faring as well as the public might think. The current and future prospects of these children, and the prospects of the nation as a whole, are reduced as a result. The nation needs to consider the significance of statistics such as these and adopt prudent policies to improve children's health if it is to successfully maximize the potential of all its children and ensure the future health of the nation.

Even more distressing than the absolute numbers are the sustained and marked disparities between white children and racial and ethnic minority children, and between children in poorer families and wealthier families. For example, blacks have higher infant mortality (Centers for Disease Control and Prevention, 2002d) and adolescent mortality rates, with the death rate for adolescent males increasing from 1985 to 2000 (125 to 130), while the rate for white adolescents males decreased (105 to 86) (Federal Interagency Forum on Child and Family Statistics, 2003). Teenage pregnancy rates have fallen but blacks still have higher rates than other population groups (Ventura et al., 2003). Hispanic children are more likely than both black children and white children to lack health insurance (Institute of Medicine and National Research Council, 1998) and twice as likely to drop out of school (Martinez and Day, 1999). These and other substantial disadvantages for some groups of children during childhood have major effects both on child health and on adult health outcomes and subsequent health care costs and productivity. These discrepancies are particularly disturbing given projected population changes over the next several decades. While the proportion of children is projected to stay relatively constant (24 percent), the non-Hispanic white child population is projected to decrease from 64 to 55 percent by 2020, while the percentage of Hispanic children is projected to increase from 16 to 22 percent (U.S. Department of Health and Human Services, 2001b).

The health of the U.S. population generally, and children's health in particular, lags behind that of many Western industrialized countries (Shi and Starfield, 2000). For example, while the infant mortality rate has decreased by more than 50 percent in the past two decades, the United States still has an infant mortality rate that is higher than all but 5 other Organisation for Economic Co-operation and Development (OECD) nations (Hungary, Mexico, Poland, the Slavic Republic, and Turkey) (Organisation for Economic Co-operation and Development, 2002). While this might be partly attributable to the more inclusive definition of live birth used in the United States, data suggest that this is not the only factor. An in-depth comparison involving 13 industrialized nations in the mid-1990s showed that the United States ranked worst (13th) in rates of low birthweight. Similar poor rankings for postneonatal mortality (11th) indicate that the poor infant mortality ranking is not a result solely of the high percentage of low-birthweight infants. Postneonatal mortality is less sensitive to low birthweight and more sensitive to receipt of good basic (primary) care (Starfield, 2000b).

In another international comparison, the United States ranked lowest among major industrialized nations on equity of child survival (to age 2) and had the highest probability of dying before age 5 (World Health Organization, 2000). The United States also ranks poorly (23rd) in child (ages 1–14) death rates from injuries among 26 OECD countries (1992–1995 data). Among a subset of 15 of these countries (including Mexico, a developing country by OECD standards), the United States ranks in the worst 5 on 3 of the 5 categories of injury deaths: 11th for motor vehicle injury deaths, 15th for deaths resulting from fire, and 14th for deaths due to homicide (United Nations Children's Fund, 2001).

WHY MEASURING AND USING CHILDREN'S HEALTH DATA ARE IMPORTANT

Measurement and appropriate use of data on children's health and influences on health can help ensure that federal, state, and local policies are based on good information and are designed to enhance the health of children. This will reap benefits for both today's children and the adults they will become. The use of child health reporting systems can improve awareness among policy makers and other stakeholders about the complex needs of children and their families (Halfon, Newacheck, Hughes, and Brindis, 1998). Good measurement and reporting of data as well as judicious integration of data help to target public expenditures and interventions toward identified problem areas and identify areas for further research. Comprehensive tracking systems can help to identify changes in patterns in children's health and to develop appropriate public health responses. For example, recognition of obesity and asthma as significant public health issues might have been facilitated by more comprehensive data collection and monitoring systems that identified changes and the likely correlates of these changes.

At the state and local levels, combining data from multiple sources can increase planning efficiency and provide a more useful picture of children's health. States and localities have used child health tracking systems to target public health insurance enrollment activities (Box 6-4 is one example), to increase immunization rates and receipt of other preventive health services, to identify areas with particularly high incidence of such diseases as cancer, to facilitate case management among the many medical and other service providers sometimes involved in children's lives, and to improve communication across agencies and with legislators and other policy makers (Association of State and Territorial Health Officals, 2003). Measurement systems that consider the relationship of various factors in the family, community, and physical environments also serve as early warning systems about things like toxic neighborhoods, risky family situations, and poor school environments. Monitoring of such influences can help identify the need for policy or other interventions early and, if implemented, avoid poten-tial long-term negative consequences.

Good measurement systems also allow comparison within and across juris-dictions. They facilitate identification of specific geographic areas where health problems are concentrated. The establishment of state and local data systems allows these areas to compare their progress with that of other comparable areas and to identify areas that need improvement. Finally, good data systems at the local, state, and national levels provide early evidence of failures and successes so that more rapid and more targeted modifications can be made in interventions and public policies.

THE COMMITTEE'S STUDY

In 2000, Congress responded to concerns raised about risks to children's health by directing the U.S. Department of Health and Human Services[1] to fund a study by the National Academies. Congress requested the National Academies to conduct "an evaluation on children's health [that would] assess the adequacy of currently available methods for assessing risks to children, identify scientific uncertainties associated with these methods, and develop a prioritized research agenda to reduce such uncertainties and improve risk assessment for children's health and safety."

The Board on Children, Youth, and Families of the National Research Coun-cil and Institute of Medicine in consultation with the Department of Health and Human Services and expert advisers developed a statement of task that expanded this basic charge. The Committee on Evaluation of Children's Health: Measures of Risk, Protective, and Promotional Factors for Assessing Child Health in the Community was formed to examine key issues regarding the definition and mea-surement of children's health, influences that affect children's health, and the optimal use of data on children's health. Specifically, the committee was charged with considering these questions:

1. How is children's health defined? Are these definitions appropriate? If not, what is an appropriate definition of children's health?

2. What data and methods are being used to assess and monitor children's health at the federal, state, and local levels? Are these data and methods adequate and appropriate? If not, what types of data and methods are needed and what are the strategies for their development and application? How could new technolo-gies be used to link individual, family, community, and clinical data to assess and monitor children's health? What are the technical challenges and limitations for linking such data?

---

[1]The Consolidated Appropriations Act 2001 (P.L. 106–554).

3. What are the risk, protective, and promotional factors to children's health, safety, and well-being? What data and methods are used to assess and monitor these factors? Are these data and methods adequate and appropriate? What new assessment tools or methods are needed and what are the strategies for their development and application?

4. Ideally, how should data be used to inform both policy and practice to ensure children's health, safety, and well-being? What are the ethical considerations in obtaining such data and in their application?

The study committee included 13 members with expertise in key areas related to children's health. The committee heard from a range of stakeholders active in various aspects of the field to benefit from a wider range of viewpoints and to obtain input on our charge. The committee's first tasks were to (1) define what is meant by children; health, safety, and well-being; and risk, protective, and promotional factors and (2) determine how to approach the task of reviewing federal, state, or local data and methods.

Children

The committee adopted the term "children" to refer to groups of individuals from the time of birth to their 18th birthday. Surveys and other data sources employ differing age ranges, and the committee recognizes that, from a developmental perspective, there is no exact age at which childhood definitively ends. Numerous factors can affect the timing of one's transition from adolescence to adulthood and, as a result, individuals transition from child to adult roles at different rates. For some, adult roles are assumed during adolescence, while for others this does not occur until the middle of the third decade of life. Nevertheless, many datasets and systems consider individuals before and after they reach legal majority, so the committee has chosen age 18 as a *minimum age* for ending childhood. However, while the committee asserts that data on children's health should extend at least to that point, collection of data for those older than 18 should be an important data collection priority for the nation. The committee also recognizes that myriad factors affect the developing fetus prior to birth that impinge on and influence the health of children at birth. In this report these prenatal factors are considered and discussed as influences on children's health.

Although the terms "youth" or "adolescents" are often used to refer to older children and the terms "infants" and "toddlers" refer to very young children, for ease of reference, this report uses the term "children" to encompass all these groups. If a statement is intended to refer to a subset of the child population (e.g., infants, adolescents) the relevant descriptive term is used in the text.

Children's Health, Safety, and Well-Being

The committee was asked to assess definitions of health and questions related to children's health, safety, and well-being. This section provides a brief overview of the committee's approach to children's health and outlines how safety and well-being were considered in the report. Chapter 2 discusses these issues in more detail.

Health: Most available definitions or conceptualizations of health have been developed for adults. In the committee's view, these approaches do not account for issues particularly salient for children and do not reasonably transfer to children's health. Definitions of children's health must account for their special characteristics, particularly rapid development during childhood. They also must consider multiple influences that interact over time in different ways as children develop and change. The committee proposes a new definition of children's health that embraces health conditions, functioning, and health potential in a new conceptual model that considers multiple interrelated factors as influences.

Safety: Safety generally refers to aspects of the environment that contribute to health, including the physical environment (e.g., absence of toxins or pollutants in ground water, use of car seats and bicycle helmets), social environment (e.g., low neighborhood crime rates, low rates of risky behaviors either by the children or adults), and psychological environment (e.g., the perception of not being in personal danger). Some environmental and behavioral influences might be conceptualized as contributing to less safe situations, while others might be viewed as health-promoting, safety-related, or protective.

At any given moment in time, children are exposed to a range of risk and protective influences. To the extent that one or the other predominates (assuming this could be determined), it may be possible to characterize children's social or biological environments as relatively safer, health-promoting, or risky. More often it is possible to characterize an environment as risky or safe with respect to a single influence or single set of variables. Such factors can be used to make statements about the likely current or future health of a given population and, in effect, are often used as "proxies" for the actual health of a given population. In this report, children's safety is considered to be those influences that result in an environment that contributes positively to health and is discussed primarily in Chapter 3.

Well-Being: Well-being is commonly considered to be the sense of self as appraised by the individual. Concepts such as quality of life, fulfillment, and ability to contribute constructively to society and one's own family are important aspects of well-being. Well-being inherently involves comparisons with how one feels one should be, given one's age, preexisting health status or the health status of other persons in the social network, and physical status. For example, some children with attention deficit disorder and asthma that is controlled by medication, who are able to participate in a range of extracurricular activities and have many friends, may perceive themselves as healthy and fortunate, whereas others may not. Or children with no obvious physical illness but a subjective sense of poor well-being might be conceived to be in good physical health but potentially in compromised psychological health or in physical peril. Thus, one's sense of well-being is an important component of overall health that has been shown to affect one's overall functioning and prognosis, at least in adult health (Berkman and Syme, 1979).

In the developmental literature, well-being is often considered to be a state broader than health that incorporates social, psychological, educational, behavioral, and economic dimensions. The term "health and well-being" is used to recognize that aspects of children's life beyond traditional health considerations are important to both their current condition and to their future potential as adults, as well as to capture positive aspects of health. The committee contends that behavioral, psychological, and social well-being are core aspects of health and has incorporated these within the domain of health termed "health potential," discussed in the next chapter. As used in this report, the term "health" therefore inherently embraces health-related aspects of well-being.

Risk, Protective, and Promotional Factors
(Influences on Children's Health)

A multitude of biological, behavioral, and environmental factors can either pose a risk to children's health or act in a protective or health-promoting capacity. For example, children's social environments can be characterized by a number of influences that can be viewed as safe, health-promoting, risky, or detrimental. Many factors (e.g., peers) can be either a risk to health or a protective factor, depending on the specific circumstances. Given this uncertainty, the committee adopted the term "influences on children's health" to refer to risk, protective, and promotional factors.

The distinction between *health* and *influences on health* is usually straightforward. In a few instances, however, the distinction is ambiguous. For example, risk behaviors are considered an influence in this report, although a strong case could be made that daily alcohol use by an adolescent indicates poor health in terms of functioning. Likewise, an individual's genetic endowment is considered an influence because in most instances gene expression interacts with other factors before it causes disease or impairment in functioning.

The committee recognizes that children's health is the result of a dynamic set of factors. In a few cases, randomized, controlled trials or experimental studies (or both) have demonstrated a causal link between a particular influence and health. In other cases, while there is evidence to suggest a link between the influence and health, a direct causal link has not been established. In determining whether to include a given influence in this report, the committee included factors that meet at least two of these three criteria: (1) the existence of randomized control trials or experimental studies that demonstrate a causal link; (2) longitudinal prospective studies plus other nonexperimental or quasi-experimental evidence that supports a link; and (3) observational studies, plausible theory, or animal studies that support a link. Furthermore, inclusion required a substantial body of evidence with replicated studies and multiple, independent laboratories or researchers reaching the same conclusions.

Typically, current research assesses the effect of a single or a small set of influences but does not allow an assessment of the relative importance of multiple influences in relation to one another. *In the committee's view, the relative lack of research on children's health generally, and the interaction of various influences specifically, precludes a reliable ranking of influences.* Instead, we have included all factors that meet a defined threshold of evidence and excluded those that, while plausible, do not yet have sufficient evidence to support their effect. The committee calls for research to allow refinement of the influences and their relative effect.

Data and Methods

Numerous federal, state, and local surveys and administrative data sources are used to inform policy and programmatic decisions. In specifying available data sources, the committee chose to focus on national data sources or state-level sources that are available in all or most states. Conducting a comprehensive review of the innumerable data sources that measure children's health or a component of it in individual states or localities was not feasible. Instead, the committee highlights state or local examples to illustrate strategies proposed in the report.

THE COMMITTEE'S PREMISES

The committee approached its charge based on several underlying assumptions related to the importance of measuring and using data on children's health:

- children are vital assets of society;
- critical differences between children and adults warrant special attention to children's health;
- children's health has effects that reach far into adulthood;
- the manifestations of health and definitions and causes of ill health vary for different communities and different cultures; and
- the tracking of data on children's health and its influences is an essential part of efforts to improve children's health and the health of the adults they will become.

Children Are Vital Assets of Society

Children have intrinsic value in their own right. In the committee's view, fully protecting the health and growth of children is one of society's primary responsibilities. Optimal health and development are necessary preconditions to provide the opportunity for all children to reach their inherent potential. The reality that some children do not have the opportunity to grow up healthy and become productive members of their communities and the nation has enormous ramifications for all. Failure to optimize the health and development of children will result in future burdens of dependence that come from an unhealthy and unskilled workforce and dysfunctional families. Furthermore, growing scientific evidence demonstrates that disparities in health have their origins in early childhood and, if not addressed, are compounded over the life course (Ben-Shlomo and Kuh, 2002; Hardy, Kuh, Langenberg, and Wadsworth, 2003; Halfon and Hochstein, 2002; Institute of Medicine, 2001b). Therefore, the committee undertook its task with the conviction that it is important for the whole of society to be committed to ensuring that children are as healthy as possible and that all children are afforded an opportunity to optimize their individual health and development. In the committee's view, maximizing children's health will provide immediate benefits to them as well as determine their capacity to contribute to society and the common good over the long term.

Critical Differences Between Children and Adults

Many other reports have examined issues related to the health of Americans generally. Thus, a legitimate question is: Why should a report focus specifically on the health of children? The answer is that there are many differences between children and adults. Therefore, it is inappropriate to assume that what enhances or impedes adult health translates directly into children's health. While many factors may be relevant to both child and adult health, a wide range of factors affect them differentially.

Developmental Differences

Children's physiology and behavior differ in ways that require a different view of their health that is sensitive to rapid developmental change and unique developmental considerations. The particular patterns of gene expression, the relative sizes and growth of children's organs, the injuries to which they are susceptible, and the manner in which they interact with their environments differ in many ways from adults. For example, the surface area of their skin and lungs is proportionately greater in comparison to their weight than at any other time of life. This makes children more vulnerable than adults to certain types of environmental exposures (National Research Council, 1993). Children's behavior also differs in significant ways from that of adults. Children are by nature exploratory and many of their exploratory behaviors, hand-to-mouth behaviors, crawling, climbing, testing the limits of their capacity, and experimentation involve activities that are not normative for adults. As a result, children have greater exposure to a number of hazards in their physical world. In addition, they lack the cognitive mastery and behavioral inhibitions that are normally associated with adults and consequently they may exhibit behaviors that place them at significant risk for negative long-term consequences.

In addition, children grow more rapidly, most notably during the early years and again during adolescence, and change body and organ sizes and proportions at faster rates than at any other time of life. Furthermore, development occurs at different rates in individual children, and it is heavily influenced by a wide range of factors, from nutrition and nurturance to experiences and opportunities for learning (National Research Council and Institute of Medicine, 2000). The manner in which a child grows cognitively, emotionally, socially, and physically are key components of children's health that are not routinely part of assessments of adult health. As a result, indicators of a healthy 6-week-old, 6-month-old, and 6-year-old will be different. Given these dynamic elements, in general, it is necessary to look at changes over time, rather than a point assessment to distinguish among different levels of health.

Dependence

Childhood is characterized by children's dependency on their families and communities (Jameson and Wehr, 1994; Halfon, Inkelas, Wood, and Schuster, 1996). A newborn infant cannot survive without adult caregivers. Children are not free agents who can access services, determine diets, or change the environments in which they are raised. They lack voice and control of their own destiny. While autonomy increases with growth and development, during most of their childhood children are fundamentally dependent on the adults in their environment for the prevention of disease and the promotion and protection of their health and development.

Different Manifestations of Poor Health

The distribution of disease in childhood and the nature and types of health threats that affect children are different than in adults. Children have a lower prevalence than adults of chronic illnesses that require expensive, high-tech interventions and a higher prevalence of repeated acute illness. They also experience an array of congenital problems and inborn errors of metabolism that may not be seen in adults. What especially distinguishes the majority of children from adults is their greater resilience, less rapid biological deterioration, and continued ability to develop and grow in the face of negative health conditions. As a result, in many cases, interventions are more possible and more effective with children than with adults.

Childhood Has a Long Reach

What happens to children early in their lives can have profound implications for later health and well-being during adulthood (Wadsworth, 1999). A great deal of information is emerging on the high degree to which early events and conditions of childhood serve as precursors of adult disease. *From Neurons to Neighborhoods*, a recent report of the National Academies, states: "What happens during the first months and years of life matters a lot, not because this period of development provides an indelible blueprint for adult well-being, but because it sets either a sturdy or fragile stage for what follows" (National Research Council and Institute of Medicine, 2000, p. 5). Experiences early in life establish a physical, psychological, and social foundation on which future development and adult health are based. This can include prenatal and perinatal insults as well as exposures in childhood that lead to negative adult health outcomes. For example, early exposure to ultraviolet light has implications for the development of melanoma in adulthood. Habits and behaviors developed during childhood can also lead to health problems in adulthood. Diet and exercise habits acquired in early childhood have been shown to have cumulative effects that alter adult health outcomes in the absence of appropriately targeted interventions.

Both positive and negative influences early in life not only have direct effects on health during childhood, but also act to influence future health at each stage of development. Both negative and positive factors and health disparities compound their effects over a lifetime. At each stage, previous health affects current and future health, and the cumulative effects of early differences in health may result in profound differences in later health (see Keating and Hertzman, 1999).

Failure to influence children's health in a positive way may result in later excessive morbidity. The later consequences may be even more difficult and expensive to change than might prevention efforts put forth earlier in life. The capacity of an adult to contribute as a productive member of society may also be dramatically affected by poor health experienced as a child. This also means that there is often a long lag time between the measurable effects of interventions in childhood and changes in health later in life. This in turn makes it much more difficult to assess whether health is improving in both the short and the long run.

Community and Cultural Variation

Although there are some absolute notions of health (e.g., absence of disease), the manifestations of health differ across social and cultural groups. This is reflected in the differing notions of health across human societies and within societies over time. Common and technical use of terms like "disease," "illness," and "impairment" is embedded in a cultural context, which will determine whether certain symptoms, signs, or disease manifestations are considered normal or worthy of distinction in either a positive or negative way. For example, notions of normal body size differ substantially in different parts of the world and over generations. Aspects of health, social, and cultural norms influence concepts of health as well as understanding of the causes and consequence of the variety of its aspects. When these notions translate into individual and group behaviors and attitudes, they can have a major effect on health.

Culture also provides a framework for the use of home remedies. For example, in some Hispanic and Asian communities, health is a balance between "hot" and "cold," and an imbalance in favor of one can cause illness necessitating a remedy from the other to restore harmony (Risser and Mazur, 1995). Other cultural variations that can be misconstrued are the traditional practices of cupping and coining, which can be mistaken for child abuse (Hansen, 1998), and home remedies for such folk illnesses as caída de mollera (fallen fontanelle), mal ojo (evil eye), and empacho (intestinal blockage).

In addition, social or cultural views on health, as well as the circumstances of a given community, may affect the priorities of that community in terms of what is considered important. It is therefore critical for specific societies and communities to define the measures they deem most salient to their local circumstances and for those working to improve health to take into account cultural differences and the priorities of that community. For example, a low-income community in which food is scarce and healthy children are defined by carrying extra weight may not consider obesity a priority health problem compared with reducing other more immediate threats to health, such as crime.

Use of Data to Improve Children's Health

How can the nation assess whether movement toward the goal of optimizing children's health society-wide is being achieved? Without the capacity to measure and monitor progress, there is no way to know whether changes in policy make a difference toward improving children's health. Lack of valid and reliable information impedes comparisons across time or place or in response to interventions. Without data to measure and monitor children's health, the effect of changes in the social, cultural, and physical environment will remain unknown.

What is measured is often what gets attention. Conversely, aspects that are more difficult to assess are more likely be ignored. This report addresses the questions of whether what is measured is what ought to be measured; whether it is being measured in an appropriate manner; and whether information is being used in a way that will optimize children's health.

THE COMMITTEE'S VISION

Although the committee views the findings in this report as relevant to multiple audiences, federal, state, and local decision makers are considered to be the primary audience. The committee proposes strategies to address gaps in knowledge about children's health and influences on it, tools available to measure both, and ways to use data about children's health and influences on children's health to inform policy decisions. The committee's recommendations aim to focus on action and results, address future health measurement needs, and improve understanding of children's health and influences on children's health through specific research priorities.

To make the report as practical as possible and facilitate its use, the committee focuses on feasible next steps such as integrating existing datasets, and outlines strategies by which children's health might be improved. The definition of children's health and the conceptual framework presented in this report have important policy implications for the ultimate health of the nation, as well as the health of the nation's economy, its workforce, and its viability as a future leader among nations.

Given the rapid strides in the development of new technologies, such as electronic information systems and the Human Genome Project, the committee has addressed future information needs both in terms of specific types of indicators as well as the types of systems and infrastructures necessary to make better data available at national, state, and local levels.

Where indicators, measurement tools, and measurement systems are not available, the committee has identified research to address gaps in knowledge. Research to examine the interaction of multiple influences and improve understanding of the dynamic nature of children's health is also identified.

STRUCTURE OF THE REPORT

This report has seven chapters. The next chapter focuses on our definition and conceptualization of children's health. It outlines a definition of children's health that reflects the committee's view that children's health is a developmental, multifaceted state that is socially and culturally defined and specifies its components. The chapter presents the conceptual framework adopted by the committee for thinking about both the internal and external influences that affect children's health.

Chapter 3 reviews the scientific evidence pertaining to the ways in which various influences have been shown to affect children's health. It outlines influences specific to children including their biology (their genetic make-up and internal biological environment), and the behaviors they exhibit as they interact with their surroundings. The chapter also outlines influences external to the child, including the family, community, culture, and physical environments as well as policy environments and services systems.

Chapter 4 outlines the available tools and data for measuring children's health and the adequacy of these methods, including specifying gaps based on the committee's definition of health. Chapter 5 provides a similar review of tools, data, and gaps for measuring the influences discussed in Chapter 3. Chapters 4 and 5 focus primarily on available national data.

Chapter 6 discusses data systems, outlines the value of data integration, and presents strategies to begin to develop improved data systems, including discussion of the ethical, technical, and political challenges inherent in these strategies. This chapter introduces the potential value to state and local policymakers of improved use of available state-level data.

Chapter 7 presents the committee's conclusions and recommendations. This chapter focuses on what can be done at the federal, state, and local levels to improve children's health by advancing efforts to measure and use information on children's health and its influences. This final chapter also outlines the committee's recommendations aimed at improving knowledge of how various factors interact to affect health and their relative importance.

Finally, several appendixes follow the body of the report. Appendix A provides short descriptions of existing core datasets for measuring children's health and compares them based on periodicity, age, and geographic level surveyed. Appendix B examines the extent to which current major surveys capture data on children's health and its influences and provides a comparison across surveys in both narrative and tabular form. Appendix C presents information on national-level syntheses that use secondary data to track multiple indicators over time and examples of the indicators they track. The glossary in Appendix D defines frequently used terms, Appendix E identifies acronyms referred to in the text, and Appendix F provides biographical sketches of the committee members and staff responsible for the report.

2

Children's Health:
A New Conceptual Framework

Historically, the definition of children's health has received little consideration separate from that of adults. Although views of adult health have evolved from a focus on morbidity and mortality to consider broader aspects of health, considerations specific to children have generally been excluded. This chapter lays out a new definition and conceptualization of children's health. It reviews the ideas that led to the committee's definition and puts forth a model of how health evolves in children. It summarizes the principles underpinning the model and the ways that different influences operate. Finally, the chapter outlines the domains of children's health that serve as a basis for measuring it.

Although many of the principles outlined in this chapter also apply to adults, they are particularly salient for children. The committee's charge calls for a focus on children, an emphasis the committee thinks is warranted given the historic lack of attention to children's health in relation to adult health. However, those involved in population health issues more broadly may want to consider the potential applicability of the definition and conceptual model outlined in this report to adults.

VIEWS ON CHILDREN AND CHILDREN'S HEALTH

The roles of children have changed throughout human history and across different levels of social organization. Children in agrarian and early industrial societies were expected to participate in the work of the family from early childhood, helping other family members in household activities and caring for one another. Many died while still very young, and those who survived were expected to contribute to the family's economic situation and, eventually, to the support of their aging parents. There was little collective commitment to the provision of education or services to improve health and only limited knowledge of the environmental factors that influence healthy development. Modern societies generally have less urgent need for children to enter the workforce, and the technological age demands a longer period of schooling and greater skill level from its workforce.

Awareness of and commitment to protecting the health of children and to their nurturance has increased in recent decades (see Zelier, 1994). Observational and empirical research in the 20th century, led by individuals such as John Watson (behaviorism), Arnold Gesell (maturational stage theory), Sigmund Freud (psychoanalytic theory), Jean Piaget (cognitive development theory), Erik Erickson (psychosocial theory), John Bowlby (attachment theory), Urie Bronfenbrenner (ecological theory), and Arnold Sameroff (transactional theory), created the concepual basis for understanding the cognitive, emotional, and social importance of childhood and the roles played by both family and societal forces.

The social transformation of childhood in modern societies reflects a retreat from the view that parents have full and unlimited jurisdiction over their children to one in which the welfare of children is increasingly understood as a shared social responsibility which requires investments in education, health care, and other institutions. At the same time, there has been a growing body of evidence that children's development is influenced both by their families and by the social forces and cultural norms that society produces. Thus, children's health, development, achievements, and social attainments have come to require the interest, guidance, and protection of both families and society—not just for the intrinsic value of children but for society's collective future. This view of childhood is embedded in the very foundation of such social institutions as schools and the health care system, which play important roles in preparing children for the challenges of modern times and ensuring that, as they grow and develop into adults, they are prepared for life in an increasingly complex world.

From a public policy perspective, this emerging view was crystallized in the major social changes that took place in the 19th and 20th centuries and was manifested in national policies for providing health care to indigent populations, free and compulsory public education, mandatory immunizations that both protect individual children and provide group immunity against widespread epidemics of infectious diseases, policies for protection of the welfare of children, and the creation of the juvenile justice and child welfare systems (Katz, 1997; Cravens, 1993; Levine and Levine, 1992).

In the United States, these policies resulted in the creation of the Children's Bureau in 1913, which later evolved into the present-day Maternal and Child Health Bureau (Hutchins, 1997); a federal agency to oversee education; later the establishment of the National Institute of Child Health and Human Development; and the creation of subsidized health care benefits for particularly needy children. In more recent years, such collective concern for the health and welfare of children has increased the commitment to improve children's health services, as reflected in the passage of Medicaid, extensions of Medicaid, and legislation creating the State Child Health Insurance Program. Although the sustainability of some of these initiatives remains in doubt and the trajectory of public interest in children has not been one of continuously increasing concern and commitment, over the course of the past three centuries there has been considerable progress in increasing societal commitment to children.

EVOLVING CONCEPTS OF HEALTH

Notions of health have also evolved over the last century. At the turn of the 20th century, when infectious diseases posed the greatest threat to health, health was viewed as the absence of disease or injury. Disease causation was usually described using simple causal models, epitomized by the germ theory (i.e., an infectious agent alone was responsible for disease) and theories of Mendelian inheritance (i.e., a single gene alone produced the effect observed), in which cause and effect were immediate. Even if not always observable, the mechanisms were simple, singular, and presumably understood.

Public health monitoring and surveillance systems instituted at the beginning of the 20th century focused on measures of survival and used mortality rates for different conditions and age groups (neonatal, infant, and child) as the predominant measures of health. During the first half of the 20th century, the growing and changing medical profession and the health care delivery system also defined health as the absence of disease. Common indicators of health included the numbers or rates at which a disease affected members of a population. The International Classification of Diseases and Related Health Problems (ICD), which dates back to an 1891 international statistical congress, was originally codified as a standard for health measurement by classifying causes of mortality. The ICD was adopted by the World Health Organization (WHO) in 1948 and has been revised every 10 years. It is used as the basis for diagnostic coding in the United States and throughout the world. It makes possible systematic recording, analysis, interpretation, and comparison of both morbidity and mortality data across geographic, national, and temporal boundaries (Chatterji et al., 2002).

This classification continues to develop with evolving notions of health. The new International Classification of Functioning, Disability, and Health focuses not only on impairments of body parts and systems, but also on individual participation in daily activities and on the interaction between disorders and environments that alter functioning (Chatterji et al., 2002).

Changing patterns of morbidity and mortality, routine treatment of infectious diseases, and the increased prevalence of chronic conditions caused shifts in ideas about health. Models of health promotion and disease prevention began to account for the influence of dietary and exercise behaviors, as well as for exposures to multiple influences over longer time frames. This is well illustrated in how various behavioral influences (e.g., poor diet, lack of exercise) interact with genetic influences to affect the development of obesity and how multiple influences (e.g., genes, exposure to allergens and antigens, family behaviors, physical and social environments, health services) affect the development and severity of childhood asthma (Evans and Stoddart, 1990, 2003).

In the United States, the high cost of chronic conditions and the high proportion of elderly people who have one or more of these conditions have led to a primary focus on these aspects of health. As multiple influences on health became better understood, the notion of health as a positive capacity and a prerequisite for a range of human accomplishment took root, elevating the importance of both disease prevention and health promotion (Breslow, 1999).

Precise definitions of health, emphasizing negative, normative, and positive notions of health, have been debated for centuries (Institute of Medicine, 2001b, p. 21). Over time, there has been growing recognition that health is more than the absence of disease. This concept was most dramatically articulated in 1948 by WHO with the following definition (which remains their current definition): "Health is a state of complete physical, mental, and social well-being, not merely the absence of disease or infirmity."

Several recent reports from the National Academies have reviewed issues in the definition and measurement of health for various specific purposes. These include studies focused on (a) better understanding of the interplay of biological, behavioral, and social influences on health outcomes (Institute of Medicine, 2001b); (b) improving performance monitoring of community health services (Institute of Medicine, 1997); and (c) defining the future research agenda in the behavioral and social sciences for the National Institutes of Health (National Research Council, 2001). Each of these previous reports, as well as several others, highlights the advantages and disadvantages of various definitions, but in none has the primary focus been directed toward children's health issues. Each, however, emphasizes the importance of notions of positive health and the interplay of multiple individual and environmental factors.

Many critiques of previous definitions focus on their breadth: what is included and what is excluded. For example, while the WHO's broad and comprehensive definition of health has been used extensively to exhort and advocate for new health interventions and policies, it has also been criticized as being overly inclusive of all human endeavors and very difficult to apply for the purposes of health measurement (Institute of Medicine, 2001b; Young, 1998; Evans and Stoddardt, 1990). Similarly, while there are advantages to biologically based definitions of health, including the specification of precise biomarkers, such definitions cannot capture all the important and commonly understood components of health, such as the capacity to respond to stress or resist disease.

From a medical perspective, health is still defined largely as freedom from injury, disease, or disability. However, the medical community is increasingly concerned that definitions of health that focus on the absence of disease ignore other aspects of health as well as future health. This void has become more of an issue as the knowledge base and the capacity to measure influences on health have increased.

From a population health perspective, operational definitions of health that focus on measures of morbidity and mortality have also been criticized, because they do not account for the intersection of health and behavior (Evans and Stoddardt, 1990; Institute of Medicine, 2001b). They also fail to incorporate mechanisms for linking health to the multiple influences on health outcomes. The Institute of Medicine (1997) concluded that a broad definition of health that embraces well-being as well as the absence of illness is necessary for effective community efforts aimed at improving health.

Building upon the abundant evidence that children's health has special characteristics, the committee sought a comprehensive and integrative definition and conceptualization of health that reflects the dynamic nature of childhood, is conceptually sound, is based on the best scientific evidence, and provides a basis for both measuring and improving children's health. A recent collaborative effort of the 15 member states of the European Union Health Monitoring Programme came to a similar conclusion. Although the specific elements of their model differ, CHILD—Child Health Indicators of Life and Development—proposed an approach to measuring children's health that embraces the importance of development, the need to consider a range of influences in order to adequately understand and measure it, and the need for data to stimulate action (Rigby and Kohler, 2002). Policy makers in the United States may want to consider possible adaptation of the CHILD system to the context, priorities, and data mechanisms available in the United States.

The committee was also cognizant of the increased emphasis on the prevention of health threats and impairments in children, as well as on the increasingly broad mandate for child health professionals in the United States to involve themselves with multidisciplinary efforts to maximize health. Such efforts are reflected in the publication of Bright Futures, a guideline for the care of children (Green and Palfrey, 2002). Bright Futures has designed training and education for families, health professionals, and communities on health promotion and prevention strategies. Recognizing that health and well-being are a result of interactions of many biological, psychological, social, cultural, and physical factors, it strives for comprehensive health promotion and a productive relationship between the child health professional, children, parents, and the community.

A NEW DEFINITION OF CHILDREN'S HEALTH

For the purpose of this report, health is a characteristic of a child or group of children, whether current, past, or future, and is defined by the committee in the following way:

Children's health is the extent to which individual children or groups of children are able or enabled to (a) develop and realize their potential, (b) satisfy their needs, and (c) develop the capacities that allow them to interact successfully with their biological, physical, and social environments.

The definition proposed echoes the principles developed at the Ottawa Charter in 1986 that embraced positive aspects of health and declared that to "reach a state of complete physical, mental and social well-being, an individual or group must be able to identify and realize aspirations, to satisfy needs, and to change or cope with the environment. Health is, therefore, seen as a resource for everyday life, not the objective of living. Health is a positive concept emphasizing social and personal resources, as well as physical capacities" (Ottawa Charter for Health Promotion, 1986). The committee refined this perspective in its definition of children's health to reflect the heightened importance of a developmental perspective and the fact that health results from the interplay of multiple influences.

The committee's definition views health as a positive resource that gives children the ability to interact with their surroundings and to respond to life's challenges and changes. Moreover, it incorporates development in the definition and specifies a fundamental principle of development—the optimization and maintenance of function over time. At the same time, it focuses on the intrinsic characteristics of children and their resources for interacting with the environment.

DOMAINS OF HEALTH

Based on the committee's expertise, current conceptualizations reflected in various internationally endorsed classification schemes, and current research, the committee defined three domains of health as fundamental to the assessment of children's health: health conditions, functioning, and health potential. This section discusses the conceptualization of these domains. Chapter 4 outlines current approaches to measuring the domains.

The process of developing a vibrant, flexible, and responsive measurement strategy for representing the health of children in the United States depends not only on a definition of health and the conceptual and theoretical underpinning of that definition, but on how the nation operationalizes health in the assessment of an individual child and populations of children. Specifying and relating the multiple domains of health are the central challenge of health measurement (Chatterji et al., 2002). This section specifies the domains that should be considered part of a national framework for measuring children's health.

The concepts draw on various frameworks that have been proposed to account for the multiplicity of influences on health over the past several decades (Canadian Government, 1974; Laframboise, 1973; Epstein, 1996; Wilkinson, 1992; Marmot and Syme, 1976; Marmot et al., 1984, 1997; Berkman and Syme, 1979; Evans and Stoddart, 1990; Institute of Medicine, 1997, 1999; Halfon and

Hochstein, 2002; Black et al., 1980; Acheson, 1998; Starfield and Shi, 1999). Several previous attempts to develop a way to measure health have been reviewed. Most were developed primarily for adults rather than for children and focus on negative aspects of health. The concepts proposed by the committee take a broader view of health and are consistent with the conclusions of other recent Institute of Medicine committees and the pioneering work in other nations to reconceptualize children's health and to measure and monitor it (Institute of Medicine, 1997, 2001b; Eiser, 1997; Eiser and Morse, 2001).

Domains to Consider and Criteria We Have Used

Measuring the multifaceted nature of health requires distinctions among domains of health in order to assess and track its different aspects. Because health is dynamic (i.e., both changing and changeable), constantly developing, and affected by multiple factors concurrently, it is inherently difficult to measure. This has important implications for defining and depicting domains and subdomains. The components of health are not easily slotted into self-contained and non-overlapping categories.

The committee viewed several criteria as crucial for identifying domains to guide the measurement of health. These include the need to:

- Use current scientific evidence about the domains and the influences on health and be responsive to new knowledge about influences on health.
- Be comprehensive in capturing multiple aspects of health.
- Allow for comparisons across diverse populations and developmental stages. That is, the domains should be consistent across developmental stages although different measures may be used for assessment.
- Be useful for assessing the nature and magnitude of the effects of different policies and interventions on health outcomes of children.
- Recognize that previous and current health status influence subsequent health.

Given the extended time frames and latent effects of different exposures and changes in individual characteristics, some aspects of health may not be amenable to immediate accountability and manipulation. Therefore, in some areas it may not be practicable, credible, or possible to assess the effect of policy, program, or process changes on morbidity, mortality, and the incidence of health conditions. Instead, it may be necessary to rely on validated intermediate outcomes as proxies for such ultimate outcomes, such as measuring known influences on health. Finally, it should be self-evident that measures must accurately reflect all of these qualities of the model.

The committee proposes that health be viewed as having three distinct but related domains: *health conditions,* a domain that deals with disorders or illnesses of body systems; *functioning*, which focuses on the manifestations of individual health in daily life; and *health potential*, which captures the development of health assets that indicate positive aspects—competence, capacity, and developmental potential (see Table 2-1). Ideally, the science, if sufficiently advanced, would guide the measurement of the individual's ability to respond successfully to future threats to health.

Health Conditions

Health conditions refer to alterations in health status reflected as disease, injuries, or impairments or as pathophysiological manifestations of disorder (signs and symptoms). Health conditions are usually classified using the ICD, which is currently in its tenth edition (ICD-10). Developed for epidemiological purposes, the ICD system permits standardized and systematic recording and analysis of health conditions, injuries, and many common symptoms. Different categories are used in the ICD to classify certain conditions. They may be acute and self-limited, acute but likely to recur, or chronic; they may be anatomical, physiological, or psychosocial. They include a wide range of specific as well as nonspecific conditions and syndromes.

Functioning

The functioning domain reflects the direct and indirect effects of one or more health conditions and their treatments as well as problems resulting from multiple health problems on the daily life and activities of the child. It includes all aspects of physical, psychological, cognitive, and social functioning as they express themselves in children's daily activities and behavior.

Alterations in functioning have been used informally by health care providers to measure the significance of injuries and to gauge the effects of acute and

TABLE 2-1 Domains of Health

Health Conditions	Functioning	Health Potential
Alterations in health status due to disease, disability, or injury	Physical, cognitive, emotional, and social functioning and deficits	Competency and capacity in physical, cognitive, emotional, social well-being, and developmental potential
Symptoms	Functional deficit, disability (disability days, bed days)	Resilience
	Restriction in activity (total and by specific conditions), morbidity burden	

chronic health conditions. While measures of physiological function fall within the realm of health conditions, not all physiological alterations have a significant health effect in terms of altering functioning (e.g., changes in the pigmentation of the hair) (Ustun et al., 2002). There is rarely a one-to-one correspondence between a diagnosis and its translation into a level of impairment in daily life. Two individuals with the same abnormal laboratory value or radiological finding may have very different life experiences, with one unaffected or only mildly affected in his or her daily life and the other experiencing major dysfunction.

In addition, the functional expression of a condition is heavily influenced by the various ways in which it is modified by other factors intrinsic to the child (e.g., personality, comorbid conditions, genetic endowment) and the environment. For example, a child who lives in a one-story house will experience fewer limitations in function when experiencing joint or muscle disease than one living in a five-story walk-up apartment.

Similarly, the level of compensatory mechanisms and treatments available (e.g., durable medical equipment, implants, medications) will change the expression of the condition in terms of the child's functioning. Measures of functioning also have great meaning because of their implications for caregiving, dependence, and the ability to participate in social roles. Another advantage of these measures is that they permit a look at the effects of multiple conditions as well as the effects of the conditions and their treatments, including side-effects. They provide a common measure for assessing the health of children across conditions (Stein et al., 1987; Stein and Jessop, 1990).

Limitations in mobility, usual activities, or full participation in school are important aspects of physical function. Psychological function includes a wide range of functions, both cognitive (e.g., alertness, confusion, problem-solving ability, receptive language ability) and emotional (e.g., affect, mood, temperament). Given the profound developmental growth that takes place over the life course of a child, these subdomains constantly change, which creates significant challenges for accurate measurement of psychological deficits. For example, a specific disease can cause a child to regress in emotional or cognitive capacity. However, without repeated measurement of that child's function, it would be difficult to determine whether a regression had taken place.

Social functioning refers to limitations imposed on children in the realm of their usual activities and relationships. For a young child, the subdomains of social role function include the ability to engage in ordinary play and the ability to attend school and participate in all school-related activities. Social functioning also includes measures of social integration and social connection, including the ability to make and keep friends and to play a supportive or instrumental role in the lives of others. Culture contributes in major ways to the definition of appropriate social functioning, and thus this domain may have different meaning for different subgroups.

Alterations in function include physical, cognitive, emotional, and social impairments and measures of functional disability (e.g., disability days, bed days, limited activity days) and diminished developmental opportunities due to disadvantage caused by health condition, stigma, and social valuation. Measurement of these alterations in functioning may include gross and fine motor deficits; oral motor skills in a young child; alterations in physical growth and weight; and restrictions in activity, mobility, and self-care, as well as impairments in psychological functioning (i.e., cognitive functioning, such as problem solving, receptive and expressive language) and in social roles, such as attachment, relational capacity, affect, mood, behaviors, and school dropout rates.

Health Potential

Health potential includes both health assets that provide the capacity to respond to physical, psychological, and social challenges and risk states that increase vulnerability to other aspects of poor health. Health potential includes subdomains that the research literature has indicated are important measures of a child's capacities and reserves. Included in this domain are positive developmental assets and health capacities that provide and indicate ability to form positive relationships, regulate emotional and cognitive states, and respond to multiple challenges, including exposures to disease and psychological and physical stress, among others. While to some extent this might be looked on as the positive aspect of functioning, that is, the capacity to function in the face of threats to one's health, we have chosen to distinguish this domain as unique because of the inherent bias toward defining functioning only as normal or deficient. Few if any measures of functioning capture this more positive aspect of a person's assets and resources and of the characteristics that make them resilient.

Other characteristics described as resilience factors that fall within this domain include curiosity, responsiveness, reflection, imagination, self-efficacy, problem-solving ability, self-sufficiency, optimism, and disease resistance and recovery (Starfield et al., 1993). All are characteristics that add to a child's ability to deal with and bounce back from adversity.

EVOLUTION OF THE COMMITTEE'S MODEL

The committee sought to develop a model of health that depicts how a variety of influences interact over time to produce health. One model that reflects considerable progress in this regard is put forward in *Healthy People 2010* (U.S. Department of Health and Human Services, 2000) (see Figure 2-1). It shows the interaction of biology and behavior and the interactions of the physical and social environments on both. It also reflects the influence of public policies and interventions and of access to quality health care on the health of individuals and groups.

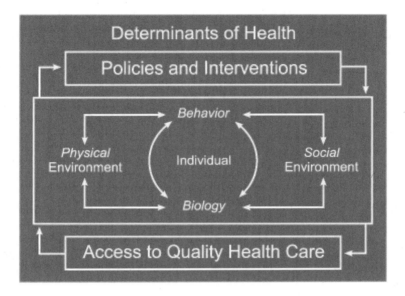

FIGURE 2-1 Model used by the *Healthy People 2010* report.
SOURCE: U.S. Department of Health and Human Services (2000, p. 30).

For the committee, the model falls short for use with children because it does not reflect the dynamic and developmental nature of children's health and is too narrow in its view of determinants or influences on health; for example, it fails to articulate the importance of cultural factors or to recognize the importance of services other than health care. Health results from complex interactions of many aspects of the child's environment, genetic endowment, and behavioral responses that constantly influence and affect one another. Several principles of this dynamism are critical to a full model of children's health.

Health and Development

Development is important in the biological and behavioral processes that determine health capacities, optimize function, preserve health, and lead to the presence or absence of disease throughout life. Cumulative experience, inherent adaptive capacities, dynamic interactions with physical, social, and cultural environments, and genetic predisposition all interact to determine developmental trajectories (Institute of Medicine, 2001b; National Research Council and Institute of Medicine, 2000; Hertzman, 2000; Halfon and Hochstein, 2002). A growing body of scientific research specifies the biological mechanisms and physiological pathways that determine the way health develops (Halfon and Hochstein, 2002; Keating and Hertzman, 1999). Early health is an influence on future health. Health and health influences interact throughout childhood. Several considerations relevant to children's health are developmental in nature: critical and sensitive periods in children's development, the importance of timing and multiple time frames, the age-specific patterns and distributions of children's health influences, the importance of transitions, and the long reach of childhood.

Sensitive and Critical Periods

Children's development includes both sensitive and critical periods. Sensitive periods refer to times when a child is especially receptive to certain kinds of environmental influences or experiences, good or bad, and the ideal time to provide or to avoid them. Critical periods refer to times when certain experiences or influences have a deterministic (positive or negative) effect; the health effect would not occur from the same exposures at other times (Ben-Shlomo and Kuh, 2002).

Many examples of influences on children's health have vastly differing effects at different developmental ages and stages. Although the terms sensitive and critical are used interchangeably in this report, the committee recognizes that there are relatively few, if any, critical periods outside the biological area. Examples of critical developmental periods include exposure to specific influences during fetal development (e.g., rubella, folic acid, ionizing radiation) or during adolescence (e.g., mumps). The need for appropriate stimulation and interaction in infancy and early childhood in order to develop appropriate vision, language skills, and attachment is an example of a sensitive period. The timing of experiences and exposures to certain health influences are important considerations when assessing children's health. In addition, exposures and experiences during sensitive and critical periods affect not only the current health of children but also their future health and functional capacities.

Timing and Multiple Time Frames

The timing of specific influences on the development of health conditions and health trajectories is important to consider when measuring children's health (Halfon and Hochstein, 2002). Assessment of health at a single point in time provides only a snapshot of a dynamic process. It is also important to consider the developmental trajectory of the health of a child over time, both for individuals and within groups. What may appear as good or impaired health at one stage may change over time. Some influences may exert their effects rapidly, while others remain latent and alter subsequent health or cumulate (often in conjunction with other influences) to manifest their effects much later in life.

Patterns and Distribution of Children's Health Influences

The patterns and distribution of children's health influences are age specific. A child's development occurs explosively in the first years of life, gradually becomes slower with advancing age, and again accelerates during adolescence, so that their relative salience varies with age or developmental stage (Bogin, 2001). For example, in young children, family-related influences are a major factor on health and development, with neighborhood, schools, and peer group playing a greater role as individuals age (Nordio, 1978; Rutter et al., 1997; Wadsworth, 1999; Halfon and Hochstein, 2002).

Transitions

Transitions present special challenges and windows of opportunity. As children move from one stage to another, new demands and stresses may influence their health. At several points (e.g., birth, entry into school, puberty) children must negotiate new environments that challenge adaptive mechanisms in new ways. At the same time, transitions provide an opportunity for growth and mastery and are critical times for interventions (Baltes, 1997; Brazelton, 1995; Graber and Brooks-Gunn, 1996).

The Long Reach of Childhood

There is growing awareness that childhood has a long reach on future health. Several recent reports have emphasized the importance of prenatal and early postnatal development on lifelong health and well-being (Institute of Medicine, 2001b; National Research Council, 2001). For example, birthweight has been shown to be directly related to later cardiovascular disease (Barker, 1998; Ben-Shlomo and Kuh, 2002).

Influences on Health Are Multiple, Interactive, and Changing

In the committee's view, another set of changes to the model of children's health should adequately represent the multiple and interacting influences on health.

Multiple Influences

At any given time, multiple present and past influences affect children's current health. Health results from the interaction of genetics and children's environments. As discussed in Chapter 3, there are many ways in which the environment interacts with and affects the expression of genetic potential, or vice versa. While biological, psychological, behavioral, social, cultural, economic, and physical influences are individually important, these factors usually do not operate alone, but interact with one another over time (Engle, 1977; Sameroff and Fiese, 2000). Factors in the social, physical, and cultural environments can influence individual biological and behavioral manifestations of health, suggesting that biology and behavioral outcomes are not often independent (Institute of Medicine, 2001b). Our model presents the multiple influences on children's health in the following categories: children's biology and behavior; their social environments, including family, community and culture; their physical environments; services; and policy.

Influences Interact

Multiple influences co-occur and interact over time. Individuals influence and are influenced by their families and the social networks and organizations in which they participate (e.g., child care, schools, places of worship), the community of which they are part, and the society in which they live (Institute of Medicine, 2001b). This concept of intertwined influences (Bronfenbrenner, 1979; Bronfenbrenner and Ceci, 1994; Boyce et al., 1998) also captures the dynamic interactions among these constantly changing and interacting contexts.

Evidence from research on human development indicates that these multiple contexts broaden and deepen for individuals as they age, serving to channel and reinforce influences into developmental pathways (Boyce et al., 1998; Dawson et al., 1994, 2000; Halfon and Hochstein, 2002). Many influences co-occur, so that the effects of poverty, for example, may occur through multiple factors, such as poor nutrition, educational opportunity, and neighborhood violence (Bronfenbrenner and Ceci, 1994). The nature and strength of such interactions differ across the life span, and early influences may set in place a series of vulnerabilities and strengths that change the effects of later influences.

A NEW CONCEPTUAL MODEL

To more accurately reflect the dynamic process of multiple, interacting influences from which children's health evolves, the committee proposes a new conceptual model. Our model builds on the categories of *Healthy People 2010* but adds to them and views them as a kaleidoscope. In a kaleidoscope, individual pieces of colored glass are arrayed in a fixed form but in a variety of colors and shapes based on how the specific colors and shapes of glass interact when the kaleidoscope is turned. So too do the results of specific influences on health change as the influences change and interact over time and throughout development to produce health (see Figure 2-2).

In our model, the various influences are presented as overlapping circles that interact within the broader context of policy and services. The relative importance of individual influences varies over time as children move into new developmental stages and the influences interact; the pattern of health that emerges

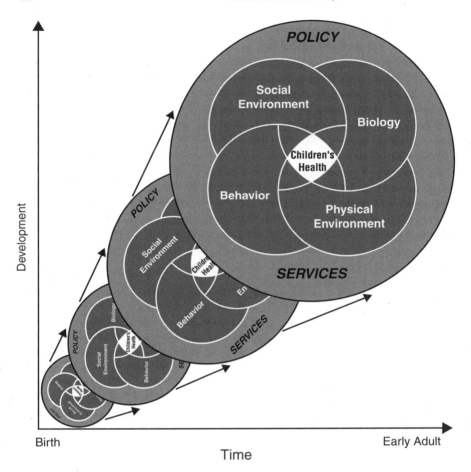

FIGURE 2-2 A new model of children's health and its influences.

also varies. The model illustrates that the effect of influences will vary based on both time and stage of development. Since development is an uneven process, with periods of rapid growth and periods of relative quiescence, it is not synonymous with time, nor is it the same from child to child, and the interaction of various influences changes with both time and developmental stage.

As children age, the kaleidoscope turns and the patterns change, reflecting their changing health. At some ages, these turns are very rapid, reflecting substantial developmental change; at others they are less so (though still more rapid than in adults). Each turn incorporates the previous elements, including the child's former health, and casts them in new light. All affect the child's present and future health into adulthood and old age. Because this notion of health is not static, multiple time frames must be addressed. With each turn of the shaft, the pattern will be altered, if only slightly; some effects may not manifest until later in a child's life. The spheres, representing influences, overlap each other so that the final pattern is not just a collection of distinct health influences, but rather a display of the interactions among the spheres of influence. The relative salience of different influences also varies by developmental stage. Although the figure shows each sphere to be of equal size, the relative sizes of the spheres are dynamic.

Criteria for the Measurement of Children's Health

The criteria used in other national, state, and local health measurement initiatives can inform understanding of how health is and should be measured. Certain common criteria emerge from a review of several of these other efforts as useful guideposts for selecting individual domains and indicators as well as in selecting a set of indicators (Institute of Medicine, 1999, 2001b; National Committee for Quality Assurance, and others). The committee has adopted a common set of criteria for guiding the selection of domains and indicators and for assessing the gaps that currently exist in the information collected on children's health. Thus, measures of children's health (domains and indicators) should be important, valid and reliable, meaningful, culturally appropriate and relevant, sensitive to change, and feasible to collect.

- Important—the domains and indicators should account for all important aspects of current or future health outcomes.
- Reliable and valid—measures should be reproducible over repeated measurements and observers. Validity implies that a measure has meaning in terms of the intended concept in a way that meets several different types of scrutiny.
- Meaningful—domains and indicators should capture the special health attributes of children including their developmental vulnerability and potential, patterns of morbidity and mortality that distinguish children from adults, as well as their evolving independence. They should also provide a way to assess and track disparities that may start in childhood and be compounded over time.
- Culturally appropriate and relevant—measures should reflect the full array of health as understood by different subgroups and should be psychometrically demonstrated to assess comparable domains across groups.
- Sensitive to change—measures should be sufficiently sensitive to measure meaningful changes. For example, a measure that would distinguish only between alive and dead would have relatively little use in assessing the changes in health of a child or group of children over time.
- Feasible to measure—measures should be sufficiently useful and practical for information collection that they generate a constituency that has the political will to use them.

Measurement of Children's Health

Additional features are crucial for the measurement of children's health to be useful from a policy perspective. In the committee's view, any approach to measurement should:

- Contend with the relationships between health at one point in time and future prospects (health expectancy).
- Allow for gradations of measurement, as well as thresholds that can be used to facilitate decisions about which individuals or populations are in need of intervention. Thus it should be useful at different points on the spectrum, for example from excellent to poor health.
- Track changes in children's health over time and consider developmental stages.
- Be developed in a manner that protects privacy and confidentiality.

As this report makes clear, few measures currently meet these standards.

3

Influences on Children's Health

Children's health is determined by the interaction of a multitude of influences, reflecting complex processes. We divide these influences into biological, behavioral, and environmental (physical and social) even though our model of children's health views their effects as highly intertwined and difficult to isolate. This chapter provides a summary of published literature and a framework for understanding those influences.

OVERVIEW

Biological influences as discussed in this chapter include genetic expressions, prenatal influences, as well as biological constraints and possibilities created by perinatal and postnatal events plus prior states of health. Behavioral influences include the child's emotions, beliefs, attitudes, behaviors, and cognitive abilities that affect health outcomes. Environmental influences are wide-ranging and include infectious agents, toxins such as lead and air pollution, and social factors such as loving interactions with caregivers, socioeconomic resources in the family and community, and peer relationships, segregation, racism, culture, the availability and quality of services, and policies that directly or indirectly affect these other interactive influences (see Box 3-1).

The role and effect of biological, behavioral, and environmental influences change as children grow. For example, a pharmacological agent like thalidomide is highly toxic within a narrow window during pregnancy but not afterward, an attachment to a caring adult is especially critical during infancy, and peer influences appear to grow steadily from toddlerhood through adolescence. Even within

---

BOX 3-1
Organization of Influences on Children's Health

Children's biology

Children's behavior

Physical environment
- Prenatal exposures
- Childhood exposures
- Home, school, and work settings
- Child injury and the provision of safe environments
- The built environment

Social environment
- Family
- Community
- Culture
- Discrimination

Services

Policy

---

a childhood stage, health influences can act in very different ways because of the differing cultural interpretations that families attach to them.

While biology, behavior, and environmental categories are useful for organizing our discussion, it is important to understand that healthy development is not the product of single, isolated influences or even types of influences. Warm and nurturing parenting is an important family influence, but prematurity or visual impairment can make an infant unresponsive to a mother's initial nurturing. Mothers may react with apathy or disinterest, which produces even more withdrawal on the part of the infant (Lozoff, 1989). While simplified schematics or models help to organize understanding of the influences on children's health both during childhood and beyond, life is not as simple as these models suggest.

One caveat should be kept in mind in reading through the following review of evidence. Few of the cited studies drew their evidence from randomized experiments. And few if any of the nonexperimental studies included all relevant variables in their data and analyses. Thus, the findings reported in these studies are likely to suffer from exclusion of potentially important categories of influences, so that the associations that are reported as being important may be due to their associations with a more important or equally important characteristic, or due to interactions with other types of factors so that their effect may be manifested primarily or only in certain population groups. A related problem is that few of the cited studies include data that represent the whole population of children. Thus, the findings that are reported as significant may be significant only in the population studied or similar populations. Nonetheless, the committee found the evidence to be sufficiently compelling to warrant inclusion when there was a plausible, well-supported connection between the influence and health.

Moreover, inferences about the relative importance of the variety of influences are heavily dependent on the nature of the theoretical models that underlie statistical analysis. If more proximal influences are mixed with more distal ones, they may appear to have stronger effects, even in situations in which more distal factors are operating on a multiplicity of proximal influences and therefore have cumulatively greater effect overall. Thus, future research should adapt more appropriate pathway techniques to help to sort out the patterns by which the influences interact to produce different states of health.

Finally, the relative lengths of the following sections are not meant to signify the relative importance of the influences. For some, the prevalence is less well known than for others. From the viewpoint of influences on population or subpopulation health, the relative frequency of the different influences is at least as critical as the degree of the risk that they pose to individuals. Additional research is needed to refine understanding of the relative contribution of each of the influences and the relevance of each across a variety of social and cultural groups.

CHILDREN'S BIOLOGY

A child's biology determines how physiological processes unfold and how organ systems adapt to outside influences. Biological response patterns, including responses to stress, novel situations, and primary relationships, can directly and indirectly influence other biological, cognitive (learning), and behavioral processes. The term "biological embedding" has been used to describe how the external environment influences and shapes the biological environment (including the central nervous system), which in turn changes the way the individual interacts with the external environment (Hertzman, 1999).

Genes

DNA provides the blueprint for life. The units of heredity, or genes, are specific sequences of DNA that code for proteins that affect the particular physiology and anatomy of an individual. All cells contain the full array of genes but, depending on the cell type, some are expressed while others are not; for example, certain genes coding for proteins in the retina are expressed in the cells of the eye, but not in the pancreas cells.

Disruptions in genes can be caused by events before, during, or after conception and may produce disorders immediately or later in life. A parent can pass on a defective or abnormal gene or set of genes, a malfunction can occur during combination of maternal and paternal DNA, or exposure to an outside substance or condition can occur after conception that alters the genes in the fetus. Physical and social environments (e.g., family, community, school, culture) interact with and influence these biological processes.

Influences of Genes on Responses to Different Environments

Classically, genes have been considered to be the "instructions" for building proteins, although it is clear now that they have other functions as well. A gene may affect health as a result of the interaction of its protein product with another aspect of a child's biology. The combinations of these interactions may result in an enhanced, worsened, or inconsequential change in health status. For example, sometimes an alteration in the gene (i.e., mutation) is identified due to the presence of a particular disease state, or it can be deduced that an individual with the mutation has a high probability of developing a particular disease. Understanding the biological pathway of the disease and its interactions with other biological processes facilitates treatment options by modifying the causal path. In the case of Huntington's disease, for example, the disorder appears to be in part mediated by glutamate excitotoxicity; giving patients a substance that blocks this effect (glutamate receptor antagonists) interrupts this pathway and may retard the manifestation of the disease (Ferrante et al., 2002). The influence of genes on health always exists in an environmental context; in the next sections we describe how genes affect behavior and the physical and social environments.

Genes and Behavior. That genes affect behavior has been amply demonstrated in honeybees (Ben-Shahar et al., 2002) and higher animals (Ruby et al., 2002; Chester et al., 2003; Hendricks et al., 2003). Examples in humans are being rapidly discovered, including genes that influence the relationship between exposure to trauma and susceptibility to posttraumatic stress disorder (Stein et al., 2002), genetic polymorphisms that protect against alcoholism (Wall, Carr, and Ehlers, 2003), mutations that result in sleep disorders (Wijnen et al., 2002), and several genes that are associated with simple phobias (Gelernter et al., 2003).

Genes and the Physical Environment. The physical environment includes ubiquitous agents (e.g., ultraviolet light, amino acids and sugars in the diet, noise, speech) and somewhat less universally encountered ones (e.g., loud music, medications, pollutants). Some genes result in poor outcomes following common environmental exposures (e.g., phenylketonuria with phenylalanine, galactosemia with galactose, xeroderma pigmentosa with ultraviolet light exposures). Individuals with these genotypes are likely to be affected by the disease because they have a high chance of being exposed to the physical environmental agent. In some cases, the physical environment can be modified to improve outcomes (e.g., a phenylalanine-free or galactose-free diet may improve IQ, no sunlight or ultraviolet exposure may reduce skin cancers). There are also gene alterations resulting from uncommon physical environmental exposures that affect health. Examples include a higher risk of lung cancer in individuals lacking glutathione S-transferase mu who smoke (Perera et al., 2002) and noise-induced hearing loss in some individuals exposed to high levels of noise—the gene or genes in this case are just being discovered (Kozel et al., 2002). These genes are known as *susceptibility genes.* An example of a positive susceptibility gene to a physical environmental agent may be that for perfect pitch. It appears that individuals with exposure to music and a family history of perfect pitch are more likely to acquire perfect pitch (Alfred, 2000).

Genes and the Social Environment. The identification of genes that confer susceptibility to adverse or beneficial responses following exposure to diverse social environments has only just begun. In one study, abused children with a genotype conferring high levels of neurotransmitter-metabolizing enzyme monoamine oxidase A expression were less likely to develop antisocial problems in adulthood (Caspi et al., 2002). The risk of developing alcohol abuse or dependence also appears to have both a genetic susceptibility and a family influence (Macciardi et al., 1999; McGue et al., 2001), as does the risk for relapse and poor outcomes with schizophrenia (Campbell, 2001).

Characteristics of Gene-Environment Interactions

The expression of certain genetic characteristics depends on the environment in which they occur. Thus, gene expressions that lead to a disease in one context may not lead to a disease, or may result in a different disease, in another context (Holtzman, 2002). Inheriting a single copy of the hemoglobin S gene makes an individual resistant to malaria (Aidoo et al., 2002). However, inheriting two such genes gives the individual sickle cell anemia, a severe disease. Outside of malaria-endemic areas, sickle cell trait, the inheritance of one copy of hemoglobin S, has no known adaptive benefit and may be maladaptive. A single cystic fibrosis gene has been postulated to be protective against diarrheal diseases such as cholera, conferring a survival advantage to individuals who carry one copy of the gene (Rodman and Zamudio, 1991). However, individuals with two such genes have cystic fibrosis, a severe disorder with altered pulmonary and gastrointestinal function. Other examples of genes with positive influence also exist in given environments. The gene or genes that confer protection from cancer (Gonzalez et al., 2002; Reszka and Wasowicz, 2002) have been described.

Genes may confer susceptibility only during a specific span of time, referred to as a critical period. For example, 20 percent of children are extremely sensitive to thalidomide during a critical 15-day period from day 20 to day 35 of gestation, although the gene or genes responsible for this enhanced sensitivity have not yet been identified (Finnell et al., 2002). Presumably there are narrow windows of rapid development throughout childhood, including puberty, but critical windows of sensitivity to disruption have not been adequately described (Selevan et al., 2000). The complex interrelationships between genetics and environmental stimuli are not clearly defined and are an active area of current research.

Gene Expression

Understanding of the genome has rapidly expanded the study of the ways in which genes interact with diverse influences (e.g., physical and social environments) to affect health. Expression of genes (the amount of the protein encoded for by the gene) has a profound influence on the health of the individual. Gene expression is determined by many factors, such as promoters, regulators, mutagens/carcinogens/teratogens, X-inactivation, message stability, rate of protein degradation, prior exposures, all of which are affected by the environment. Interactions between genes and the environment influence different physiological pathways and adaptation (Holtzman, 2001) and may lead to adaptive or maladaptive phenotypes. An interesting example is the hygiene theory of childhood asthma, which postulates that children living in hygienic, low-pathogen environments develop an imbalance between two types of immune cell classes (TH1 and TH2). Children with an imbalance of TH1 and TH2 are more likely to develop allergies and asthma when confronted with allergens. When children live in low-hygiene, high-pathogen environments, they develop a strong system of immune regulators (a balance between TH1 and TH2 cells), and they are less likely to develop allergies or asthma (Yazdanbakhsh et al., 2002). Children living on farms or in homes with at least two cats or dogs in the first year of life have been shown to have significantly lower rates of allergic sensitization tested at 6–7 years (Ownby et al., 2002).

Healthy development depends on gene expression being responsive to changes in the environment. For example, the radical change in the environment at birth is responsible for changing the expression of genes to enable the baby to make the transition from intrauterine to extrauterine life. These include the production of proteins that close the ductus arteriosus (Kajino et al., 2001), alter lung liquid absorption (Matalon and O'Brodovich, 1999), produce barrier function in the skin (Harpin and Rutter, 1983), produce immunoglobulins, and alter gene expression in brain development. Thus, to be healthy, newborns must make profound changes in gene expression as they transition from intrauterine to extrauterine environments.

Converging findings from genetics and molecular biology demonstrate that a host of internal and external signals can stimulate or inhibit gene expression, including subtle factors such as the light-dark cycle (Hegarty, Jonassent, and Bittman, 1990) and tactile stimulation (Mack and Mack, 1992). This pattern of contingency is now recognized as part of the normal process of development in embryology and developmental biology, and there is a growing body of literature demonstrating how factors, including internal neural and hormonal events and external sensory events, activate or inhibit gene expression during individual development (see Davidson, 1986, 2001; Gilbert, 2000; Holliday, 1990).

Body Stores

Chemicals in the environment (air, water, dirt, dust, food) move into the body across such biological barriers as skin, lungs, and the gastrointestinal system. Exposure is considered to be contact of the agent with the biological barrier; following exposure, the agent crosses the barrier and is found inside the body (the internal dose). After uptake or absorption across the barrier, chemical agents (including drugs) are distributed throughout the body, metabolized, and eliminated (U.S. Environmental Protection Agency, 2003; Atkinson et al., 2001).

The rate of elimination varies substantially for different agents; some are eliminated in a matter of minutes; others may be found in the body for years following exposure. The amount of chemical/biochemical/vitamin/mineral stored or measured in the body is called the "body stores" or "body burden" of that agent. The committee has adopted the term "body burden" in this report. Body burdens of a chemical or drug represent the amount of cumulative exposure and, in some instances, can be transferred to another individual (e.g., from a mother to the fetus or infant through the placenta or in breast milk).

Body burdens can improve or harm health, based on their biological characteristics and presence during certain periods of development. Maternal body burdens of either lead or polychlorinated biphenyls (PCBs) impair the cognitive function of offspring if present during critical periods during fetal development (Gomaa et al., 2002; Lai et al., 2002). A body burden of lead in the bones of young children has been associated with poor social behavior (Needleman et al., 2002; Wald et al., 2001), poor cognitive performance or development (Lanphear et al., 2003; Rogan and Ware, 2003), and impaired pubertal progression (Selevan et al., 2003). The relative impact of body burdens varies with developmental stage. Relatively lower body burdens of organic mercury will reduce cognitive development in young children more than at older ages (U.S. Environmental Protection Agency, 2000c; National Research Council, 2000).

Some body burdens can have positive impacts on healthy development. For example, maternal body burdens of folate during the early first trimester of pregnancy significantly reduce the risk of a baby with a neural tube defect (Wald et al., 2001). Adolescents with higher levels of folate also have a significantly decreased risk of juvenile hypertension (Kahleova et al., 2002), and adults with high folate stores appear to be at substantially lower risk of cardiovascular disease (Wald, Law, and Morris, 2002). Some body stores that are beneficial at lower levels can become harmful at higher levels: a baby's appropriate body burdens of iron will improve cognitive outcome, but an inappropriately high body burden of iron potentiates oxidative stress (Rao and Georgieff, 2001) or can cause iron overload disease. Low maternal or fetal levels of vitamin A are associated with developmental disease, as are high levels.

The impact of some body burdens vary across time and, to be understood, must be assessed at different times. For example, a maternal body burden of PCBs causes exposure to both the fetus and to the newborn via breast milk. Body burdens at one time may also impact measures of health in later time frames. A child who has received treatment for Hodgkin's lymphoma, increasing the genotoxic body burden, is at risk for secondary cancers (Hack et al., 2002).

Early Programming

While not without controversy (Huxley et al., 2002), there is a growing literature on the potential role of "perinatal programming," referring to the processes in which specific influences during critical or sensitive periods of development can have lifetime consequences by altering metabolic pathways and other physiological systems. This appears to be a special case of the more general phenomenon of how environmental influences can be embedded in biology during critical and sensitive periods of development.

In humans, the relationship between fetal growth, postnatal growth, and the risk of such diseases as hypertension, coronary heart disease, and non-insulin-dependent diabetes have been frequently studied (Bertram and Hanson, 2002; Barker, 1998). Both human epidemiological and animal experimental studies support the hypothesis that relative undernutrition in the fetus results in significant and relatively permanent changes in important physiological systems (Nathanielsz, 1999). Perinatal programming indicates that sensitive or critical periods of development may have lifelong effects and influence the development of chronic diseases later in life (Ingelfinger, 2003). However, it does not discount the potential effect of the external environment (Seckl, 1998; Ingelfinger and Woods, 2002; Falkner, 2002; Roseboom et al., 2001) in modifying the effects.

Fetal undernutrition is believed to induce persistent changes in several metabolic pathways, but the exact mechanisms are only now being pieced together through a range of animal experiments and human measurement studies (Seckl, 1998; Barker, 1998). Because it is likely that events occurring at other times modify prior influences, there is a growing interest in understanding the predisease pathways and biological changes that occur prior to the recognition of a vast array of clinical outcomes. Currently many of these predisease markers are either below current limits of detection or produce changes that are not currently measured on a routine basis (Lucas et al., 1999; Keller et al., 2003; Ingelfinger, 2003).

Examples of such programming during particular sensitive or critical periods of development are coming to light. For example, low numbers of nephrons are associated with hypertension, and it has been shown that individuals whose mothers experienced severe protein-calorie malnutrition during the third trimester, when nephron development takes place, are most at risk of hypertension (Roseboom et al., 2001; Keller et al., 2003). Outcomes associated with programming early in life may also promote health. For example, rats receiving high levels of licking and grooming as pups are less fearful compared with rats that received low levels of licking and grooming (Francis et al., 2002). The mechanism for this change in behavioral programming appears to be the influence of maternal licking on gene expression during a critical period of development and subsequent changes in the development of synaptic receptor sites for specific neurotransmitters (Francis et al., 1999).

Similar environmental influences on the development of behavioral pathways have been described in rhesus monkeys (Champoux et al., 2002), and studies of premature human infants show substantially greater increases in body weight after introduction of massage therapy (Field, 2002). In contrast, disruption of maternal bonding during infancy has been shown to have profound negative effects on later relationships (National Research Council and Institute of Medicine, 2000).

CHILDREN'S BEHAVIOR

As used in this report, behavior refers to a child's emotions, beliefs, cognitions, and attitudes, as well as his or her overt behaviors. Some behaviors are planned and deliberate; others are reflexive, impulsive, and contingent on environmental circumstances. A child's emotions, beliefs, and attitudes affect health, principally through the way they modify a child's explicit and overt behaviors, such as his or her health and life-style choices. These in turn alter the child's eventual health outcomes. Examples include social and interactional behaviors (e.g., compliance with parental requests, peer interactions), health preventive behaviors (e.g., avoiding smoking, driving with a seat belt, choosing good friends), or illness-management-related behaviors (e.g., behavioral adherence with a treatment regimen or health care appointments).

Health-related behaviors may be health promoting (those that increase the likelihood of future health, such as regular balanced diet and exercise) or health impairing (those that adversely cause actual morbidity or mortality, such as smoking, drinking, or reckless driving). A body of recent research suggests how these behaviors develop and describes the role of family, peers, and social environment, including media, in shaping this developmental process (Tinsley, 2003). While behaviors like smoking, drinking, and exercise are known to affect later health, it is not clear how these behaviors develop in childhood (McGinnis and Foege, 1999).

Often these health behaviors are considered proxies for health, even though they may not necessarily constitute health per se. Some health policies attempt to change youth behaviors that are thought to affect health. An example is the requirement for regular school attendance, which may both reflect current health and exert effects on a given child's likelihood of future health.

Behavioral influences on children's health are often reciprocal, both influencing and influenced by parents, peers, and others. For example, parenting style, family traditions, and peer influences affect not only fairly simple youth behaviors, such as compliance with behavioral requests or participation in health prevention programs (Patterson and Fisher, 2002), but also more complex behaviors, such as participation with disease management regimens. This section focuses on the internal psychological factors that underpin children's behavior, with implications for subsequent health outcomes.

Emotions, Attitudes, and Beliefs

In addition to the influence of explicit behaviors on health, a child's internal emotional, attitude motivation, or belief states may exert effects on health. For example, research on both adults and children has shown direct relationships between internal attitudinal and personality factors and health outcomes, perhaps through mechanisms that link internal emotions, attitudes, and beliefs with stress reactions and immune responses (Berry and Worthington, 2001; Herbert and Cohen, 1993; Kiecolt-Glaser, 1999, Lawler et al., 2000). Thus, external events perceived as stressful by a child may function as triggers for an asthma or inflammatory bowel disease flare, over and above any biological exposure or adherence to therapy (Rietveld and Prins, 1998; Santos et al., 2001). Presumably such effects are conveyed through a child's emotional arousal states, which in turn result in physiological changes, such as increased pulse and elevated blood pressure, glycemic, and immune responses. This research has solid empirical support in both the adult human and animal research fields (McEwen, 1998; Seeman et al., 1997), but it is less firmly established for children.

Behavioral Adaptations

The hallmark of childhood is the constant exposure to new developmental challenges. As children acquire new physical and cognitive skills and experiences, their behaviors change. They explore, practice, and experiment and as a result they change and are changed. The resulting behaviors are both manifestations of their health and have significant implications for it. At each new exposure, the child may respond in a variety of ways that in turn unleash a variety of reactions in his or her caregiver and in others around him.

From birth, infants recognize, prefer, and are soothed preferentially by their mother's voice (Mehler et al., 1978; DeCasper and Fifer, 1980). They suckle more in response to it (Mehler et al., 1978), and mothers in turn are gratified by their ability to sooth their children (Klaus et al., 1972). Thus the beginnings of attachment are initiated. As an infant continues his or her explorations and trials, which themselves influence health, they produce reactions from caretakers that in turn further affect the infant's behavior and health. One of the first developmental challenges faced by an infant is adaptation to extrauterine life. Low-birthweight infants experience more difficult transitions and are more likely to be fussy during social interactions and less likely to smile and vocalize (Beckwith and Rodning, 1992; Barnard and Kelly, 1990). These infant reactions in turn impose stresses on the parent, which may affect the child's health through impaired attachment. If the parent responds in a fashion that induces further stress in the infant, the increased stress in turn may affect the infant's ability to secrete adequate amounts of growth hormone (Skuse et al., 1996), potentially leading to growth impairment or failure to thrive.

Attempts to make this transition are met with a variety of parental and cultural responses, all of which influence infants in ways that facilitate or impede their development. Nearly a quarter of infants respond to new stimuli in a negative fashion (Kagan et al., 1998); their early infancy imposes a series of challenges that are especially daunting and many are found to still be socially wary and exhibit evidence of physiological stress at age 6 years (Kagan et al., 1987).

Emotional development and the establishment of social relationships are among the greatest challenges of infancy and early childhood. Emotions are fundamental for human attachments, social interactions, and self-satisfaction. Therefore, the extent to which infants evoke sympathetic and empathetic emotions in others and eventually develop these emotional expressions themselves greatly influences their subsequent health. Children who do not attain these skills are more likely to encounter rejection from caretakers and peers (Dodge et al., 2003; Schultz et al., 2000). The complex interplay of genetics, parenting, and societal reactions illustrates just how precarious the early years are and how central infant behavior is for subsequent health (Rutter, 1998).

Attitudes, Beliefs, and Circumstances

The effects of individual, family, and community attitudes and beliefs on health behavior have been well described. A substantial body of research has been conducted on issues related to adherence to treatment regimens, both among parents of younger children and among adolescents (McQuaid et al., 2003; Volovitz et al., 2000; Davis et al., 2001). This work focused initially on asthma and diabetes and more recently on substance use and HIV/AIDS treatment (Manne, 1998). Current research is informed by several related theoretical models of behavior, all of which take into account youths' attitudes, beliefs, and subjective perceptions about the risks of negative outcomes, as well as the perceived benefits and difficulties of treatment (Hochbaum, 1956; Ajzen, 1991; Rogers, 1983; Bandura, 1994).

In accordance with these models, data suggest that both parents' and youths' attitudes are moderately predictive of subsequent health care behaviors, whether in the context of seizures (Kyngas, 2001; Kyngas et al., 2000), asthma (Kyngas, 1999), diabetes (Wysocki et al., 2000; Ott et al., 2000), or sexual risk avoidance (Stanton et al., 1996; St. Lawrence et al., 1995; Jemmott and Jemmott, 1994).

These conceptual considerations lead directly to specific interventions, such as motivational enhancement strategies to encourage youths' substance abuse treatment compliance (Carroll et al., 2001), engaging them in sexual risk prevention activities (Stanton et al., 1996; St. Lawrence et al., 1995), and using collaborative goal-setting strategies in enhancing adolescent diabetes self-care (Delamater et al., 2001). In addition, these theories help explain why and how child compliance may be positively (or adversely) affected by peer and family support (LaGreca and Bearman, 2002; LaGreca et al., 2002; Liss et al., 1998), as well as the support available through a good relationship between the youth and his or her health care team (DiMatteo, 2000; Kyngas et al., 2000). The effect of and the need for support may vary as a function of age (Steinberg, 1999).

Research has documented the impact of chronic illness on child and adolescent adjustment (DiMatteo, 2000; Kyngas et al., 2000). Not infrequently, depression, anxiety, low self-esteem, or other adjustment difficulties may ensue as a result of the underlying illness, increasing risk for treatment nonadherence (Wise et al., 2001; Murphy et al., 2001; Davis et al., 2001) or worsening the outcome of the primary illness (Kuttner et al., 1990; Hauser et al., 1990). Available evidence suggests that good communication skills and the development of positive relationships with the clinical team may offset the effects of negative emotions on health care adherence (Buston, 2002; García and Weisz, 2002; Shaw, 2001).

Emotion, Cognition, and External Influences

The importance of cognitive ability and understanding inappropriate health-related behaviors must also be considered. Children's ability to understand safety rules and health behaviors increases with age (Morrongiello et al., 2001). Over time they acquire the capacity to conceptualize and understand the longer term consequences of their behaviors on their health (Thomas et al., 1997). Conversely, children with developmental disabilities or impaired language ability often show increased difficulties in adhering to necessary behaviors, including health-maintaining ones (Stansbury and Zimmerman, 1999).

While attitudinal, motivational, cognitive, and emotional factors may all exert direct effects on health-related behaviors, the role of environmental factors in these behaviors should not be underestimated. For example, under some circumstances, behavioral factors may contribute less to youths' actual health care behaviors than making available a more easily used medication, such as a long-acting form of medication in the case of birth control (Stevens-Simon et al., 2001; Omar et al., 2002) or providing more stable living situations in the case of adolescents' likelihood of adhering to an HIV/AIDS drug regimen (Conanan et al.,

2003). In addition, children's behaviors may directly affect parents' ability to adhere to a treatment regimen (Searle et al., 2000), just as parental response styles may affect the likelihood of a child's complying with specific requests (Patterson and Fisher, 2002).

Cultural construction of health and disease may also affect compliance with certain treatments by both parents and children. For example, in many cultures, so-called teething diarrhea is considered to be a normal part of growth and development and thus health-seeking behavior or adherence to treatment regimens for the "illness" would be unlikely (Stanton et al., 1992).

In sum, all these psychological factors, whether a child's perceptions of peer norms, self-efficacy beliefs, attitudes about health and health care, or level of motivation to pursue specific health care behaviors, contribute to health-related choices and behaviors. With increasing age, children's behaviors, such as substance use, academic performance, violence, suicide, and auto accidents, constitute a major influence on future health. According to findings from the Global Burden of Disease study, these behavioral aspects of health are likely to exert even greater prominence in coming decades, as behavioral and life-style-related health conditions (e.g., auto accident injuries, consequences of smoking, depression) increase in their relative effect on children's health and illness (Murray and Lopez, 1996).

Complicating this point, however, is the fact that certain behaviors and emotions can serve both as health influences and outcomes. Determining when a behavior is an influence rather than a health outcome can be difficult, because children's current behaviors can affect both future behaviors and subsequent health outcomes. Regardless of the classification and especially due to the inability to distinguish behaviors as health influences or outcomes, data on children's health behavior are an important component of a system that seeks to track child health and health behaviors.

PHYSICAL ENVIRONMENT

The physical environment affects children's health by exposing them to a wide variety of external conditions. These include chemical, biological, and physical influences that exert their impact by being taken into the body (e.g., lead, methyl mercury, persistent organic pollutants) or interacting with body surfaces (e.g., ultraviolet light, physical abuse, particulate matter in air pollution) or the senses (e.g., noise, odors). The built environment affects the ways in which children are differentially exposed to some of these influences. Exposure is the sum of all exposure factors over the course of time, including the home, school, child care, and play areas. Exposures during the prenatal period can also affect children's health.

Prenatal Exposures

Although exposures of the ovum or the sperm prior to conception may have profound health effects on a child, including development of an abnormal fetus,[1] in this section we focus on prenatal influences. In most cases, exposures of the fetus are from maternal exposure. Exposures of the mother during pregnancy can come from many sources; common sources include maternal occupation, substance use, diet and water consumption, and paraoccupation (occupational chemicals or other hazards brought home by other family members). The strongest workplace exposure associations are lead, mercury, organic solvents, ethylene oxide, and ionizing radiation and poor reproductive outcome, including birth defects (Agency for Toxic Substance and Disease Registry, 1993; Schardein, 2000).

Use of tobacco, alcohol, and illicit drugs also have harmful effects. Tobacco use during pregnancy is a major cause of fetal and newborn morbidity and mortality (small for gestational age, persistent pulmonary hypertension, sudden infant death syndrome, poorer intellectual functioning) (Nicholl, 1989; Golding, 1997; Day et al., 1992; Kline, 1987; U.S. Environmental Protection Agency, 1992; Bearer et al., 1997). Heavy drinking during pregnancy is the cause of fetal alcohol syndrome (FAS), the leading known cause of mental retardation (Abel and Sokol, 1987; Sokol, Delaney-Black, and Nordstrom, 2003). Conservative estimates place the incidence of FAS at 0.33/1,000 live births (Abel and Sokol, 1991). More common effects include alcohol-related birth defects, alcohol-related neuro-developmental defects, and subtle effects on a variety of behavioral, educational, and psychological tests resulting from low to moderate levels of drinking during pregnancy (Institute of Medicine, 1996). While the effects of maternal prenatal use of cocaine, opiates, and methamphetamines on infant cognitive development and behavior remain controversial (owing to confounding environmental factors) (Bays, 1990; Tronick and Beeghly, 1999), the effects on maternal-infant interactions are more established (Breiter et al., 1997; Singer, 2000).

There are multiple short critical periods during the development of a fetus when a short, acute exposure may cause a problem. For this reason, exposures need to be tracked as highs and lows on a daily basis rather than as monthly averages. For example, water quality is regulated by monthly averages. However, a daily peak may exceed a threshold of concern and still be within the regulatory limit.

A recent review concluded that neural tube defects and small-for-gestational-

---

[1]For example, prematurity (Herbst, 1980; Kaufman et al., 2000) and hypospadias (a congenital abnormality in which the urethral opening is not at the tip of the penis) (Klip et al., 2002) increased among the grandchildren of pregnant women who took DES (diethylstilbestrol), and sperm exposure resulting from occupational exposures increases the risk of cancer (Feychting et al., 2001; Colt and Blair, 1998) and birth defects (Chia and Shi, 2002) in offspring.

age births are moderately associated with contaminated drinking water (i.e., trihalomethanes) (Bove et al., 2001). Oral clefts, cardiac defects, and complete nasal obstruction (choanal atresia) were found in studies evaluating trichloroethylene-contaminated drinking water (Bove et al., 2001). Food may also contain environmental teratogens. A well-known example is the epidemic of cerebral palsy that followed maternal consumption of fish contaminated with organic mercury in Minimata Bay, Japan (Harada, 1978).

Childhood Exposures

Characterization of exposures over time depends on developmental stage and the mechanism by which the agent produces its effect (EPA exposure guidelines, 2003). Multiple types of exposure may interact to produce their effect by the same mechanism, as for example the exposure to multiple insecticides that interfere with cholinesterases (National Research Council, 1993). Children have unique susceptibilities to chemical exposures (see Box 3-2).

Air Pollutants

Six outdoor air pollutants are regulated by the Clean Air Act: ozone, respirable particulate matter, lead, sulfur dioxide, carbon monoxide (CO), and nitrogen oxides. The effects of repeated or long-term exposure to outdoor air pollutants on the developing lungs of children are not well understood. Indoor air pollution, which is generally not regulated (one notable exception being laws prohibiting indoor smoking in public spaces), results primarily from (1) the products of combustion, such as CO, nitrogen dioxide, particulates, and sulfur dioxides; (2) volatile organic compounds, such as formaldehyde, benzene, and trichloroethylene; (3) the products of tobacco smoking (approximately 3,800 chemicals); and (4) molds.

Health effects from these diverse indoor air pollutants include respiratory irritation with cough and wheezing, exacerbation of asthma, allergic responses, cancer, and central nervous system effects (headache, nausea) (American Academy of Pediatrics, 2003). Exposure to asbestos, leading to lung cancer, is also a concern due to the prevalence of asbestos in schools and some homes (U.S. Environmental Protection Agency, 1987; American Academy of Pediatrics, 1987).

Water Pollutants

Some water pollutants are biological agents, some are chemical agents, and some are radionuclides (physical agents). Biological agents generally come from fecal contamination and include such bacteria as salmonella and *E. coli*, such viruses as hepatitis A and rotavirus, and such parasites as *Cryptosporidium parvum*. Chemicals in water include such metals as lead, mercury, and arsenic, such natu-

BOX 3-2
Children's Unique Susceptibility to Chemical Exposures

Children are more susceptible than adults to chemical exposures, and their exposure varies, depending on their physical location, breathing zones, oxygen consumption, types and amount of food and water consumed, and normal behavioral development. Specific exposures over time depend on developmental stage and the mechanism by which the agent produces its effect (EPA exposure guidelines, 2003). Estimates of chemical exposure are often retrospective, because it is difficult and costly to monitor exposures as they occur. Even if the total duration or dose of exposure is the same for two children, different patterns and timing of exposure may result in different health effects. For example, ingestion of nitrates in well water may reduce hemoglobin to methemoglobin, which is incapable of transporting oxygen (Lukens, 1987). However, if the nitrates are ingested at a slow enough rate for enzymes to change methemoglobin back to hemoglobin, no deleterious health effects occur. This is an example of a threshold effect; the health effect will not occur until the dose from the exposure reaches a particular level in the body.

Physical location. The newborn is usually held by or near the mother, or spends extended periods in a single environment (e.g., a crib), rather than several different environments. Infants and toddlers who are frequently placed on the floor, carpet, grass, or a blanket are exposed to chemicals associated with these surfaces, such as formaldehyde and volatile organic chemicals from synthetic carpet (Bernstein, 1984), pesticide residues from flea bombs (Fenske et al., 1990), dust mites, pet dander, and detergent residues. Preambulatory children also may experience sustained exposure to noxious agents because they cannot remove themselves from their environment. For example, the premobile infant must be protected from sunburn by the caregiver (Lowe et al., 2002).

Breathing zones. The breathing zone for a child, which varies based on height and mobility, is typically much lower than that of an adult. Chemicals that are heavier than air, such as methyl mercury, large particulates (Leaderer, 1990), and radon (Blot et al., 1990) accumulate in lower breathing zones. The presence of mercury in latex house paint in a child's breathing zone results in acrodynia, a hypersensitivity reaction to mercury, also known as pink disease, and prompted legislation mandating the removal of mercury from house paint (Centers for Disease Control and Prevention, 1990b).

ral toxins as *Pfiesteria* toxins, organic chemicals including pesticides, PCBs, trichloroethylene, and chlorination by-products, such inorganic ions as nitrates, and such radionuclides as radon. Systems affected by these contaminants include the central nervous system, the gastrointestinal system, and the hematological system. Many of these chemicals are also carcinogens. Children have been found to be at higher relative risk of gastrointestinal illness from contaminated water (Wade et al., 2003). In addition, children are both more highly exposed and more susceptible to the contaminants found in water. For example, lead in drinking

Oxygen consumption. Because children have a larger surface-to-volume ratio, they also have a higher metabolic rate and greater oxygen consumption (twice as much for a 6-month-old child as an adult) and minute ventilation, which is volume times respiratory rate (more than three times greater for a newborn than an adult). Exposure to any air pollutant is therefore greater on a weight-adjusted basis. For example, if radon is present, a 6-month-old child will receive twice the exposure of an adult (World Health Organization, 1986.) The increased respiratory exchange is also associated with increased vulnerability to CO poisoning.

Quantity and quality of food and water consumed. Children need to consume more calories and water per pound of body weight than adults given their higher metabolic rate. An average infant consumes 5 ounces of formula per kilogram of body weight (equivalent to an adult drinking 30 12-oz cans of soda a day). If the food or liquid contains a contaminant, children may receive more of it relative to their size than adults, making them particularly vulnerable to pollutants in water. Even the most natural of foods, breast milk, whose salutary benefits have been universally acknowledged (World Alliance for Breastfeeding Action, 1992), is affected by environmental pollutants (Ong et al., 1985; Pluim et al., 1994; Rogan et al., 1986). The diet of children is less diverse and contains more milk products and certain fruits and vegetables than the typical adult diet, and, as a result, children may be exposed to more dangerous levels of pesticides and other chemical residues than adults (Zeise et al., 1991; National Research Council, 1993).

Normal behavioral development. Children's normal behavioral development also influences environmental exposures. Children typically pass through a stage of intense oral exploratory behavior from about age 6 months to 2 years. This also places children at risk in environments with high levels of lead dust, such as houses painted with lead-based paint (Chao and Kikano, 1993), wood used in playground equipment that is treated with arsenic and creosote (Kosnett, 1990), and toxic ingredients in sand or arts and crafts materials. Given their exploratory nature, ambulatory children may wander into unusual situations for play, such as used drums, mud puddles, and empty lots, environments that have the potential for dangerous exposures. As they become adolescents, they gain more and more freedom from parental authority, often having their physical strength and stamina peak before they acquire the ability to think abstractly (Campbell, 1976). Adolescents often misjudge or ignore risks (Perry and Silvis, 1987), which may result in their placing themselves in situations with greater risk than an adult would willingly face.

water was found to be the cause of lead poisoning in several infants whose blood lead exceeded 10 mcg/dl (Baum and Shannon, 1997; Shannon and Graef, 1992).

Food Contaminants

Food contaminants can be broadly categorized as either pathogenic or toxic. Pathogenic agents include bacteria, viruses or parasites, bacterial toxins, aquatic organisms that elaborate toxins, and toxins that accumulate in the food chain, such as domoic acid. Toxic chemicals in food can be divided into three categories: (1) pesticides that have been deliberately applied to the food source; (2) colors, flavors, or preservatives deliberately added to food during processing; and (3) chemicals that inadvertently enter the food chain, such as PCBs, heavy metals, and persistent pesticides such as DDT. Particular effects of food contaminants on children include such behavior changes as hyperactivity (Carter et al., 1993) and developmental neurotoxicity from pesticide exposure in food (National Research Council, 1993).

Infectious Agents

Children also are a demographic subgroup prone to infectious diseases because of their exploratory behavior, lack of prior exposure to most infectious agents, and association with other children. Substantial advances in vaccines have reduced rates of many infectious diseases during the past decades. Nonetheless, infectious agents remain a major threat to children's health, particularly with the increase in antibiotic resistance among various infectious organisms and the emergence of new infectious agents (i.e., new strains of flu).

Children are highly exposed and susceptible to some infections that are spread by droplets from coughing and sneezing. Respiratory syncytial virus, the leading cause of serious upper and lower respiratory tract infection in infants and children, accounts for 125,000 hospitalizations and 450 deaths annually in the United States, and it may predispose children to asthma later in life. Annual epidemics occur from November to April, and virtually all infants are infected by age 2 (Black, 2003). Cytomegalovirus infection is spread in child care centers through both urine and saliva containing live virus; rates for preschool-age children in the United States range from approximately 5 to 30 percent (Centers for Disease Control and Prevention, 1985). Children are also particularly susceptible to other infectious agents, such as rotavirus and Norwalk virus, salmonella, and *E. coli* O157:H7, which cause diarrhea and dehydration and sometimes severe complications.

Children are also more highly exposed to vector-borne (e.g., via ticks, fleas) or certain zoonotic (e.g., hosted by dogs, cats, horses) pathogens due to their increased time outdoors, play activities, and behaviors. Vector-borne pathogens include Lyme disease, highest among 5–9-year-olds (Centers for Disease Control and Prevention, 2002a), and Rocky Mountain spotted fever, most prevalent under age 10 (Centers for Disease Control and Prevention, 2000b). Some arboviruses, which are transmitted by different species of mosquitoes, preferentially infect the young (e.g., La Crosse encephalitis carried by a woodland mosquito; Centers for Disease Control and Prevention, 1990a, 1998a). Cat scratch disease, carried by cats, has an estimated annual incidence of 22,000 cases, with the highest age-specific incidence in children less than age 10. Up to 25 percent of these cases result in severe systemic illness (Centers for Disease Control and Prevention, 2002a).

Noise

Few studies have estimated children's exposure to noise or the effect of noise on children's health, but there is suggestive evidence of its effect. Children appear to be routinely exposed to more noise than the recommended upper limit proposed by the U.S. Environmental Protection Agency in 1974 (De Joy, 1983; Roche et al., 1982). Noise-induced hearing loss in one or both ears among children ages 6 to 19 was found to be 12.5 percent (or 5.2 million children) (Niskar et al., 2001) and more frequent among high school students actively involved in farm work compared with peers not involved (Broste et al., 1989). In a sample of 1,218 children, 1 in 20 school-age children had minimal sensorineural hearing loss and 37 percent of the children with this hearing loss failed at least one grade (K–12) (Bess et al., 1998). Even mild hearing loss is associated with increased social and emotional dysfunction among school-age children.

Noise exposure in childhood is associated with a stress response (Tafalla and Evans, 1997—in male college students), headaches (Odegaard et al., 2003), sleep deprivation (Corser, 1996; Cureton-Lane and Fontaine, 1997), elevated blood pressure and heart rate (Matheson et al., 2003; Evans et al., 2001; Regecova and Kellerova, 1995), and poor performance including reading comprehension and long-term memory (Matheson et al., 2003; Stansfeld et al., 2000).

Radiation

Exposure to ultraviolet B radiation from sunlight exposure and the use of tanning equipment during childhood can result in substantial morbidity and mortality later in life. Health risks from exposure vary with skin type and include sunburn, skin cancer (the most common malignant neoplasm in the U.S. adult population), phototoxicity and photoallergy, skin aging, and cataracts. Approximately 80 percent of lifetime sun exposure occurs before the age of 18. Episodic high exposures sufficient to cause sunburn, particularly during childhood and adolescence, increase the risk of melanoma (Saraiya et al., 2003).

Ionizing radiation comes from both natural and manmade sources. Natural sources include radon, cosmic radiation, and ingested radon and fallout. Manmade sources include medical X-rays and some consumer products. The consequences of exposure for children's health include birth defects from prenatal exposures (microcephaly, mental retardation), neurological damage in younger children, and cancer (American Academy of Pediatrics, 1998).

Home, School, and Work Settings

The quality of their housing influences children's health. Housing conditions can contribute to the incidence of asthma, injuries, and lead poisoning (Manuel, 1999). As children age, they spend more time in physical locations outside the home, such as child care, school, and workplace settings that expose them to new physical environments. Thus, parents' choice of child care facility may affect both indoor and outdoor (e.g., playgrounds, backyards) exposures. For example, child care exposure to cigarette smoke may differ from exposure in children's own homes (Wright et al., 1989).

School-age children spend 35 to 50 hours per week in and around school buildings. In some communities, schools have been built on relatively undesirable land, such as landfill sites like Love Canal. Schools are often located on old industrial sites or near highways, resulting in exposure to auto emissions and air pollution (Frumkin, 2003). Many school buildings are old and poorly maintained, leading to exposures to air pollutants, radon, asbestos, pesticides, and lead (Etzel and Balk, 1999). The U.S. General Accounting Office reported that 20 percent of primary and secondary schools had indoor air quality problems; more than half had environmental pollutant or building ventilation problems that could affect air quality (U.S. General Accounting Office, 1995). Radon above the EPA's action level was found in 2.7 percent of schools surveyed during the 1990–1991 school year (U.S. Environmental Protection Agency, 1992). Asbestos, used extensively in schools until the 1970s, was still present in more than 8,500 schools in 1980, potentially exposing over 3 million students (U.S. Environmental Protection Agency, 1987).

Many adolescents have jobs that may expose them to occupational hazards (Pollack et al., 1990). Every year, at least 70 children die from work-related incidents (Centers for Disease Control and Prevention, 1996) and more than 65,000 are injured severely enough to seek care in emergency departments (Brooks et al., 1993). Under the Fair Labor Standards Act of 1938, which regulates work hours and safety, children younger than 18 are prohibited from working with hazardous chemicals in nonagricultural jobs. Prohibitions on chemical work in agriculture extend only to age 16, and work by children and adolescents on their own family farms is unregulated at the national level. During 1992–1995, 155 deaths were reported among agricultural workers age 19 and younger; 64 (41 percent) of these youths were working in their family's business (Derstine, 1996). For each death, many more experience nonfatal injury (Rivara and Barber, 1985), usually from farm machinery or exposure to toxins.

Child Injury and the Provision of Safe Environments

Injuries are the leading cause of death among children between ages 1 and 19, accounting for more deaths than homicide, suicide, congenital anomalies, cancer, heart disease, respiratory illness, and HIV combined (Centers for Disease Control, 10 leading causes of death, 1997). Although the total number of unintentional injury deaths has declined by more than 40 percent during the past 20 years (CDC Injury Mortality Stats), the rates of childhood injury are much higher in the United States when compared with other developed countries. In 2001, unintentional injuries consttuted 70 percent of all injury deaths to children and adolescents (0 to 20 years) in the United States (National Center for Health Statistics, 2004).

The enormous impact of injury on children's health is manifest by the fact that approximately 18 hospitalizations and 233 emergency department visits occur for every injury death (Grossman, 2000). As injury deaths continue to decline, nonfatal injuries continue to be important causes of child morbidity and disability and substantially reduce quality of life, especially among adolescents. However, it should be noted that data collection on nonfatal injuries is incomplete.

The elements of a safe and healthy physical environment differ according to a child's developmental stage. The American Academy of Pediatrics has conducted extensive reviews of the literature to establish the evidence-based recommendations in The Injury Prevention Program, an age-appropriate prevention education program (www.aap.org/family.tipmain.org/) for physicians and families. Recommendations include counseling parents on use of infant car seats, never leaving infants and toddlers alone in pools or bathtubs, the use of safety equipment for in-line skating and skateboarding, and firearm safety.

The use of playground equipment is the leading cause of injuries to children in school and child care environments, with 211,000 children receiving emergency department care annually for injuries sustained on playgrounds (Centers for Disease Control and Prevention, 1999a). Factors influencing playground injury prevention include supervision, age-appropriateness of equipment, suitable fall surfaces, and equipment maintenance. Supervision has been shown to be inconsistent, age appropriateness is infrequently indicated, and many playgrounds have had equipment with significant safety issues (Sibbald, 2002).

Automobile crashes are the leading cause of death among children over a year old. In 2000, 2,343 children under age 15 were killed in traffic crashes, including 1,668 who were passengers, 469 who were pedestrians, and 175 who were on bicycles. That same year, 291,000 children under 15 years of age were injured in traffic crashes, including 248,000 who were passengers and 22,000 who were pedestrians. On an average day, 6 children are killed and 797 are injured in motor vehicle crashes.

The determinants of motor-vehicle-related injuries and fatalities are well recognized. Some relate to behavioral issues, such as speeding, failing to yield to pedestrians at crossings, and driving while intoxicated; others relate to automobile design and features, including impact absorption, seat belts, air bags, and similar features. Still others relate to roadway features. Public health interventions addressing these factors, from seat belts to traffic signals and from law enforcement to public education and the development of bike paths, have achieved dramatic reductions in injury and fatality rates (Rivara, 1999).

The Built Environment

The built environment may be defined as the part of the physical environment created by human actions—buildings and parks, roads and trails, neighborhoods and cities. This section illustrates the importance of the built environment by describing how land use and related transportation patterns that characterize an entire metropolitan area affect injuries, air quality, and physical activity patterns (Frumkin, 2003).

Injuries

The built environment contributes to motor-vehicle-related morbidity and mortality among children by creating places that rely heavily on increasing driving time in cars and by developing certain kinds of roads that may be unusually hazardous for drivers, pedestrians, or both. Modern suburban roads may be especially dangerous. Major commercial thoroughfares and feeder roads that combine high speed, high traffic volume, and frequent "curb cuts" for drivers entering and exiting stores may pose a special hazard. In general, the prevention of injury by one-time structural changes, such as highway or automobile engineering, is more effective than actions that require repeated use, such as bicycle helmets (Layde et al., 2002).

The epidemiology of pedestrian injuries among children has been well studied and includes several factors that relate directly to the built environment: high traffic volume and speed, absence of play space, and possibly one-way streets (Pitt et al., 1990; Roberts et al., 1995; Schieber and Thompson, 1996; Rivara, 1999; Wazana et al., 2000; DiMaggio and Durkin, 2002). Large boulevards are riskier than residential streets (Kraus et al., 1996), and denser census tracts are safer than those with low density (Lightstone et al., 2001). However, the effect of residential density is complex (Rivara and Barber, 1985; Rao et al., 1997; Posner et al., 2002).

Across the country, the pattern seen for driver and passenger fatalities is repeated for pedestrian fatalities, with lower annual rates in denser cities (National Highway Traffic Safety Administration, 2001). Data from Atlanta show that as that city has sprawled in recent years, the pedestrian fatality rate increased even as the national rate declined slightly (Centers for Disease Control and Prevention, 1999a). The most dangerous stretches of road were those with multiple lanes, high speeds, no sidewalks, long distances between intersections or crosswalks, and roadways lined with large commercial establishments and apartment blocks (Centers for Disease Control and Prevention, 1999a).

Reviews of injury prevention from motor vehicles in children focus almost entirely on seat belts, car seats, air bags, and other engineering approaches or on law enforcement and education (Pitt et al., 1990; Durbin, 1999; Towner and Ward, 1998; Rivara and Aitken, 1998; Rivara, 1999). Primary prevention, in contrast, includes strategies for traffic calming (Roberts et al., 1994; Liabo et al., 2003) and strategies to reduce driving or children's time in and near motor vehicles. These strategies all relate directly to features of the built environment.

Air Quality

In environments where automobiles and trucks are the principal means of transportation, the emissions from these mobile sources figure prominently as a source of air pollution. Although vehicle engines have become far cleaner in recent decades, the sheer quantity of vehicle miles releases large amounts of carbon monoxide, carbon dioxide, particulate matter, nitrogen oxides, and hydrocarbons into the air. Nitrogen oxides and hydrocarbons, combined with sunlight, form ozone. Cars and trucks account for a substantial amount of the emissions of such chemicals.

Ozone levels do not vary over a small scale, from block to block. A child in the suburbs may sustain ozone exposure that is as high as, or even higher than, the exposures of an inner-city child. In contrast, particulate matter less than 2.5 microns diameter (Pm2.5), which can affect respiratory function, may vary from block to block. A child living near a busy intersection or near a heavily traveled truck route may sustain considerably more particulate exposure than a child living in a quieter neighborhood several blocks away.

Children who live, attend school, or play near busy roads or in crowded urban areas, where they are exposed to the exhaust from automobiles and trucks, may experience acute and chronic respiratory effects. In addition, children who live in metropolitan areas with heavy traffic, especially in parts of the country conducive to ozone formation for biogeophysical and meteorological reasons, may be exposed to high levels of ozone during the warm months of the year.

Physical Activity

The built environment plays a major role in promoting or hampering physical activity in children. Schools, parks, and even sidewalks that are integrated into the design of a community can encourage physical activity. For example, physical activity among youth increases when schools offer such facilities as basketball courts and sports fields (Frumkin, 2003). A considerable body of research shows that sprawl—as measured by low residential density, low employment, low "connectivity"—is associated with less walking and bicycling and with more automobile travel than denser communities (U.S. Environmental Protection Agency, 2001; Holtzclaw et al., 2002; Cervero, 2002; Cervero and Ewing, 2001).

SOCIAL ENVIRONMENT

Humans are social creatures. While social influences are important for children of all ages, their nature and form change over the course of childhood. In this section we describe the dynamic nature of the constituents of children's social environment and illustrate how these environmental influences manifest themselves.

Family Influences

Families are fundamental to children's well-being and have a profound direct and indirect influence on the challenges they encounter and the resources available for their needs. The range of needed inputs is broad and includes material resources, time, interpersonal connections, and institutions that parents and communities may use to promote children's development (National Research Council and Institute of Medicine, 1995b). Culturally, differing beliefs about normative development, appropriate parenting roles, and gender roles are important influences on the family (García Coll and Pachter, 2002) (see Box 3-3).

Family influences include both family demography and processes. Family demography consists of the readily measured facts of family life—composition (e.g., one versus two biological parents), financial status, and parental education. Family processes consist of the ways in which family influences operate to affect children's well-being. They include parenting styles, the provision of family environments, and health habits that may be beneficial or detrimental to children's heath. We also include in this category two parental characteristics that affect parenting—mental health and substance abuse.

Family and other environmental factors can be sources of either risk or resilience for the developing child, and it is crucial to understand that the child's response to a specific stressor is influenced by a confluence of other influences. Thus, while in general a specific influence may be negative or positive, may be of greater or lesser impact at a given developmental stage, and may show its effects at the time or at some time in the future, it is often the presence and absence of other

---

BOX 3-3
Family Influences

Family demographics
- Socioeconomic status
- Family composition and size

Family processes
- Parenting
- Family learning environment
- Parental mental health
- Parental substance abuse

risk and resilience factors that determine how an individual child will be affected (Rutter, 1990).

Although the nature and degree of family influences on children change over time, both experimental and nonexperimental evidence indicates that the family continues to have direct influence on a child's decision making well into adolescence (Larson, 1974; Romer, 1994). Two studies have shown that parental monitoring has positive effects not only on their children's performance in the classroom, but also in terms of positive health outcomes; these children had higher grades, greater self-reliance, lower rates of sexual risk behaviors and substance abuse, and also less anxiety, depression, and involvement in delinquent behaviors (Wu et al., 2003; Steinberg et al., 1991).

Family Demography

Socioeconomic Status (SES). Poverty in the United States is disproportionately concentrated among children (U.S. Census Bureau, 2002). The health and development of poor children are compromised relative to U.S. children living in higher income families (Brooks-Gunn and Duncan, 1997). Mortality from infectious diseases is 2.5 times more common and accidental deaths are twice as common among U.S. children in the poorest than among the richest 10 percent of the population. Overall mortality and cancer-related mortality are twice as high among the lowest income quintile compared with the highest income quintile (Shah et al., 1987).

Underlying most explanations for the link between low SES and impaired health are the diminished resources available to families living in poverty. Case et al. (2002) use U.S. data from national health surveys to show that children in higher compared with lower income families are healthier and appear less likely to have their childhood health conditions (e.g., asthma) manifested as poorer general child health, although Currie and Stabile (2002) found that the links between poverty and disease progression appear to be weaker for Canadian than U.S. children.

Low-income parents are also at greater risk for depression and other forms of psychological distress, such as low self-worth and negative beliefs about control, which can impair their ability to use available assets (Gazmararian et al., 1995; Pearlin and Schooler, 1978; Rosenberg and Pearlin, 1978). Nationally representative survey studies show that psychological distress is more prevalent among low-income populations because they experience more negative life events and have fewer resources with which to cope with adverse life experiences (Kessler and Cleary, 1980; McLeod and Kessler, 1990).

The relationship between poverty and child health has been a focus of attention for decades (Egbuonu and Starfield, 1982), and a relationship between low SES and poor health has been well known at least since the beginning of the 18th century. However, only recently have we come to realize that increments to socioeconomic position are positively associated with health at virtually all social levels (Marmot, 1999).

While this social gradient in health is now certain for nonelderly adults, evidence for its existence in children and youth is less well documented. A recent review of evidence from studies of younger children and adolescents indicates the existence of gradients in some but not all aspects of health (Starfield et al., 2002a). Case et al. (2002) documented increasing income gradients in health across childhood in several U.S. national surveys. Currie and Stabile (2002) found similar patterns in Canadian data.

Family Composition and Size. All families do not look alike. One-third (33.2 percent) of all births in America in 2000 were of children born to an unmarried mother (Centers for Disease Control and Prevention, 2000a), and 22.4 percent of all children live with a single parent (Centers for Disease Control and Prevention, 2000b). Longitudinal national survey studies reveal that children reared in families with two biological parents tend to complete more schooling and engage in less risky behavior (McLanahan and Sandefur, 1994), particularly if their SES is high. In a large birth cohort observational study conducted in Great Britain, children of single mothers or living with stepfathers were 50 percent more likely to have been admitted to the hospital and more than twice as likely to have had multiple admissions than children living with both biological parents (Butler and Golding, 1986).

How much of the difference can be attributed to family structure itself in contrast to the prior and often continuing stress of a divorce or separation is not clear. Intact marriages are associated with higher incomes, more male role models, fewer residential moves, and more discipline and supervision than marriages that break up (McLanahan and Sandefur, 1994). Amato and Keith's (1991) meta-analysis of 92 studies addressing the impact of divorce on children found that its impact depends on their ages. Among preschool children, divorce generally had small negative effects on their social adjustment but no effects in other domains. By contrast, children of primary school age appeared to suffer greater negative effects from divorce. The authors note that the better designed studies included in the meta-analysis found smaller effects from the divorce.

Economic and other family resources available to children also vary by family size, since more children often mean less time and money expenditure per child. Although the simple correlations between number of siblings and a host of positive outcomes are almost universally negative (Blake, 1989), the extent to which these negative correlations represent causal impacts remains in dispute (Guo and VanWey, 1999). For some aspects of development, larger families may confer advantages, as when the presence of siblings allows a child to gain experience with relations among "peers."

Family Processes

Parenting. Much has been written regarding the effect of parenting style on child development, how parental challenges and tasks change with maturation of the child, and how parenting style varies by ethnicity, which in turn influences the impact of parenting style on outcome. Baumrind (1971) proposed the prevailing conceptual framework, which applies throughout childhood and has facilitated understanding of the effect of three different styles of parenting: permissive (warm and undemanding), authoritarian (cold and demanding), and authoritative (warm and demanding).

Authoritative parenting is associated with social responsibility and self-assertion among children (Dornbusch et al., 1985) and lower levels of adolescent risk behavior and higher levels of achievement during the adolescent years (Steinberg et al., 1989). Harsh, punitive disciplinary practices are thought to feed into the cycle of anger and aggressive behavior developed by some children and youth (Petit, 1997). Patterson's theory of the socialization of aggression, well supported by decades of research, argues that aggressive children are trained to be competitive and parents are trained to encourage their competitiveness (Patterson, 1995; Patterson et al., 1991, 1992).

While a substantial observational and intervention literature supports this general framework, important variations in these elements of parenting are manifested in different cultural contexts (Steinberg et al., 1992; Wu et al., 2003). For example, in the context of Chinese immigrant families, Chao (1994) argues that parental control efforts are related to the goals of training children to have harmonious relations with others, which is considered essential to maintain the integrity of the family. In the context of black families, Brody et al. (1998) argue for the concept of "no-nonsense" parenting, which is thought to protect youths from dangerous surroundings.

Although these basic approaches to parenting appear to apply throughout a child's life course, the tasks facing parents change as the child develops, and thus parenting must change. For example, beyond tending to the infant's biological needs, the task for the parent of infants and young toddlers is the establishment of secure attachments (Rutter, 1998). Later in childhood and adolescence, parental monitoring (knowledge of the child's activities and friends) assumes greater importance, along with the other tasks of employing discipline for antisocial behavior, employing effective problem-solving skills, and supporting the development of prosocial skills (Patterson, 1982; Patterson and Stouthamer-Loeber, 1984).

There is some evidence that religiosity among adolescents contributes to lower rates of violence, substance abuse, and emotional distress; it has also been related to more health-promoting behavior, such as proper nutrition, exercise, later onset of sexual intercourse, increased academic competence, and higher levels of life satisfaction (Resnick et al., 1997; Wallace and Forman, 1998; Wallace et al., 2003; Barnes et al., 2000). It is unclear to what extent these effects are related to religion or religiosity rather than parenting, community values, or attributes of youth who tend to be religious.

Family Learning Environments. All children do not enter school equally equipped to master its associated challenges. A substantial literature demonstrates the extent to which parental practices can augment or impede the development of language and reading skills in young children and that acquisition of these early skills predicts later success in school (Hart and Riseley, 1995; Senechal and LeFevre, 2002; Zill, 1996). The quantity of speech directed toward children is a strong correlate of the child's subsequent vocabulary and emergent literacy skills (Hart and Risley, 1995; Huttenlocher et al., 1991; Dickinson and DeTemple, 1998). The literature linking parental reading to infants and toddlers with emergent literacy skills led the American Academy of Pediatrics to recommend that pediatricians "prescribe" reading to parents beginning when their children are 6 months old.

Seminal work by Bradley and Caldwell (1980) identified important aspects of the home environment that are related to children's well-being. Their widely used Home Observation for Measurement of the Environment (Bradley and Caldwell, 1984) scale assesses the type and frequency of interactions and learning experiences that parents provide for their children, both inside and outside the home. Stimulation, emotional support, structure, and safety are associated with the well-being of both low-income and high-income children (Bradley et al., 1994).

Parents and family environment represent an important determinant of childhood eating patterns and childhood obesity (Hart et al., 2003). Although relatively little research has assessed the nutritional environments provided by parents (especially obese parents) for overweight children, existing data suggest a strong environmental contribution confounded by genetic interactions. While the need to design effective family-based eating programs is clear, the evidence base for the effectiveness of such programs in the prevention or reduction of childhood obesity is limited (Birch and Davidson, 2001).

Parents' cultural backgrounds have been associated with the learning environments provided to children of all ages. Parents tend to promote not only those skills that they value, but also those they have mastered (Moll et al., 1992). In a recent study, immigrant parents of different cultural backgrounds—Cambodian, Dominican, and Portuguese—differed significantly with regard to the areas of their children's education in which they were involved (García Coll and Weisz, 2002). These differences existed even when a large majority of parents in all groups reported valuing education and having high aspirations for their children's educational attainment.

Parental Mental Health. Parental depression and psychological distress can have powerful negative effects on child well-being. Depression has been estimated to affect about 10 percent of all mothers and 20 percent of poor mothers (Dickstein et al., 1998). Depressed mothers are more likely to respond to their children with withdrawal, diminished energy, or emotion or to express feelings of hostility and rejection toward their children (Frankel and Harmon, 1996; Field, 1995). Depression appears to be a robust influence irrespective of family income (Miller, 1997; Radziszewska et al., 1996).

Reviews of observational studies suggest that children of depressed mothers compared with those of nondepressed mothers are more likely to show higher levels of aggression, sociobehavioral problems including poorer peer relations and reduced ability for self-control, and poorer school performance (e.g., Cummings and Davies, 1994). Other reviews have found that children of depressed parents are at substantially greater risk to develop depression themselves (Downey and Coyne, 1990). Not all children of depressed mothers manifest adverse outcomes (Cummings and Davies, 1994), leading to the hypothesis that the adverse effects of maternal depression are most evident when compounded by other sources of stress, such as physical abuse, marital discord, and substance abuse (Seifer, 1996; Sameroff and Fiese, 1989). Numerous studies have documented a positive relationship between parental stress levels and rates of child abuse and neglect (Sachs et al., 1999; Hall et al., 1991; Luttenbacher, 2002; Wind and Silvern, 1994; Rodriguez and Green, 1997).

Parental Substance Abuse. Many studies have documented associations between maternal alcoholism and child developmental outcomes. In one study, drinking by female caregivers predicted a less cohesive and organized family environment and higher levels of domestic violence (Jester et al., 2000). Parental substance use also affects a parent's ability to nurture and supervise. Although in the past women have been less likely than men to use illicit substances, rates have been increasing in women (National Institute of Justice, 1989; Ebrahim and Gfroerer, 2003).

Environmental tobacco smoke has been shown to cause many different health effects in exposed children, including cancer, asthma, increased severity of respiratory syncytial virus, and increased incidence of ear infections (U.S. Environmental Protection Agency, 1992). Parental tobacco use is one factor associated with children's starting to smoke (Nichols et al., 2004; Andersen et al., 2004). Recent studies also demonstrate an interaction between maternal smoking and genetic predisposition to increased rates of attention deficit hyperactivity disorder in children (Kahn et al., 2003).

Maternal infant bonding appears to be key mechanism; a recent review of 23 articles showed that 14 found recognizable negative impacts on maternal-child interactions among substance-abusing mothers, and three found a dose-response relationship with impact or an accentuation of impact related to continued substance use postnatally (Johnson, 2001).

Community Environment

Moving beyond the family, there is considerable evidence that community conditions can affect children's healthy development, especially in the case of children growing up in the most dangerous and socially disorganized communities (National Research Council and Institute of Medicine, 2000; Brooks-Gunn and Duncan, 1997). Community influences can originate in neighborhoods, schools, or other organizations and can operate through children's peer groups, the adults with whom children come into contact, or the larger set of social and cultural practices in neighborhoods. Specifically, ethnic enclaves differ not only in socioeconomic characteristics but also in their adaptive culture (García Coll et al., 1996—see Box 3-4).

As with our discussion of family influences, we organize our discussion of neighborhood and community influences using the distinction between demography and processes. Community demography consists of readily measured characteristics (e.g., poverty, adult unemployment, crowding). Processes consist of the ways in which neighborhoods and communities operate to affect children's well-being.

There are many definitions of a neighborhood or community environment (Brooks-Gunn and Duncan, 1997). In empirical studies, it is typically a geographic area defined by the Census Bureau (tracts, which are locally defined community areas). But there are social definitions of communities that transcend geographic boundaries and can vary across families and ethnic groups (Jarrett, 1997).

Community Demography

Neighborhood Demographic and Economic Characteristics. The socioeconomic characteristics of a community have a strong association with such indi-

---

BOX 3-4
Community Influences

Community demographics
- Neighborhood demographics and economic characteristics

Community processes
- Schools and early education programs
- Violence
- Social organization of neighborhoods and schools
- Peer influences

vidual health outcomes as infant mortality, birthweight, mental health, and cardiovascular status (Diez-Roux, 2002; Ellen et al., 2001). Several studies in various locations have found that even when controlling for important risk factors, such as income, race, smoking, body mass index, and alcohol consumption, residents of lower SES communities had higher rates of poor health than residents of higher SES communities (Malmstrom et al., 1999; Yen and Syme, 1999).

Yet a striking result in broad-based studies of neighborhood effects on children is that there are many more differences in families and children *within* neighborhoods than *between* them. Chase-Lansdale et al. (1997) found that, at most, 2 percent of the variation in behavior problems among 5- and 6-year-olds can be explained by a collection of neighborhood demographic and economic conditions, such as poverty, male joblessness, and ethnic diversity. Duncan et al. (2001) have shown that less than 5 percent of the variation in youth delinquency can be explained with knowledge of the neighborhood of residence. These findings must be tempered by the way in which more proximate and more distal influences are interpreted statistically.

Community Processes

National Research Council (1990), Coulton (1996), and Sampson et al. (2002) provide general summaries of ways in which neighborhood and community processes may affect children's development, including:

• institutional explanations, in which the neighborhood's institutions and resources (e.g., schools, quality of food markets, health care facilities, public health, and police protection) rather than neighbors per se make the difference;
• stress theory, which emphasizes social and psychological conditions, such as community violence, as well as the importance of exposure to such physical toxins as lead in soil and paint;
• social organization theory, based on the importance of role models and values consensus in the neighborhood, which in turn limit problem behavior among young people; and
• epidemic theories, based primarily on the power of peer influences to spread problem behavior.

Since adolescents typically spend a good deal of time away from their homes, explanations of neighborhood influences emanating from peer-based epidemics, role models, schools, and other neighborhood-based resources would appear to be more relevant for them than for younger children. However, interactions between preschool children and their kin, neighbors, religious communities, and child care and health systems suggest that neighborhood influences begin long before adolescence (Chase-Lansdale et al., 1997).

Schools and Early Education Programs. Among community institutions, formal schooling plays a major role in shaping children's development. Completed schooling is a strong correlate of such successful adult outcomes as longevity, career attainments, and avoiding crime (Fuchs, 1983), as well as such two-generation outcomes as successful parenting (Hoff-Ginsberg and Tardiff, 1995).

Nevertheless, researchers have long worried about the potentially spurious nature of these associations. Are they truly the result of the schooling, or do they instead reflect the greater ability or motivation that leads some children to complete more schooling? The most sophisticated studies strongly suggest causal impacts of schooling on earnings as well as other positive outcomes, with the apparent social rate of return to investing in additional years of schooling averaging around 10 percent (Card, 1999). Roughly speaking, this means that investing $10 in interventions that successfully promote the attainment of an additional year of schooling produces a $1 annual increment to participants' earnings. The relative roles of schooling, income, and occupation in affecting adult health are a matter of considerable debate (Krieger, Williams, and Moss, 1997; Daly et al., 2002).

Education prior to school entry appears to matter as well. Reviews of experimental evaluations of high-quality early childhood education programs have concluded that intensive programs improve children's short-term cognitive development and long-term academic achievement, as well as reduce grade retention of children in special education (Barnett, 1995; Farran, 2000; Karoly et al., 1998) and rates of academic failure, delinquent behavior, and adolescent pregnancy rates (Hawkins et al., 1992). Furthermore, some of these programs also improve children's long-term social behavior, as indicated by fewer arrests and reports of delinquent behavior. Indeed, the payoffs to early education programs may well exceed those of formal schooling (Heckman, 1999).

Schools can also have an effect on student behaviors, the ability to arrive at school ready to learn, and overall health. School health programs have increased substantially over the past several decades in recognition of the connection between health and learning. The Institute of Medicine recommended in 1997 that all students in elementary, middle, and junior high school receive sequential health education to help shape their behaviors. The report noted that skills training, peer involvement, social learning theory, and community involvement have the greatest effect on school health education.

Finally, research has confirmed the direct relationship between physical activity and long-term health. School physical education programs over the past decade have in fact shifted toward an emphasis on physical fitness rather than competitive sports. Although there is limited research on the effect of physical education on health, there is some evidence that participation among middle and high school students is below national objectives (Lowry et al., 2001; McKenzie et al., 2000).

Violence. Children's exposure to community violence in the United States, particularly among poor children living in urban settings, is strikingly high (Osofsky et al., 1993; Purugganan et al., 2000). The most extreme form of community violence, reflected in homicide rates, reached its peak in the early 1990s and has since been on a decline (Cole, 1999). Between 1985 and 1991, the homicide rate among youth ages 15–19 increased 154 percent, surpassing that of other age groups (Buka et al., 2001). Although the United States is experiencing a welcome decline in violence (Cole, 1999), homicide rates for youth remain among the highest compared with other age groups (http://www.ojp.usdoj.gov/bjs/homicide/teens.htm). Moreover, investigators estimate that homicide rates reflect only a small fraction (1/100th) of the violence witnessed or experienced by today's youth (Rosenberg and Mercy, 1986).

An emerging literature suggests that the long-term consequences of childhood exposure to community violence are similar to those noted for child victimization. Children's exposure to violence has been linked to a number of adverse health consequences, including depression, withdrawal, anxiety, posttraumatic stress disorder, fatigue due to sleep disturbance, poor school performance, participating in harmful events, having negative beliefs and attitudes toward others, and aggressiveness (Dyson, 1990; Pynoos et al., 1987; Kendall-Tackett, 2002; Buka et al., 2001; Zuckerman et al., 1995; Groves et al., 1993; Martinez and Richters, 1993). It is important to note, however, that this emerging literature lacks specificity, as it is currently not clear which types of exposure to violent events pose the greatest threat to children in terms of resulting in impaired social and emotional development and functioning.

Social Organization of Neighborhoods and Schools. Communities vary greatly in the degree to which people know each other, care about each other, and even share responsibility for each others' children. These connections among people—social networks and the norms of reciprocity and trustworthiness that arise from them—are sometimes referred to as "social capital." A higher level of social organization in a neighborhood is associated with better family and child outcomes (see National Research Council and Institute of Medicine, 1995b, p. 13; Sampson et al., 2002). Neighborhoods in which parents frequently come into contact with one another and share values are more likely to monitor the behavior of and potential dangers to children (Sampson, 1992; Sampson and Groves, 1989; Sampson et al., 1997).

Social organization is affected by the degree of sprawl in a community; increased sprawl restricts the time and energy people have available for civic involvement and reduces the opportunities for spontaneous, informal social interactions. Sprawl also is associated with decreased use of public facilities, reducing opportunities to mingle with other people, segregating people, and disrupting continuity of community across the life span. There also is evidence that mixed-use, walkable neighborhoods contribute to social capital, as measured by knowing one's neighbors, participating in political life, trusting other people, and being socially active (Frumkin, 2002, 2003; Leyden, 2003).

The basic ingredients of neighborhood social organization can also be present in schools, although the ratio of ingredients differs (National Research Council and Institute of Medicine, 1995b). Schools can serve both as protective influences and as risk factors. Students may feel connected to the class, and a well-run class may in turn increase their feelings of connectedness (National Research Council, 2001). When students feel cared for at their school, they are less likely to use illicit substances, engage in violence, or initiate sex and are more likely to report higher levels of emotional well-being (Resnick et al., 1997).

Peer Influences. Peers and friends are important throughout childhood. Poor social acceptance is problematic for children during childhood and beyond. Socially rejected, aggressive 3–5-year-old children have demonstrated stress hormone levels in the top third of their class, often spiking to the "stress" level (National Research Council and Institute of Medicine, 2000). And children demonstrating difficulties with aggression and peer rejection in middle school are more likely than other children to have demonstrated such problems during their toddler years (Rutter, 1998). Children who were rejected during the school years are disproportionately represented among adults with psychiatric problems (Coie et al., 1992) and among those with subsequent legal altercations (Kupersmidt and Coie, 1990), although the pathway of influence is not well established in these studies.

Middle adolescence is the age of the adolescent subculture. The importance of the peer group increases, as well as the pressures to conform to it. At this time, the adolescent is seeking a stable (affiliative) rather than a distinct identity (Greydanus et al., 1990). Risky behaviors become important during this time both as a means to bond to a peer group and for youth who desire to confront adults (Greydanus et al., 1990). But peer group association can also be positive; for example, the strong orientation toward academic achievement among Asian Americans has a stronger association with having Asian peers than with Asian parents (Steinburg et al., 1992).

Multiple datasets spanning several decades and across cultural and geographic niches underscore the importance of peers, peer influence, and the selection of peers as friends as factors associated with adolescent behaviors and perceptions of the world (Jessor and Jessor, 1977; Stanton et al., 1994; Romer, 1994). Thus, for adolescents, like their younger counterparts, peer relations continue to play a role in both adolescence and beyond.

Electronic Media

Electronic media (television and video, video and computer games, and the Internet) have become an integral part of everyday life for many children in the

United States and thus warrant explicit discussion. Children spend more time watching television than in any other single activity except sleep (Huston and Wright, 1997). Children between the ages of 2 and 17 spend an average of 4.5 hours a day in front of screens, watching television, playing video games, and using the computer (Woodard and Gridina, 2000). The potentially adverse consequences of television viewing led the American Academy of Pediatrics to recommend that children under 2 years old should not watch television, and older children should not have television sets in their bedrooms (American Academy of Pediatrics, 1999b).

Violent Media Content and Aggressive Behavior. The association between viewing violent television programs and aggression has been well established (Bushman and Huesmann, 2001; Friedrich-Cofer and Huston, 1986; Huesmann and Eron, 1986). Across methodologies (laboratory experiments, field studies, and longitudinal studies) and measures, research has converged on findings that viewing television violence affects both short-term and long-term aggressive behavior (Friedrich-Cofer and Huston, 1986). A comprehensive meta-analysis of 217 studies of the association between antisocial behavior and media violence revealed the correlation between the two to be sizable: .31 (Paik and Comstock, 1994), a correlation only slightly smaller than that between smoking and lung cancer (Bushman and Anderson, 2001).

Because of the interactive nature of video games, both researchers and the public are particularly concerned about the effects on children of violent content in such games (Calvert and Tan, 1994). As with television, research has converged to suggest that playing violent video games contributes to aggressive behavior (Anderson and Bushman, 2001; Bensley and Van Eenwyk, 2001; Sherry, 2001), but in this case the research is mainly drawn from smaller (i.e., Ns of 50 to 150), largely white and middle-class convenience samples.

Media Use and Obesity. Not all empirical studies have established a positive association between television or video game use (or both) and increased weight or obesity in youth. The most widely cited study is by Dietz and Gortmaker (1985), who report that the prevalence of obesity in a large epidemiological sample of adolescents ages 12–17 increased 2 percent for each additional hour of television watched per week. Subsequent studies have confirmed this relationship (Dietz and Gortmaker, 1985; Robinson and Killen, 1995; Robinson et al., 1993; McMurray et al., 2000; Durant et al., 1994).

One way in which television viewing or video game use is thought to be related to increased weight in children is that time spent with these media displaces physical activity. Evidence for the displacement of physical activity by television is mixed, with some studies documenting decreases in participation in physical activities following the introduction of television into small, mainly rural, communities (Brown et al., 1974; Williams, 1986), but more representative observational studies reporting little or no relationship between physical activity and television viewing (Robinson and Killen, 1995; Robinson et al., 1993; Durant et al., 1994).

A second hypothesis links television viewing, in particular, to increased caloric intake either from eating during viewing or as a result of food advertising on television, which tends to emphasize high-calorie, high-fat foods with poor nutritional content (Story and Faulker, 1990). There is some evidence that amount of television viewing is related to children's requests for, and parental purchases of, highly advertised foods (Taras et al., 1989) and that television advertising may produce incorrect nutritional beliefs in children (Ross et al., 1981). There is also experimental evidence that there are direct effects of exposure to advertising for high-calorie foods on children's snack choices and consumption (Gorn and Goldberg, 1982; Ross et al., 1981).

Effects of Sexual Messages and Sexual Content. Throughout childhood, adolescence, and young adulthood, people continually learn more about sex, with media being a major source of information (Brown et al., 2002; Dorr and Kunkel, 1990; Wartella et al., 1990). The average child will have viewed over 14,000 sexual simulations and sexual innuendos each year (Derkson and Strasburger, 1994). Experimental studies conducted largely with convenience samples of white, middle-class young adults (often college students) have documented negative effects of nonviolent but dehumanizing pornography, especially on attitudes toward women (Kenrick et al., 1989; McKenzie-Mohr and Zanna, 1990; Weaver et al., 1984). However, the evidence is particularly disturbing in the case of violent pornography. Two major reviews of the literature, one using meta-analytic techniques (Allen et al., 1995a) and the other a conceptual review (Malamuth and Impett, 2001), both conclude that sexual violence has been found to be arousing to sex offenders, force-oriented men, and sometimes even to "normal" young men if the woman is portrayed as being aroused by the assault.

Media Use, Cognitive Development, and Academic Skills. Theory and popular perception have proposed that because television viewing involves so little mental effort, it retards cognitive development and the development of such academic skills as reading (Healy, 1990; Winn, 1985). In the case of television, there is a large body of theory and empirical data showing that both the content and form of television programs affect children's intellectual development and social behavior (Huston and Wright, 1997). Longitudinal studies have found that watching general-audience entertainment programming can have deleterious consequences on both academic and social outcomes (Anderson et al., 2001; Friedrich-Cofer and Huston, 1986; Huesmann and Eron, 1986). But both field experiments and longitudinal studies indicate that watching educational programming in early childhood is positively related to cognitive skills (Ball and Bogatz, 1970; Rice et al., 1990; Zill, 2000), school readiness (Wright et al., 2000), and adolescent academic achievement (Anderson et al., 2001).

Much less is known about the effects of video games and computer technologies, but some theorists have proposed that the interactive character of these activities makes them more potent than television as sources of sensorimotor skill, intellectual stimulation, and messages about violence and other social behaviors (Calvert and Tan, 1994; Cocking and Greenfield, 1996; Greenfield, 1994). Researchers have demonstrated academic gains in young children of both genders, using developmentally appropriate software (i.e., software allowing children to control the program and make decisions) in academic settings in such skill areas as verbal ability, problem solving, and creativity (Haugland and Wright, 1997).

Cultural Environment

Culture is often defined by the ideas, beliefs, and values coupled with the rituals and practices of social groups, including but not limited to families. Betancourt and Lopez suggest that culture refers to "a distinct system of meaning or a cognitive schema that is shared by a group of people or an identifiable segment of the population" (García Coll and Magnuson, 2000, p. 97). Miller and Goodnow define cultural practices as "actions that are repeated, shared with others in a social group, and invested with normative expectations and with meanings or significances that go beyond the immediate goals of the action" (National Research Council and Institute of Medicine, 2000, p. 60). Thus, practices to prevent and promote health and provide treatment have to make sense and be congruent with these systems of meanings and practices. In addition, any self-report on health is embedded in these cultural constructions.

In the United States, the relationship of culture to health outcomes and their measurement is particularly significant because of the growth in diverse populations. It is estimated that by 2050, children of color will account for a majority of children in this country (Institute of Medicine, 1997). Consequently, dominant notions of health—mostly based on middle-class, northern European beliefs and practices—are increasingly out of alignment with the traditions, customs, and beliefs of those with other ancestries.

Culture affects health in many ways. One is by promoting daily activities and routines that reflect culturally defined goals and values that interact and influence developmental processes, inclusive of health (Gallimore et al., 1993; Rogoff, 1990). These routines can include, for example, health-promoting habits such as culturally prescribed foods and activities that provide adequate nutrition and caloric intake or patterns of mother-infant interaction (e.g., Harwood, 1992).

Culture also affects health by providing caregivers (and eventually children themselves) with an understanding of development and health: culture offers the context for defining what is a problem, explaining why the problem exists, providing possible treatments, and indicating who should respond (Groce and Zola,

1993; Harwood et al., 1999). Similarly, culture also provides a framework for the use of home remedies. There are studies on the use of cupping and coining, traditional practices in some cultures that have been confused with child abuse (Moy, 2003; Bullock, 2000; Hansen, 1998). Cupping, a practice used by various cultures including Chinese, Arabic, and Jewish, involves attaching cups on one's back and creating a vacuum to evacuate a malady and increase blood flow to the region, leaving marks that can be confused with the result of trauma to the area. Similarly, coining is the practice of rubbing the edge of a coin on one's skin as a treatment for an illness. Other examples of the importance of cultural meaning of health and disease definitions are the "empacho" theory used by Latin Americans (food is claimed to be "stuck" to the intestines causing vomiting, diarrhea, or early satiety—many families seek the help of folk healers or home remedies consisting of such dangerous substances as lead and mercury) and the use of "hot-cold" remedies, which were mentioned in Chapter 1 (Nuñez and Taft, 1985; Risser and Mazur, 1995).

In the United States, variables such as language proficiency, acculturation level, and recency of migration have all been identified as important sources of variability within cultures (Gutierrez et al., 1988) with significant impact on health. Biculturalism (identifying simultaneously with two cultures) rather than linear acculturation (adopting a single cultural identification over time) has been found to be related to better outcomes (Gil et al., 1994; Szaponick et al., 1981).

An interesting finding in the health literature is what has been termed the "Latino epidemiological paradox" (Markides and Coreil, 1986) or "the immigrant paradox" (Fuligni, 1997; Portes and Rumbaut, 2001), whereby recent immigrants who tend to be more economically deprived and less acculturated, or individuals from Hispanic backgrounds in general, tend to have better health outcomes than other groups from the same ethnic backgrounds or non-Hispanics (Hayes-Bautista et al., 2002; Hayes-Baustista, 2003). The mechanisms behind these surprising findings are not well understood. One possibility is that of selection bias; that is, first-generation immigrants to the United States may be the healthiest and most motivated subset of potential immigrant families. But it has also been hypothesized that traditional cultural practices serve as protective factors.

These and other findings have led investigators to posit cultural differences as sources of both risk and resilience (García Coll et al., 1996; García Coll and Magnuson, 2000). In other words, culture does not constitute a source of vulnerability or risk per se, but cultural differences can become a source of risk when (1) cultural differences are seen as deficits that need to be remedied or fixed, (2) cultural differences lead to mismatches between caregivers or the child themselves and members of dominant institutions, and (3) cultural differences lead to experiences of discrimination and diminished life opportunities due to segregation. There is evidence that these sources of stress are not limited to low-income populations but are experienced by groups with higher socioeconomic backgrounds as well (McAdoo, 1981; Tatum, 1987).

Discrimination

A sparse but growing literature on discrimination, particularly regarding race and ethnicity, documents its effect on health. Krieger (2000) reviewed 20 research articles that used instruments to measure self-reported experiences of discrimination: the most common association with discrimination (10 studies) was with mental health; the second (5 studies) was with hypertension. Unfortunately, all studies concerned adults only.

A more recent review confirmed the findings of a substantial association between racial/ethnic discrimination and mental health, with additional associations with various physical health measures (Williams et al., 2003). In one study, simulated racial discrimination was associated with physiological dysfunction, which was associated with subsequent poor health (Harrell et al., 2003); again, the studies included adults only.

Van Ryn and Fu (2003) proposed a pathway through which health provider behavior in clinical or public health settings contributes to discrimination. In this case, the pathway would be as relevant to children as to adults, as adults generally accompany children in health services encounters and act as proxy for them. Nazroo (2003), reviewing evidence on ethnic discrimination from the United Kingdom, concluded that social and economic inequalities, underpinned by racism, are a fundamental source of ethnic inequalities in health across population subgroups. Chaturvedi (2001) suggested that recognition of different kinds of effects from racism, including on children, could help to sort out the pathways by which the multifactorial and interacting influences affect various aspects of health. To that effect, a recent review (McKenzie, 2003) provided added evidence for an effect of racism on health, including the documentation of racism as well as the mechanisms by which it operates.

SERVICES

Although few would debate the relevance of health services to improving individual health, many have actively debated the contribution of health services to the health of populations. In recent decades, writers such as Thomas McKinley have made strong arguments that improvements in population health have come more from improvements in other spheres (particularly nutrition) than from interventions provided by health services (McGinnis et al., 2002). Although there is increasing recognition of the effect of services in the behavioral and social arenas on health (Institute of Medicine, 1997, 2000), evidence regarding specific outcomes of these programs is limited.

In contrast, the medical literature is replete with reports of the effectiveness of specific biomedical interventions that influence the course of particular diseases. John Bunker has gone further and estimated that health services in general account for about half of improvements in health (measured as increases in life expectancy) in the most recent half-century (Bunker, 2001). While his monograph demonstrates the important role of health services, it reinforces the simultaneous importance of other influences.

The effect of social factors on health, and the possibility of their remediation, does not detract from the importance of health services, at least in part because one of the correlates of social factors is differential access to and appropriate use of health and other services. Documentation of the overall effect of services specifically on children's health is more limited. A 1985 publication on the importance of health services on the incidence, prevalence, and severity of 16 important conditions in childhood (Starfield, 1985b) illustrated the importance of access to health services. However, this study provided no quantitative estimates of the total magnitude of effect of health services on the child population, and it predated numerous new vaccines and other general environmental improvements that have further reduced morbidity and mortality. It was also based on a model of health that was more disease-oriented than the multifaceted conceptualization of health proposed in this report.

In more recent years, it has become clear that the nature of health services, rather than simply their presence, is important. For example, an accumulating number of studies, both in the United States and abroad (as well as international comparative studies) have shown the importance of a strong primary care orientation in health services systems (Starfield et al., 1998). The benefits of a strong primary care orientation are even more salutary for children than for adults (Shi and Starfield, 2002).

Comprehensive, high-quality center-based early education has been demonstrated to improve a range of educational outcomes (National Research Council and Institute of Medicine, 2000). A growing literature supports the ability of early intervention services to intervene and modify developmental health trajectories in children who are at risk of developing developmental, behavioral, and mental health conditions (Ramey et al., 1992; Karoly et al., 1998; Olds and Kitzman, 1993; Olds et al., 1997, 1998, 1999). The availability and configuration of services in a given community can be logically assumed not only to affect a range of children's health outcomes, but also to create a context for and to affect the range of other influences.

Figure 3-1 presents a theoretical framework modified from Halfon and Lawrence (2003) to illustrate how services can direct or modify a course of healthy development; modify predisease pathways; and minimize the risk of exposures before they occur, thereby actively promoting the development of health capacities. Services can reduce exposure to health-compromising events. For example, there is strong evidence that multiple doses of pneumococcal vaccine lead to

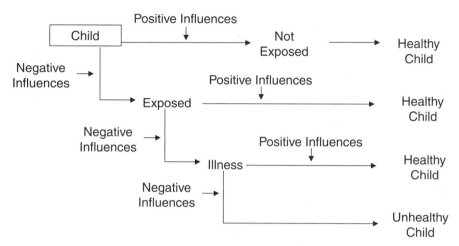

FIGURE 3-1 Where services can effect change in healthy development.
SOURCE: Adapted from Halfon and Lawrence (2003).

significant decreases in otitis media (ear infections) and subsequent hearing loss (Fireman et al., 2003). Public health activities to improve nutrition and public health education campaigns have resulted in health improvements. For example, introduction of folic acid in grain-based products decreased the risk of neural tube defects (Fletcher and Fairfield, 2002). The Back to Sleep campaign, aimed at educating adults on proper infant sleeping position, has been credited with a dramatic reduction in the occurrence of sudden infant death syndrome (Willinger et al., 1998).

Services can modify the relationship between exposure and the onset of disease once the child has been exposed—thereby altering the nature of the exposure outcome pathway. Children exposed to a case of meningitis may receive prophylactic antibiotics to avoid coming down with the disease themselves. Newborn screening identifies infants with phenylketonuria, enabling dietary modification that avoids adverse manifestations of the disorder.

Another way in which services influence health outcomes is to modify or reduce a disease or to promote a specific rehabilitation or habilitation process. For example, the lives of children with cystic fibrosis have been transformed and their prognoses improved as a result of service delivery systems that have lengthened life expectancy and improved functional capacity (Schechter, 2003).

Services relevant to children's health include a broad array of interventions, such as health promotion and preventive services, diagnostic, treatment, and rehabilitative services, educational programs, and a variety of social services. They include specific health interventions, such as immunizations, as well as programs of integrated services that systematically address prevention, promotion, treatment, and risk reduction simultaneously, as is the case in model chronic disease management programs (American Academy of Pediatrics, 2002). Services function at several different levels, including the level of the individual child, family, and community, as well as larger social, physical, and policy environments.

Table 3-1 lists a range of potential services relevant to children's health that reflects the committee's conceptualization of it. While not exhaustive, this list depicts a continuum of services designed to improve the health of children and the functions they serve. It includes services provided by the personal and public health system, as well as the environmental health, education, and social service systems. Prevention-oriented services are shown to include health promotion services that are focused at the population level (e.g., injury prevention, anti-smoking campaigns), as well as services that are part of ambulatory health care provided through the primary care system (e.g., immunizations). Treatment-

TABLE 3-1 Illustrative Services for Children, Youth, and Families

Prevention-Oriented	Treatment-Oriented	Long-Term Care, Home and Community-Based Care
Early intervention programs; early literacy	High-risk mother and infant care services	Long-term inpatient mental health care
Infectious disease control	Emergency medical services	Chemotherapy, cancer radiation treatment
Nutritional services	Smoking and substance abuse cessation programs	Convalescent and rehabilitation care
Lactation services	Acute medical care	Child protective services
Exercise programs	Mental health, behavioral treatment, and therapy	Home visiting
Safe sex education		Home health care
Injury prevention programs	Chronic disease management	Child care
Topic-specific health education targeted at schools, child care, and parenting	Medication management, rehabilitation therapies	School-based clinics
	Crisis intervention	Case management care coordination
Media campaigns	High-risk mother and infant care services	Caregiver respite
Environmental risk abatement programs (e.g., lead)	Emergency medical services	After-school programs
Vision and hearing screenings	Smoking and substance abuse cessation programs	Peer support groups for adolescents
AIDS education, testing, and counseling	Acute medical care	Social skills development, stress management
Smoking and substance abuse prevention	Mental health, behavioral treatment, and therapy	School-based special education and rehabilitation for developmental delay, learning disability, mental health problems and programs for gifted and talented students
Prenatal care; pre- and postpregnancy counseling	Chronic disease management	
Immunizations and well-baby care	Crisis intervention	
Developmental, behavioral, and mental health assessment and guidance		
Genetic screening and counseling		

oriented services include those that are provided in clinical encounters and ambulatory care settings (e.g., acute medical care), as well as those that are provided in hospitals (e.g., emergency services). Long-term, home, and community-based care includes community-based rehabilitative services designed to restore function (e.g., physical therapy), as well as habilitative services designed to maintain the development of function (e.g., speech or language therapy for children with language impairments).

Research is warranted to tease out the role that a range of services play in mediating and modifying influences so children can stay healthy, as well as supporting and promoting their optimal health. Improved specification of the effects of services, better targeting and customizing of services for specific populations, and improved monitoring of the effect of specific services on population health measures should be considered important research and analysis priorities.

POLICY

The health of children in the United States is affected by laws, rules, and regulations developed at the national, state, and local levels. These governmental actions determine the availability of publicly supported services and often regulate the provision of privately administered services. They are integral to how communities operate.

Policies directed specifically at health or health care services, such as eligibility for publicly funded insurance (Currie and Gruber, 1996a) or requiring a child to be immunized prior to starting school (Briss et al., 2000), have both intuitive and documented effects on children's health. But many improvements in children's health over the past century were also influenced by policies in areas other than health. Prominent examples include improvements in children's health as a result of the decision to include vitamins in food products (e.g., vitamin D in dairy products and folic acid in cereals and breads) and fluoride in drinking water (Centers for Disease Control and Prevention, 2001); drinking water and food quality standards (Environmental Protection Agency, 1996; Perdue et al., 2003); educational and child care standards and programs (e.g., the Individuals with Disabilities Education Act); and environmental emissions and engineering safety standards (Perdue et al., 2003).

Innumerable serious injuries and deaths have been prevented by traffic safety standards, such as car seats and speed limits (Sleet et al., 2003; Farmer et al., 1999), consumer product safety standards (Sleet et al., 2003), and such building codes as requiring fencing around swimming pools and safety protections on high-voltage electrical equipment (Stevenson et al., 2003).

The policy environment also affects children's health in less obvious ways. For example, welfare policy decisions play a role in families' SES and even child achievement (see discussion below), and education policies play a role in the availability and quality of schools in a given community (Chase-Lansdale et al., 2003).

Although many policies affect children's health, most are developed and implemented without formal consideration of their effect on children. It is beyond the scope of this report to provide a comprehensive review of all policies that have had an impact—or could have an impact—on children's health. Instead, we illustrate the importance of policy with discussions of fluoridated water, children's health insurance, and welfare reform.

Fluoridated Water

Fluoridation of drinking water has contributed to reductions in dental caries in both children and adults (National Research Council, 1993), and the Centers for Disease Control and Prevention (CDC) has highlighted water fluoridation as a significant public health achievement (Centers for Disease Control and Prevention, 1999b). Cross-sectional studies conducted in the mid-1900s showed water fluoridation to have an effect on dental caries and prompted policies to fluoridate water in many cities throughout the United States. A review of studies on the effectiveness of water fluoridation conducted in the United States between 1979 and 1989 found that caries were reduced between 8 and 37 percent among adolescents (Newbrun, 1989). There is some evidence that water fluoridation has been particularly beneficial for communities of low socioeconomic status (National Research Council, 1993; Riley, Lennon, and Ellwood, 1999), perhaps attributable to their disproportionate burden and lower access to dental care. Evidence of the effectiveness of water fluoridation in reducing dental caries has led to other approaches to introduce fluoride, including the addition of fluoride in toothpastes and topical fluoride treatment by dental professionals.

There has been some debate about whether water fluoridation increases the risk of a range of other health conditions, including cancer, osteoporosis, and Down syndrome. A review by the National Research Council (NRC) in 1993 concluded that there was no credible evidence to support these claims. The NRC is currently conducting a study to review the evidence since 1993 and advise EPA on the adequacy of its current water fluoride standards in the context of the variety of fluoride sources now available.

Health Insurance

The role of health insurance for health care access and service use[2] has been a focal point of health policy and specifically children's health policy over several

---

[2]Policies focused on improving the quality of health services available to children in the United States are equally important. Because there is an extensive literature on the importance of appropriate health care treatments to improve health in the face of disease, we do not review that here, but underscore the importance of access to care based on the information that health can be enhanced through health care.

decades. In contrast to all other industrialized nations and despite frequent incremental attempts to expand health insurance coverage, a substantial proportion of children remain uninsured, and many more have inconsistent or inadequate health insurance (http://www.census.gov/prod/2003pubs/p60-224.pdf). While health insurance is an important contributor to access to and use of health services (Starfield, 2000a; Currie and Gruber, 1996a), it is far from the only factor. The availability and distribution of providers, the functioning of the primary care system, and multiple nonfinancial barriers are also important variables that affect health care access and use (Starfield et al., 1998; Halfon, Inkelas, and Wood, 1995).

The two primary publicly funded programs that provide health insurance for children—Medicaid and the State Child Health Insurance Program (SCHIP)—require families to demonstrate initial and continuing financial eligibility. Implemented in the 1960s, Medicaid coverage increased dramatically during the 1980s and early 1990s as a result of major policy changes in laws that sought to expand Medicaid eligibility (Currie and Gruber, 1996a). Although participation in Medicaid programs is far from universal (Cutler and Gruber, 1996), and most uninsured children still receive medical care, the increased access to health care afforded by Medicaid has been associated with better birth outcomes (Currie and Gruber, 1996b), lower rates of preventable illness (Starfield, 1985a) and improved efficiency of medical care delivery (Dafny and Gruber, in press).

In 1997, SCHIP was initiated to provide further health insurance coverage for uninsured children. SCHIP provided additional funds to states to expand their health insurance coverage by either using Medicaid expansion or, alternatively, developing state-run health insurance programs for children. Despite these efforts to expand insurance coverage, far-from-universal SCHIP program take-up and other factors still left 9.2 million children without health insurance coverage in 2001 for the full year (http://www.census.gov/prod/2003pubs/p60-224.pdf; LoSasso and Buchmueller, 2002). An additional number lack insurance for part of the year. States with policies that facilitate eligibility and certification procedures have been shown to have higher rates of enrollment (Dick et al., 2003).

Health insurance of any type cannot facilitate access to health care services when the necessary resources are not present. In the absence of national health insurance, national health policy has supported the development of a safety net of services in the form of community health centers in areas with a shortage of health facilities and personnel. Currently there are about 800 such centers across the country, all of which provide high-quality primary care services. Recent evaluations indicate that the presence of these centers improves the health of children and reduces racial disparities among the populations who receive services from them (Politzer et al., 2001; Shi and Starfield, 2000).

Welfare Policy

From a policy perspective, it is important to ascertain to what extent policies directed at families or adult family members, even if not explicitly targeted on child well-being, in fact alter children's chances of healthy development. We illustrate this kind of policy analysis with the welfare reform law (the Personal Responsibility and Work Opportunity Reconciliation Act of 1996), which was directed first and foremost at increasing the employment and reducing the welfare dependence of mothers.

Evidence on the likely effects of welfare reforms comes both from random-assignment experiments and from longitudinal survey studies (National Research Council and Institute of Medicine, 2003). A key finding from the experiments is that effects on the achievement and behavior of younger children were consistently more positive in programs that provided financial and in-kind supports (earnings supplements) for work than in those that did not. The packages of work supports were quite diverse, ranging from generous earnings supplements provided alone to more comprehensive packages of earnings supplements, child care assistance, health insurance, and even temporary community service jobs. At the same time, these experiments produced evidence of negative effects on adolescent achievement across all types of programs, although a prominent nonexperimental study did not replicate the negative adolescent results (Chase-Lansdale et al., 2003). Systematic approaches to evaluate the effect of policies on children of this sort are the exception, rather than the rule, and few other systematic attempts can be identified.

CONCLUSION

This chapter provides a discussion of evidence concerning the influence of various types of characteristics on the health of children. Although imperfectly understood, the important role of interactions of these influences, which may differ in kind and amount at different ages and stages of development, is amply supported by the evidence. Notably absent from most of the discussion, however, is the relative importance of the various types of influences on children's health at different ages. For the most part, evidence for the influences comes from studies of the relative risk imposed by them. However, exposure to influences differs in frequency from one influence to another. Influences that have a high relative risk may be of only minor importance to the health of the population of children if they are relatively uncommon. In order to understand the effect of these factors on the health of children, such information is critical (see Goodman et al., 2003).

4

Measuring Children's Health

This chapter outlines the nature of existing data in light of the committee's conceptualization of children's health. It begins with an overview of the available data and outlines two types of gaps in current data collection that need to be filled in order to make them more useful: gaps in the conceptualization of health and gaps in measurement. The chapter closes with a discussion of approaches to filling these gaps and an outline of new ways of approaching the concept and measurement of children's health.

CURRENT APPROACHES

As noted in Chapter 2, children's health has traditionally been assessed by evaluating indices that include the proportion of newborns born small or too early, infant mortality rates, disease-specific incidence and mortality rates, and proxy-reported ratings of health or activity limitations. Available data come from several sources: vital statistics, surveys, and clinical and administrative datasets (U.S. Department of Health and Human Services, 1981).

Vital statistics are part of a standardized state and national system for reporting data on births and deaths. They provide information on births and on rates and causes of death in childhood and adulthood. These systems have been ongoing for more than a century and, while there are a variety of new challenges that arise in the interpretation and use of these data, they are well recognized as important both within countries as well as for international comparisons. In the United States they are used to calculate rates of birthweights, identify birth defects, and track rates and causes of death. An annual compilation of the trends in

91

these data is published (see MacDorman et al., 2002). Another source of standardized reporting of data is the mandated reporting of communicable diseases, which is required of all health care providers and laboratories, to state health departments and, ultimately, the Centers for Disease Control and Prevention (CDC). This system is used to track major infectious diseases and their state and national trends. Outbreaks involving children and patterns of sexually transmitted diseases among adolescents are regularly monitored. In addition, the Maternal and Child Health Bureau (MCHB) has established 6 standard outcome measures that are reported for all states, as well as 18 performance measures.[1]

Survey data have the advantage of providing national estimates of self-reported or, more usually in the case of children, proxy-reported conditions in childhood. The United States collects a great deal of survey data about children, but few surveys are specifically designed to focus on measuring children's health. For many decades the measurement of children's health at the national and state levels has been included in measurement systems that have focused primarily on measuring adult health. This is particularly ironic since the current national system of health statistics had its origins at the early 1900s with assessment of the health of women and the birth of their children (Hutchins, 1997) yet has evolved to focus on adults. The preoccupation of the health care system during the latter part of the 20th century with the prevalence, impact, and cost of chronic diseases in adults and the elderly led to a predominant focus on specific chronic diseases. This focus on chronic disease, along with a long preoccupation with health care costs, has centered national health data collection on their prevalence, the utilization of services for managing them, and the current health expenditures associated with them. In many disease-oriented surveys, children appear to be healthy because of their low prevalence of chronic disorders commonly diagnosed in adults. This orientation and the relatively low price tag for the delivery of child health services have led to an incomplete understanding of children's health (Schlesinger and Eisenberg, 1990). Until recently, there were only a few special one-time or periodic supplements, such as the Child Health Supplements to the National Health Interview Survey (NHIS) in 1981 and 1988 that focused on children's health.

National Child Health Data Collection Efforts

Many federal agencies are now involved in collecting regular and periodic health information about children (see Box 4-1). The National Center for Health Statistics (NCHS), which is a part of the CDC, has several ongoing surveys that concern the health and health care use of children in the United States (Brown,

---

[1]For additional information, see http//www.ahcpr.gov/chtoolbx/measure5.htm and https://performance.hrsa.gov/mchb/mchreports/Search/core/cormenu.asp.

BOX 4-1
Key National Sources of Data on Children's Health by Sponsor

DEPARTMENT OF HEALTH AND HUMAN SERVICES

Centers for Disease Control and Prevention/National Center for Health Statistics
- Vital Statistics
- National Health Interview Survey (NHIS)
- National Health and Nutrition Examination Survey (NHANES)
- State and Local Area Interview Telephone Survey (SLAITS)

Center for Disease Control and Prevention/National Center for Chronic Disease Prevention and Health Promotion
- Youth Risk Behavior Survey (YRBS)
- Behavioral Risk Factor Survey (BRFS)

Maternal and Child Health Bureau/Health Resources and Services Administration
- National Survey of Children with Special Health Care Needs (NSCSHCN)
- National Survey of Children's Health (NSCH)
- National Survey of Early Childhood Health (NSECH)

Agency for Healthcare Research and Quality
- Medical Expenditure Panel Surveys (MEPS)

National Institute of Child Health and Human Development
- National Longitudinal Survey of Adolescent Health (ADD-Health)

DEPARTMENT OF EDUCATION
National Center for Education Statistics (NCES)
- Early Childhood Longitudinal Study—Kindergarten Class of 1998–1999 (ECLS-K)
- Early Childhood Longitudinal Study—Birth Cohort (ECLS-B)
- National Household Education Surveys (NHES)

DEPARTMENT OF LABOR
- National Longitudinal Survey of Youth (NLSY)

NOTE: See Appendix A for a brief description of each of these data sources and the relevant web link and Appendix B for an outline of the data elements corresponding to the health conditions, functioning, and health potential domains for 12 of the current surveys.

2001), including the National Immunization Survey, a telephone survey that collects vaccination data on children between 19 and 35 months. Most major ongoing national data collection efforts also continue to include children in general population surveys. This is true of the annual NHIS and the National Health and Nutrition Examination Survey (NHANES), as well as other special surveys that NCHS supports or administers from time to time. NCHS collaborates with the Agency for Healthcare Research and Quality (AHRQ) to conduct the Medical

Expenditure Panel Surveys, which also include data on various aspects of children's health (as reported by proxies, usually parents). Other nationally representative data are collected directly from adolescents through the Youth Risk Behavior Survey (YRBS) conducted by the CDC and the National Household Survey of Drug Use and Health, conducted by the Substance Abuse and Mental Health Services Administration for persons 12 years and older.

A fairly recent addition to the portfolio of the NCHS is the State and Local Area Integrated Telephone Survey (SLAITS), which uses the same design approach and sampling frame as the ongoing National Immunization Survey. SLAITS is a survey platform designed to collect state- and local-level health care data. It can be used by other federal, state, or local government agencies or private organizations to conduct additional data collection by purchasing use of the platform and time for other surveys. It has been used by other federal and state government agencies as the vehicle for several new surveys for children and has produced a great deal of additional information in a fairly short time frame. This mechanism of using telephone interviews of parents has recently been providing important national and state-level estimates of children's health from families that have access to telephones in their homes.

The MCHB of the Health Resources and Services Administration, which has its administrative roots in the Children's Bureau established in 1912 (Hutchins, 1997), has been a historically consistent federal advocate for the measurement of children's health. The MCHB has recently used the SLAITS mechanism to conduct three surveys that expand national and state-level data on the health of children. In 2000, MCHB used SLAITS to conduct the largest survey to date on the health of children who have special health care needs (van Dyck et al., 2002). It is the first national survey that was designed to allow state-level estimates, in addition to national estimates, of all measures, including the number of children with special health care needs. The goal, contingent on adequate future funding, is to administer it periodically to generate trend and performance evaluation information.

Also in 2000 the MCHB, along with NCHS, CDC, and the American Academy of Pediatrics, sponsored the National Survey of Early Childhood Health (NSECH) using the SLAITS platform to assess the health of children ages 4 to 35 months, the content and quality of well-child health care, and steps parents can take to promote the health and development of their young children.[2] It was a one-time pilot survey conducted with 2,068 families nationwide (National Center for Health Statistics, 2002b).

More recently, the MCHB sponsored another survey using the SLAITS plat-

---

[2]The NSECH also assesses family income, medical insurance coverage and adequacy, day care and day care affordability, and receipt of nutritional and other low-income benefits.

form, the National Survey of Children's Health (NSCH). NSCH is designed to assess the physical and emotional health of children from birth through age 17 and, like the National Survey of Children with Special Health Care Needs will provide state-level as well as national estimates.

Another child health module that has been added to the SLAITS platform is the Child Well-Being and Welfare module, although to date it has been used by only two states, Texas and Minnesota. The National Center for Environmental Health in CDC is using the SLAITS platform to obtain national and select state-level data on predictors of asthma. Although not focused on children, the survey includes them.

Although all of the national surveys aim to obtain representative national samples, survey methodology has some inherent weaknesses. These include the inevitability of some response bias (such as the inability of the SLAITS platform to obtain information about families without telephones in their homes or of household interviews to obtain data on the homeless), issues about whether or not the interviews are conducted in multiple languages, and of cultural validation of questions across groups. In addition, since each minute of questions on large-scale surveys is extremely costly, there is always pressure to ensure that the time is used efficiently. This often leads to many areas being assessed superficially (and in some cases tailored to adults) and to a distinct preference against the inclusion of standardized psychometrically validated instruments, which contain multiple questions, to measure complicated constructs.

One notable exception to the lack of inclusion of psychometrically validated measures has been in the area of child mental health, for which behavioral inventories have been included in the Child Health Supplements in 1981 and 1988. However, overall there has been a paucity of measurement and monitoring of child and adolescent mental health, despite the fact that this is a major cause of morbidity.

In addition to the surveys mentioned above, other agencies, such as the National Institutes of Health, often fund or themselves mount national surveys, such as the National Longitudinal Survey of Adolescent Health (called ADD-Health). For the most part, these are investigator-initiated efforts. They often break new ground in measuring influences or implementing new methods, or provide detailed information about particular aspects of children's health. For example, ADD-Health provides valuable data on a range of adolescent health influences, including peers; the Fragile Families and Child Well-being Study provides the first national look at the influence of father involvement among low-income, unmarried, first-time parents and a married comparison group[3] (although the early waves of this study are not concentrated on health); and linkage of geocoded

---

[3]For additional information, see http://crcw.princeton.edu/fragilefamilies/index.asp.

survey data with census data was advanced by investigator-initiated efforts. Investigator-initiated surveys do not always take advantage of advances in government-mounted surveys, nor are government-mounted surveys quick to adopt the advances from investigator-initiated efforts. Coordination and linkage of surveys, as well as sharing of knowledge regarding survey methodology, should be improved across both government and investigator-initiated surveys. The federally sponsored Developing a Daddy Survey (DADS) initiative may have relevant lessons for such coordination efforts. DADS is a public-private effort to better understand fatherhood and father involvement in children's lives by adding questions to several national surveys.

The National Institute of Child Health and Human Development is leading an effort to develop the National Children's Study, a longitudinal study designed to examine the effects and interactions of a broad range of environmental influences on children's health (including traditional factors, such as chemical, physical, and biological factors, as well as other factors, such as family structure and economics, neighborhood factors, and local and state policy). As envisioned, the study will follow 100,000 children from before birth through age 21. A wide range of individuals, researchers, organizations, and federal agencies have been involved in the planning and design of the study. During the course of the committee's deliberations, the exact specifications of the study were not clear, and funding had not been secured.[4]

The National Center for Educational Statistics (NCES) has several noteworthy national surveys of children's well-being. The birth cohort of the Early Childhood Longitudinal Study (ECLS-B) is in the process of gathering data on children's health, development, care, and education from birth through 1st grade from a sample of 10,600 children born in 2001. The Early Childhood Longitudinal Study, Kindergarten Class of 1998–1999 (ECLS-K) focuses on children's early school experiences, beginning with kindergarten and following children through 5th grade. Its sample is also nationally representative and numbers just under 20,000. The National Household Education Surveys program provides descriptive data on the educational activities of the U.S. population, both children and adults. The ECLS-B and the ECSL-K collect substantial data on environmental factors but relatively little information on health.

Appendixes A and B list the nation's major data resources for measuring and tracking children's health and its influences. It is clear that there are many surveys that tap various aspects of health. Our review shows both the gaps and the considerable overlap and duplication. What is less apparent is that, when an aspect of health is covered, it is often covered using diverse methods, which may include unreliable ways of eliciting information or employ techniques that produce conflicting and inconsistent information. For example, although many surveys in-

---

[4]For additional information, see http://www.nationalchildrensstudy.gov.

clude a question about the overall rating of a child's health, this information may not always be obtained from someone with the same relationship to the child. In some surveys it is answered by a respondent who may not be the child's primary caretaker and in others by a parent or the person who is most knowledgeable about the child's health. Questions about the child's functioning have inconsistent wording across surveys. When wording is inconsistent over a period of time, it is difficult to know to what extent changing rates of identification are a result of those changes (Newacheck et al., 2003).

It has been recognized for some time that data could be collected and used more efficiently if they were better coordinated across agencies. The U.S. Department of Health and Human Services Data Council, responsible to the secretary of health and human services, was intended to accomplish this, but it has not focused on the need for new approaches to the conceptualization of children's health or on the consequent appropriate data collection and dissemination.

National Data Syntheses

There have been several national efforts to use secondary national data to produce annual reports on the health or well-being of children (see Box 4-2). These reports are used by policy makers at the federal, state, and local levels and by others interested in children's health issues to understand trends. Although they can be useful tools to monitor specific indicators over time, they do not enable understanding of the dynamics of children's health or the interaction of influences and health.

For the past 15 years, the MCHB has published an annual report entitled *Child Health USA* that includes data on child health indicators, as well as state-specific data on selective indicators. It also includes trends and progress toward

---

BOX 4-2
National Data Syntheses

America's Children and the Environment
America's Children: Key National Indicators of Well-Being
Child Health USA
KIDS COUNT
Child Trends Data Bank

NOTE: See Appendix C for web links for these syntheses and examples of the indicators tracked.

meeting the goals and objectives in the next decade as set out in the federal reports (Health Resources and Service Administration, 2002).

Over the past 10 years, several other federal efforts have created a greater focus on children's health, particularly on aspects of health traditionally defined as "well-being." In 1994 the Office of the Assistant Secretary for Planning and Evaluation (ASPE) created an annual publication entitled *Trends in the Well-Being of America's Children*. In the same year, a Federal Interagency Forum on Child and Family Statistics was instituted and was formally established in 1997 by executive order. The forum is a formal structure for collaboration among 20 federal agencies that produce or use statistical data on children and families. Since 1998 it has produced a report, *America's Children: Key National Indicators of Well-Being*, now produced on a biannual basis, which presents secondary data on economic security, health, behavior, social environment, and education. ASPE is currently developing a report, *Social Indicators: Measures of Children, Family and Community Connections*, to better understand family indicators in the domains of family structure; family functioning; family, work, and child care; school involvement and civic engagement; and social connections. The Environmental Protection Agency has produced two editions of *America's Children and the Environment*, which presents trend data on environmental contaminants in air, water, food, and soil; biomonitoring data; and data on childhood diseases associated with factors in the physical environment.

Another source of secondary information is the databank maintained by Child Trends, Inc., which provides ready access to a wide range of current data sources pertinent to children's health and its influences. Finally, KIDS COUNT, a project of the Annie E. Casey Foundation, uses census data to produce national and state-level indicators of child well-being. KIDS COUNT produces an annual data book, makes data available on their web site, and funds a network of state-level projects (see Box 4-3).

Healthy People 2010, a national initiative that defines objectives to identify the most significant preventable threats to health and establish national goals related to these objectives, specifies numerous indicators to track the health of the U.S. population. While there are multiple indicators specific to children throughout the numerous identified objectives, with the exception of those relevant to adolescents, there have been limited efforts to use this mechanism to develop a comprehensive focus on the health of children, and the indicators specific to children are not presented in an integrated format.

Other Potential Sources

Other potential sources of information on children's health are clinical and administrative data derived from records or billing information supplied by health care providers. There are large datasets on enrollees in private health insurance plans and in state Medicaid and the State Child Health Insurance Plan. Another

BOX 4-3
KIDS COUNT

KIDS COUNT, a national and state-level project aimed at assessing the status of children in the United States, was initiated by the Annie E. Casey Foundation in the late 1980s.

The initiative is designed "to contribute to public accountability for different child outcomes, resulting in a model for data-driven advocacy for children, their families, and their communities." KIDS COUNT publishes an annual data book that presents state-level data on the educational, social, economic, and physical well-being of children using indicators from multiple data sets. The Casey Foundation also funds a national network of state-level KIDS COUNT projects that provides a more in-depth and detailed view of children in their state.

The 10 measures used to rank states on overall child well-being include:
- percentage of low-birthweight babies;
- infant mortality rate;
- child death rate;
- rate of teenage deaths by accident, homicide, and suicide;
- birth rate to teenage mothers;
- percentage of children living with parents who do not have full-time, year-round employment;
- percentage of teens who are high school dropouts;
- percentage of teens not attending school and not working;
- percentage of children in poverty;
- percentage of families with children headed by a single parent.

The project has also published a series of special reports, such as:
- KIDS COUNT Data on Asian, Native American, and Hispanic Children: Findings from the 1990 Census;
- City KIDS COUNT;
- Success in School: Education Ideas That Count;
- Child Care You Can Count On: Model Programs and Policies;
- When Teens Have Sex: Issues and Trends—A KIDS COUNT Special Report;
- The Right Start: Conditions of Babies and Their Families in America's Largest Cities; and
- Children at Risk, State Trends 1990–2000: A First Look at Census 2000 Supplementary Survey Data.

For more information, see www.kidscount.org.

large administrative dataset is the AHRQ's National Hospital Discharge Data Set. However, these sources vary in the degree to which they are representative of conditions in the population, because they undercount individuals with poorer access, tend to be health insurer specific, and because of the considerable evidence that coding is often inaccurate. Issues related to how to interpret data for which there are no clear denominators and the unreliability of coding are serious. In the first case, there is no way of knowing how to interpret rates of diagnoses, since the population is not stable over time, with people going in and out of practices and plans. In the second, there are obstacles to overcome in order to ensure that coding is consistent. Of concern is the bias frequently introduced by the requirements for reimbursement of medical services, which often influences the ways in which diagnoses are reported. Another limitation is that some sites or plans, especially managed care plans, do not collect data on patients but, rather, on visits. Other concerns relate to how issues of cultural mistrust, perceived racism, or stereotyping may introduce measurement errors when providers and patients are from different cultural, ethnic, and racial backgrounds. Some of these latter problems exist in survey data as well.

State and Local Approaches

At the state and local levels, the measurement of children's health has been even more variable. Other than infant mortality and other mandated perinatal indicators that are collected as part of national vital statistics, as well as the recent SLAITS surveys that have sufficient power to allow state estimates, state and local data collection is inconsistent across jurisdictions. In 1998 ASPE, in collaboration with the Administration for Children and Families and the David and Lucile Packard Foundation, implemented a state-level initiative to build on the work of the Federal Inter-Agency Forum on Child and Family Statistics. This initiative funded 14 states over a 2-year period to develop and track various state-level indicators of children's health and well-being and "to institutionalize the use of indicators in state and local policymaking" (http://aspe.hhs.gov/hsp/cyp/child-ind98, accessed February 25, 2003).

Federally required reporting largely reflects categorical program funding, which often relies on measures of service utilization as proxy measures of health and is driven by funding allocation rather than a well-developed strategy to measure the health of children. In the past decade, some of that has begun to change due to new initiatives originating at the federal and local levels. First, the federal MCHB now requires that all states develop indicators of program performance and measures of the health of mothers and children as a requirement of receiving maternal and child health funding. With a specified set of indicators, states are now collecting and aggregating data on child and family health issues, but there is considerable latitude in how these indicators are measured and hence a lack of standardization. In many states, the demand for indicators has also trickled down to the local level. This move to require a common set of indicators may ultimately form the basis for a common set of metrics on children's health across states.

CityMatCH, a national organization of local maternal and child health agencies, also has facilitated the enhanced collection and reporting of local maternal and child health data. For example, CityMatCH provides city-specific data reports of national comparative data regarding specific health problems, such as infant mortality and low birthweight. Another local data collection enhancement has grown out of the recent focus on the development of healthy cities and communities, which has focused on promoting population health and launching community-wide health improvement initiatives. Similar offshoots specifically focused on children's issues have resulted in development in many localities of community health reports (Halfon et al., 1998; Fielding et al., 1999), made possible by increasing data and information processing and dissemination at the local level. Many of these community health reports focus on children and family health issues, and in many locations across the United States these reports have also been based on new data collection or data synthesis projects.

A network of children's preventive services tracking registries is now operating in six states and New York City as a result of a Robert Wood Johnson Foundation initiative, All Kids Count.[5] These data systems are developing the prototypes for a nationwide system of integrated population-based registries that could be linked with primary care providers to ensure that all children have a "medical home" and that public health officials and other policy makers have population-based data on all children. The rationale for some of these efforts is to demonstrate that local data systems could support the reports of health care providers in activities to promote the health and development of children (Halfon and Hochstein, 2002). These initiatives are very promising. However, it is important to note that only a relatively small proportion of communities are involved or assessing indicators or measures in the same way.

IMPROVING MEASUREMENT OF CHILDREN'S HEALTH

In looking at the current compilation of information about children's health in terms of the committee's conceptual framework, we outline data collection efforts by domain and then look further at the steps that should be taken to improve measurement strategies. While we have chosen to organize this discussion into three discrete domains, it must be emphasized that there is no single universally accepted approach to the delineation of domains of health. Thus to some extent the division is always somewhat arbitrary. Nevertheless, in our view the domains we identified are consistent with current thinking as reflected in the recently adopted International Classification of Functioning as it applies to children (Simeonsson et al., 2003) and with current research in this field.

Existing sources of data contain many items related to aspects of children's health as conceptualized in this report, although not organized around the specific domains suggested below. Most current indicators of health are in fact proxy measures, single items that do not clearly fall into a single domain or cannot be combined to measure the domains fully.

---

[5]For additional information, see http://www.allkidscount.org.

Health Conditions

The first domain, which we call health conditions, contains information on disease, impairment, injury, and symptoms. Most of the items come from vital statistics (in the form of low birthweight and death by cause data), from clinical or administrative data as reported on claims or encounter forms, from injury reporting systems, or from registries. Some surveys also collect data on proxy-reported (or occasionally, in the case of adolescents, on self-reported) health conditions, injuries, and impairments. There are differences in the ways that the principal data agencies (i.e., CDC, NCHS, MCHB, and AHRQ) define specific diseases and measure them. Also, agencies use different age categories, even within childhood. As a result, the country has various estimates for the prevalence of health conditions, making it difficult to compare sources of data regarding conditions and to understand reasons for the differences in estimates.

Another concern is that the cumulative data from most surveys provide estimates for prevalence, but not for the incidence, of individual diagnosed conditions, and there is little information about the overall health of individual children. That is, surveys often look at one or two disease entities, rather than a profile of how diseases cluster in groups of individuals. Diseases are not randomly distributed in the population (Starfield, 1991; Kunitz, 2002), and an accumulating literature (Starfield, 2001; Long et al., 1994) documents the magnitude of this co-occurrence (comorbidity), which is especially pronounced in childhood, when the overall prevalence of health conditions is low but unexpected co-occurrence of different types of illnesses and impairment is higher than would be expected by chance distributions (van den Akker et al., 1998).

Despite this knowledge, most data collection efforts do not describe or facilitate explanation of the clustering of health conditions in specific individuals or population subgroups. There is considerable and robust evidence that children with ongoing health conditions, such as asthma or diabetes, are more likely to have other types of conditions as well. For example, a large literature, for both adults and children, demonstrates that mental health problems are more common in children with chronic physical conditions than in the overall child population (Harris et al., 1996; Long et al., 1994; Stein and Silver, 2002). Thus another concern about the currently available data is that they focus on individual conditions, rather than on the health of groups of individuals.

Given the recent estimates by the surgeon general (U.S. Department of Health and Human Services, 1999) that approximately 1 in 10 (11 percent) of children of ages 9–17 have a significant behavioral or emotional disorder with substantial impairment in current functioning, it may be surprising that there are no assessment approaches currently in place that track child and adolescent emotional health in all of its important aspects.

Generally missing are data on physical and emotional symptoms. Both clinical records and surveys are potential sources of data on symptoms; their coding would be facilitated by more widespread use of the International Classification of Primary Care (ICPC) (Lamberts et al., 1993) or potentially by the newly adopted International Classification of Functioning, Disability and Health (ICF), discussed in the next section. The ICPC was developed by the World Association of National Colleges and Academies, an international association of family physicians, for use in the coding of presenting problems in primary care. It codes a wide variety of types of problems, diagnoses, and other types of reasons for visits (e.g., medication refill, administrative reasons, well-person care) and is compatible with the World Health Organization's International Classification of Diseases.

Functioning

The second domain, which we call functioning, is generally represented by single items or nested items in health surveys. These questions generally explore limitations in functioning related to school or play, which are considered the main functional arenas of children. The utility of existing data and a more complete range of data on physical, cognitive, emotional, and social functioning, as well as disability and restriction of activity, would be enhanced by adoption of the ICF, as it becomes better known by practitioners and survey organizations. This system is designed to inventory different aspects of participation in a wide range of daily activities and to assess the structural and environmental barriers that impede or facilitate functioning. However, it has not yet been adapted to be rapidly used in clinical care or in surveys. The domain of functioning could also benefit from more detailed descriptions of levels of functioning in a range of settings and roles.

Several measures of child functioning are available, such as Functional Status II (R) (Stein and Jessop, 1990), the Wee FIM (Msall et al., 1994), and the Rand measure (Eisen et al., 1979). Each of these measures focuses on a different part of the spectrum of functioning, from unimpaired to severely impaired. Virtually all these instruments depend on the capacity of the clinician or parent respondents to assess a child's performance of activities compared with a theoretical norm and to report accurately on aspects of health and on deviations from normal. The reporting individual must be able to observe accurately and to interpret and communicate the observations in a reliable way. Functional status measures do, however, have the advantage of being applicable to children with a wide range of conditions of varying types, and of including the effects of multiple health conditions (comorbidity) and their treatment (Stein et al., 1987; Starfield, 1992). In many ways these measures represent the summation of multiple health impairments and treatments on the daily lives of children.

Health Potential

The third domain, which we call health potential, is severely underrepresented in existing data sources. Specific indicators of competency and capacity are aspects of developmental status that are rarely measured in surveys or assessed in administrative data. While single items, such as susceptibility to illness ("seldom gets sick"), are sometimes included, most measures of health potential exist for research purposes. They have only rarely been used in clinical settings or ascertained in community surveys. The concept of resilience, until recently, has not been included as part of health. Encompassed in the concept of resilience are such characteristics as protection against (immunization or immunity to or resistance to) illness, problem-solving ability (or "coping"), health-promoting behaviors, physical fitness, and constructive peer and social relationships. These data have been collected in a few local unpublished evaluations of new health programs.

Thus, the country lacks even basic information on the frequency or distribution of characteristics of resilience and other aspect of positive health in childhood and on its variability across the population. Although there is some information on immunization status, it is not generally linkable with other health information. There is no coordinated or linkable data on other aspects of health potential.

PROFILES AND INTEGRATIVE MEASURES

When more than one dimension of health is measured, the question arises of how to compile the information about the different components of health to facilitate a population perspective. One approach is to create profiles that characterize health according to the patterns of scores in each domain of health. This allows for understanding of differences in *patterns* of health across subgroups of the population. It is a necessary component of understanding the ways that variations in health along specific dimensions affect future health over time and how influences of health may affect one dimension more than another.

The creation of profiles of health is an achievable goal. As mentioned earlier, there is potential for combining current indicators into domains and further incorporating domains into profiles that represent integrated measures at the individual level, which can be aggregated to subpopulation and population levels. Not only might such profiles describe the health of individuals and populations generically, but they also could provide the basis for describing the clustering of good and poor health within and across populations and population subgroups (Riley et al., 1998b; Starfield et al., 2002; Starfield, Robertson, and Riley, 2002). There are research tools that assess such profiles, but these are not widely known, generally have a large number of questions, and have not yet been incorporated into thinking about the assessment of well-being across diverse populations. Profiles can capture information about the health of individuals as well as the health of populations and their subgroups (Starfield, 1974; Riley et al., 1998; Riley, Green, Forrest et al., 1998).

Beyond the creation of profiles, many favor the creation of integrative measures that would in effect sum the various components into single score or index of health.[6] Such indices exist in other areas, such as in economics, and although the elements in their calculation may be controversial, they have demonstrated utility in following patterns over time and across communities. In the case of constructing an overall integrative measure of children's health, it would be ideal to incorporate the values that individuals, groups, or society assign to the duration of survival as modified by conditions, impairments, and deficits in psychological, social, or physical functioning and also to assess the individual's health potential. Integrative measures should characterize the special aspects of children's health, such as developmental capacities.

A good measure of health would include a summary score of relevant strengths and deficits that are combined across several components or constructs of development, as is the case for attempts to measure school readiness, which aim to include a child's physical and neurodevelopmental function, cognitive capacity, language function, and social emotional development. Although such measures may not routinely assess health conditions or health impairments, they may provide a composite evaluation of a child's potential to thrive in an educational setting and help forecast that child's or group of children's health, emotional, and social needs (Janus and Offord, 2000).

One approach that has gained in popularity, especially in tracking the health of children in drug treatment trials and other forms of research, is the use of measures of health-related quality of life. These instruments include a wide range of health-related elements, including some of the ones mentioned above. However, they also include a subjective (and in the case of young children, a parental) assessment of pain and other symptoms, general well-being (including some elements that are not consistently thought of as health), and in some cases even parental mental health and stress. Most are lengthy and almost all are proprietary (i.e., not in the public domain). As a result, they have relatively limited acceptability for measuring the health of populations. Thus, we have chosen not to discuss them in any detail here.

Another approach that we reviewed is the use of disability-adjusted life years. These summary scores are predicated on ascribing an economic value to the loss of active and productive contribution to society, primarily in economic terms. These techniques discount the benefits of improvements in children's health, since they place little value on the payoffs that do not result in immediate earnings. Thus they favor improvements in the health of adults who are actively contributing to the community over children's health, since the benefits of improved

---

[6]In March 2004 the Brookings Institution, in cooperation with the Foundation for Child Development and Duke University, released a new index of the well-being of American children. While the index is likely to increase national attention on issues related to children's health and well-being, it does not capture the complexity of children's health and development recommended in this report and may run the risk of overly simplifying children's health issues. Only one of the domains addresses health.

health for children often accrue well into the future, after they have become adults. To some, this leads to an unwarranted bias in favor of productive ill adults over childrearing, immunization, and other investments relevant to children's health.

With the possible exception of overall attempts to quantify a child's school readiness, few measures in current use provide actual profiles of different aspects of children's health, and there is a paucity of integrative measures that cover the age range from infancy through adolescence. Analyses of extant national surveys do not contain profiles or integrative measures of children's health. The only generic measure that is widely available comes from survey-based self- (or, more often, proxy) reports of whether health is subjectively perceived as excellent, very good, good, fair, or poor. In terms of the validity of this question, it is known that lower ratings, as for adults, are associated with poorer health. In children this is manifest by more illness in the previous 12 months and more impairments that limit participation (Alaimo et al., 2001). Children with chronic conditions and functional limitations are more likely to be rated in fair or poor health (Hogan, Rogers, and Msall, 2000; Newacheck and Halfon, 1998; McGauhey et al., 1991; McGauhey and Starfield, 1993). Recent data also indicate that reports on this single item are correlated with scores on the different domains of health when elicited from children in health surveys, and that poorer health ratings are associated with higher utilization of health services in the following year (Riley et al., submitted). However, the predictive validity of these single item ratings for both adults and children may not be the same in diverse population subgroups. One report on children suggests that it may differ in various racial and ethnic groups and that this is not entirely due to differences in other measures of health status such as chronic illness and reported disability (Siegel et al., 2004).

Overcoming Conceptualization Gaps

The approaches summarized provide some important descriptive data about the prevalence of diseases and some information on overall functioning, but these strategies provide little information about the overall health of individual people or groups of people, how their health varies over time, or even the proportion of the population who have more than one condition. They do not reflect the dynamic, multidimensional concept of health that we have proposed, nor do they assess the health potential of children. Childhood implies developmental plasticity. It follows therefore that the best measures of health should reflect this plasticity and most especially children's current and capacity for continued health. They should also detect very early or "pre-stages" of illness as represented by intrinsic and extrinsic predisposition to overt pathology and be able to assess and quantify the spectrum of health in a population of children.

Thus, the first challenge is to delineate methods for measuring the dynamic, developmental, and multidimensional concept of health, including health potential. At a minimum, this requires a consensus about the most important or critical components of health and an increased priority on the importance of monitoring children's health as a matter of national interest. It is also complicated by a number of issues: specific constituencies with a focus on subsets of issues, concerns about the stability and meaning of different domains at any given point for current health, lack of clarity about the current meaning of a given level of health across diverse populations of children, and incomplete information about the predictive validity of a given measure. However, in the committee's view, with concerted focus, resolution of these issues is possible and much of the missing data are obtainable within a reasonable time frame. Mapping trajectories through ongoing collection of data that adopts the same conceptual framework would enable rapid strides to be made in both measuring and understanding children's health and would make it possible to identify and address the needs of subgroups with poorer health.

Overcoming Methodological Gaps

The continuous changes in children as they age can complicate the measurement of their health and require altering the yardsticks used to assess health at various developmental stages. Different individual items may be required to measure domains and subdomains across developmental stages. Inconsistency of the measure or items requires that one sort out how much change reflects measurement error and how much reflects true change in the domain being assessed. This is true even when the same measurement strategy is used consistently over time, because reliability of particular measures may differ systematically between younger and older children.

Another issue that complicates measurement is the need for proxy respondents. Very young children cannot answer questions for themselves, and even school-age children may not be able to respond about some domains of health, because they have not yet developed the ability to perform the level of abstract thinking necessary to answer certain kinds of questions. Those with impairments or disabilities may develop the ability to respond for themselves at a later age than is usual. As a result, it is necessary to obtain data from adult caretakers, parents, or clinicians, at least through the early school-age period. This may produce changes in responses if parental caretakers change over time or when children become old enough to respond for themselves. Parents from diverse backgrounds may also bring different notions of health and disease and may provide different information as a function of the interviewer's background.

Improving Reliability and Validity

Measures of complex concepts such as emotional health and resilience are not often captured in single-item questions. Rather, they require a collection of items to tap the various components that are included in the concept. Well-standardized procedures must be used to assess whether the purported measure is actually doing the job of measuring the concept. This process involves collecting different types of data and subjecting them to analyses to determine if they meet customary standards of reliability (i.e., consistently measures the concept) and validity. Tests of validity are further subdivided into assessments to determine whether the measure behaves in an expected way in relationship to other measures, where they exist, and in relationship to what is known about predictors—for example, of good and poor health. In particular, issues of reliability and validity are compounded when back-translations are needed (Erkut et al., 1999b) and when cross-cultural testing is not available (Scientific Advisory Committee of the Medial Outcomes Trust) (Lohr et al., 2002).

Measures must be quantifiable and reflect the broad range of health outcomes while remaining valid, meaningful, and culturally relevant. The importance of these standards for the measurement of children's health is threefold. First, few measures of these important aspects of children's health meet these standards, and even fewer do so across the full age spectrum (infancy through adolescence) or across subpopulations of different races, ethnicity, or cultures. There is a need for more research in this area to develop better and more sensitive measures that can then be used in large-scale data collection.

Second, there is a need for brevity and efficiency in measures and hence a strong bias in designing surveys against using multi-item measures and scales in large population monitoring activities and in clinical settings because of the expense of administration of each additional question. Organizations that monitor the health of populations aim to do so with single items or with a small set of items, rather than with scales. Yet reducing complex issues to single items is problematic at best. In the area of children's health, this process is further complicated by the paucity of well-developed psychometrically sound instruments for measuring health that span the age range. As a result, with some occasional notable exceptions, primarily in the area of children's mental health, NCHS and others have traditionally used single items preferentially. Newer measurement techniques have been developed that in some cases allow for truncating the number of items that need to be obtained (item response theory) (Hays et al., 2000; Bjorner et al., 2003; Ware, 2003), but even these techniques require extensive measurement development and administration in data collection of a substantial number of items in order to measure a construct as complex as functioning (Moore et al., 2002).

Third, there has been reluctance to invest in the development of instruments and in the funding of the amount of testing that is required to refine an instrument and to determine its reliability and validity across the age spectrum and across diverse populations.

As our conceptual model and definition have highlighted, children have special health attributes that distinguish them from adults. Their unique developmental aspects mean that one must consider not only what domains of health are measured but also how and when to measure health. The timing of measurement is important relative to critical and sensitive periods of development and relative to critical transitions and turning points in children's lives.

Other Methodological Challenges

The committee noted a number of other methodological challenges to current health efforts. First, manifestations of health may vary from setting to setting (for example, in school and at home), so what is noted by an observer in one setting may not be seen in a different setting. As a result, information discrepancies are common when multiple informants are used and procedures must be employed that connect the information and observations provided by different informants.

Second, young children and even older youth tend to not be accurate reporters of their own experiences and behaviors, in part by virtue of cognitive immaturity in younger children and because of concerns about the consequences of candid disclosure in older youth.

Third, privacy concerns are also important, because some health-related phenomena may be associated with embarrassment, stigma, or even legal consequences (e.g., substance use, unprotected sex, suicidal ideation, aggression or violence, victimization).

Fourth, many health-related phenomena, whether positive or negative, are experienced by many youngsters at one time or another over the course of their development, so it may be unclear when they become important in terms of current or future health. For example, many youth experience suicidal ideation, many are intermittently depressed or anxious, and many experiment with drugs or unprotected sex, but not all of those who do have serious health issues. To distinguish what is normal from what is unhealthy or of concern, measurement experts often attempt to qualify the presence or absence of a given condition by adjectives related to severity, frequency, or duration, for example, extreme sadness, frequent drug use, ability-limiting illness. However, most qualifying terms such as "extreme" or "frequent" are also subjective and could be interpreted differently by informants of different cultural backgrounds. Even if one attempts to demarcate normal from abnormal with more specific modifiers (e.g., sadness lasting all day, most days, for two weeks or more), knowledge about what constitutes normal and abnormal is lacking and may vary by age of the child.

Meaningful measurements of health across regions and populations often require reliance on multiple informants, reconciliation of discrepant information across informants, combining different measures across informants and settings, demonstration that the measurements are not simply normal variations (e.g., extreme in terms of frequency, duration, or severity or in short- and long-term prognosis) of impairment in functioning or compromise in future health. As a result of the above concerns there should be support in all data collection activities for methodological efforts to ensure reliability and validity.

Even when longitudinal surveys have gathered health information at multiple points in time, it is rare when analyses of these data have taken advantage of the latest statistical methods. Both hierarchical linear models (Raudenbush and Bryk, 2002) and latent variable growth curve models (e.g., Duncan et al., 1999) can be applied to the problem of understanding the nature and determinants of developmental trajectories.

Appendix B indicates whether measures on the most common federal surveys deal with specific aspects of health and mental health conditions (e.g., depression), whether multiple informants are utilized, and the extent to which empirically established most-valid informants are used for particular health constructs, whether for a risk or an actual health condition. As can be seen from the tables in the appendix, the sole exception to the general failure to attend to these issues is the current iteration of the NHANES study, which is gathering in-depth information from parent and youth informants in such a manner that actual health conditions can be distinguished from high-risk behaviors. The difficulty in doing so is not simply a problem of survey design but has to do with how the mental health, education, and medical fields conceptualize mental health and illness. Many physical and mental health disorders are on a spectrum with common day-to-day problems experienced by everyone. The absence of clear, critical indicators for mental health and illness with strong face validity and an empirical basis for clear medical necessity and impairment in functioning is an important conceptual and methodological hurdle that has not been fully addressed by health researchers and policy makers.

Another methodological problem concerns the representativeness of samples (Brown, 2001). With the exception of major national surveys conducted as ongoing activities of NCHS, AHRQ, and NCES, most samples are representative only of particular communities or regions, usually with time-limited funding sources as a part of an investigator-initiated research study (e.g., National Institute of Health funding). While some of these regional studies are longitudinal, there is generally no clear ongoing commitment to funding or approach that is part of a health-monitoring strategy with explicit ties to policy. Even well-conceived and nationally representative recurring surveys (such as NHIS) are often limited (at least partly due to resource constraints) by failure to use in-depth assessment approaches, failure to use most-valid informants, and failure to link influences with health conditions reflecting disease burden and policy import.

Opportunities to Improve the Conceptual Basis for Health Assessment

The conceptualization of children's health is challenging. Health in childhood extends far beyond diseases, disabilities, and impairments that are typical indicators of adult health. Childhood health is characterized by developmental plasticity, which is not a major facet of adult health. There are critical and sensitive periods of development with major impact on future health outcomes. Early health experiences contribute heavily to subsequent health trajectories.

Measurement strategies should capture what these principles embody. In particular, strategies should capture changes in particularly sensitive periods of development and map how health during one period influences and predisposes to subsequent states of health.

Mapping the health trajectories of individual children or entire populations of children requires consideration of what measures in a specific domain can be linked across developmental periods to create a conceptually consistent measurement trajectory, and also what group of measures across domains can be assembled to account for an aggregate trajectory. Conceptual work related to school readiness illustrates what could be done for a variety of health domains (see Figure 4-1). Measuring specific dimensions of a child's health at birth and at several other ages (e.g., 1, 3, and 5) in a consistent manner could result in a composite health trajectory and a way to plot aspects of children's health in much the same way that one currently plots growth trajectories either for individual children or a population as a whole.

Without a strategy to develop composite indicators, it will not be possible to track health across developmental stages. A domain and subdomain structure should be consistent across developmental stages, even if specific individual items

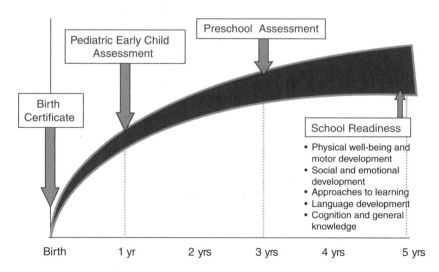

FIGURE 4-1 Systematic data collection for tracking school readiness trajectories.
SOURCE: Halfon et al. (2004).

representing the domain or subdomain differ from one developmental stage to another.

It seems especially important to develop good tools to assess the health of children at major transitions, such as entry into preschool or the beginning of adolescence because these represent critical points at which potential health problems may interfere with the developmental tasks. Measurement strategies should be devised to elicit not only important milestones in development but also the trajectory of characteristics that affect the attainment of those milestones at expected times. For example, most children babble and make simple words before they start saying phrases, and they make declarative statements before they ask questions. But it is unknown how much the variation in the acquisition of those skills affects overall language development except in the most extreme situations.

Addressing the Need for Data on Health Characteristics of Subpopulations

Vulnerable Subpopulations

Disparities in health by race and ethnicity are well documented (Institute of Medicine, 2002b, 2003) and demand national attention. A large subpopulation of children also has poorer health due to social disadvantage. Children in lower income families have more severe health problems and worse health prognoses than children in higher income families. Except for most large national surveys that collect data on family income and parental education, few or no data are collected to provide a systematic understanding of differences in health in population subgroups based on socioeconomic status.

In addition, there are specific subpopulations of children that deserve special attention because of their extra vulnerability to poor health. Localized studies and long-term follow-up studies of specific populations of children (e.g., children who are abused or neglected or in foster care) indicate that some have poorer health (including mental health) and more developmental problems and seriously compromised long-term health trajectories. At present there is limited systematic collection of health-related data on most of these subpopulations at either a local or a national level. A similar situation holds for children with special health care needs due to chronic and debilitating medical or mental health conditions, children in special education school systems, children with severe emotional and behavioral disorders, and institutionalized children. Each of these vulnerable subpopulations of children is poorly reflected in health measurement attempts. Moreover, most surveys intentionally exclude institutionalized children, many of whom have severe health impairments. The very small size of some of these special populations require targeted special studies.

Age-Related Subpopulations

In addition to gaps in the measurement of the health of subpopulations defined by current health and social adversity, there are also gaps associated with age and development, particularly a lack of data related to the middle childhood years. While the NHIS, NHANES, and other national data collection efforts include data on all children, sample size and response burden issues usually preclude the kind of detailed information that is necessary to assess the health of children relative to their developmental age and stage or membership in particular subgroup populations. The NHIS contains a few questions specific to young children, school-age children, and adolescents, and the new MCHB-sponsored NSCH will provide a few more questions relevant to age and developmental stage questions. However, neither of these surveys provides the information needed to develop a comprehensive picture of the health of young children, to better understand the role of various risk and protective factors during early childhood, to assess their access to personal or public health services, or to measure the impact of health care on health. Until the NSECH was piloted, there had not been a data collection effort targeted on the health, health care content, quality of health care, or home health behaviors of families with young children. Since the NSECH is not a part of the regular national survey series, there is no guarantee that there will be ongoing collection of such relevant early childhood health data (Halfon, Olson, Inkelas et al., 2002). Similarly, while there has been recent emphasis on the importance of early childhood and the first 5 years of life as well as considerable focus on adolescents, there has not been the same kind of focus on middle childhood. Relative to adolescents and early childhood, this is a vastly ignored developmental period with regard to the collection of information on health and health influences. Ongoing monitoring of health risk through state administration of the YRBS provides some information on health, although only for those ages 12 to 17 (Brown, 2001).

Addressing the Need for Data on Functioning and Positive Aspects of Health

Standard surveys often ask about whether children are limited in the amount of play (for children under 5 years), or school they experience, but there are few other assessments of their overall functioning. Since many children with even severe impairments are able to play, and most are able to attend school, especially under current policies, this is only a gross estimate of their overall functioning. There are currently few other attempts to assess the overall functioning of children on a population basis, in part because of the relative paucity of measures available to assess functioning, and in part because many of the existing measures require the administration of multi-item questionnaires or other assessments. More work is needed in developing tools that are efficient and valid in this domain.

Although there are some data on health risks, there are very few data on positive health measures and other health and developmental assets, including characteristics that help to ward off threats to ill health. Similarly, there are no coordinated or linkable data regarding states of "resilience," such as physical fitness and nutritional status. While many communities throughout the United States have engaged in the measurement of positive youth behaviors and developmental assets as part of their own local interest or projects, it is important to consider how measuring the developmental assets of young people can be encouraged in all communities and the data made available to public and private entities interested in fostering positive health development in their youth.

In March 2003, Child Trends convened a national conference of leading researchers to review the state of the art in measurement of positive development. The conference concluded (Child Trends, 2003) that a theory of positive development was still lacking, and that many if not most of the measures that have been developed still lack demonstration of validity. Two areas were included under the broad rubric of positive development: (1) positive feelings, attitudes, and beliefs and (2) skills, behaviors, and competencies. The role of culture in the first of these two categories was recognized as a major consideration in interpreting the value of the measures. Other major issues were related to data collection and to the choice of type of respondent. Further work on theory development and research on positive measures was recommended, a direction with which the committee concurs.

CONCLUSION

In the near future, it may be possible to determine the early origins for many significant adult health conditions, such as adult-onset diabetes mellitus, coronary heart disease, and hypertension, as well as to have information about the risk of developing common childhood diseases such as asthma, attention deficit hyperactivity disorder, and some metabolic and diet-related conditions. There is already success in predicting the likelihood of rare Mendelian diseases. Whether there will be similar success in predicting many common adult conditions remains to be seen. At present there is no mechanism for assessing the distribution of genetic risk profiles in the population or relating them to the environmental influences that are likely to determine the actual likelihood of ensuing disease and disability as well as resilience. Developing better data collection mechanisms to array environmental influences in relation to biological or genetic factors is an area in which greater gaps in measurement are likely to be felt in just a few years.

Although there are data that indicate that children are not thriving, many current measures cannot capture either their successes or their failures. The committee's view is that the nation must move ahead in developing a more comprehensive measurement strategy that captures the dynamic nature of childhood, assesses all the domains of health, and tracks composite trajectories of children's health. Strengths and deficits in the current measurement strategies have been highlighted. Measures that assess health potential and provide more comprehensive assessment of functioning, as well as for composite measurements of health, need to be developed. Deficiencies in the assessment of health and influences on health during middle childhood and of special population subgroups also need to be addressed.

Movement toward frontiers in health assessment in children will be facilitated by the development of new tools from current and recent research efforts. A variety of instruments is available, many of which have been employed to good advantage in investigations of the outcomes of research interventions. The potential to adapt these tools for use in large population surveys should be explored.

5

Measuring Influences on Children's Health

A comprehensive system to monitor children's health would contain an inclusive, continuing assessment and monitoring of the range of influences on children's health, including children's biology and behavior, social environments (family, community, culture, and discrimination), physical environments, and services and policy contexts. Development of such a system requires careful long-term consideration of which influences are important, how they are being measured, how to improve their measurement, and what additional measures might result in important benefits to children's health.

We begin this chapter with an overview of current issues and challenges in measuring the multiple influences on children's health. We then outline the current approach and particular challenges of measuring each of the influences identified in Chapter 3 and then discuss how the gaps in measurement of each influence might be improved, including potential future opportunities in light of advances in research methods. Many of the methodological problems and practical obstacles in measuring various health influences are the same as those in developing and implementing measures of health. These areas of overlap are not repeated here, although commonalities are briefly noted. Many of the current surveys that capture data on influences were mentioned in the previous chapter and are outlined in Appendixes A and B; descriptive information regarding specific surveys is not repeated here. Appendix B lists various data elements for the influences outlined in this report that are captured by 12 of the major national surveys.

For some types of influences discussed below, there is ample evidence of the effect they have on children's health. The challenge is to ensure their adequacy in date collection efforts so that differences across time and among subpopulations can be effectively monitored. For others, although there is evidence that they influence health, the challenge is to develop more adequate means of understanding the nature of their influences. In these instances, attention needs to be focused on using data collection to facilitate studies of the way in which they operation on populations and subpopulations.

OVERVIEW

The measurement of many influences poses methodological challenges that must be considered and systematically addressed in future research, surveys and evaluation studies. For such factors as biological influences on children's health, invasive medical tests may be necessary and raise potential ethical questions about risk-benefit ratios of specific assessment procedures. In other cases, the need for highly personal information raises confidentiality concerns and concerns about unintended consequences of shared information. In still other instances, such measures as policy influences may require aggregation across governmental units and agencies.

Several overall issues must be considered to improve the measurement of influences on children's health. First, how do various influences interact with one another over time to affect health? Specific influences may set in motion a chain reaction, unleashing other biological and behavioral processes than can cascade toward a specific outcome (final common pathway) or a range of potential outcomes (multiple pathways). Since each interaction in such a cascade is potentially a point to monitor and intervene, understanding and measuring such effects become important methodological challenges. As a specific developmental stage or sensitive period, exposure to a specific influence can unleash a cascade of effects with significant short- and long-term impacts, whereas the same exposure at a different stage may have a muted or minimal effect.

Another challenge is how to understand and model the effect of multiple influences for policy purposes. For example, when a child is exposed to multiple adverse influences at the biological, behavioral, family, and community levels, are these factors simply additive, or are they multiplicative (Rutter, 1994; Werner, 1993)? The most effective prevention and intervention strategies may target high-risk groups (i.e., those affected by multiple risk factors), rather than using strategies that address single risk factors. For policy purposes, which children may be most at risk for later adverse outcomes, and which may be most in need of special assistance?

Aggregation of data on influences at the individual, family, and community levels is complicated (Small and Supple, 2001) and prone to errors in the application of statistical techniques, drawing appropriate causal inferences, and estimating the relative size of influences' effects.

Apart from biomarkers, the physical environment, family demography, and results from formal medical evaluations, almost all influences require the subjective reports of people (often parents reporting for children) who must describe their perception of the presence or absence, severity, and duration of a particular health influence. Such perceptions tend to differ from person to person, raising important concerns about the validity of any single source of information, particularly when policy decisions (such as the distribution of resources) are to be based on such information.

Despite the fact that parents from different cultural backgrounds must complete these surveys, there are often insufficient data demonstrating that survey items are accurately understood by parents across different cultural contexts, and surveys are not consistently offered in multiple languages. While this challenge poses daunting obstacles to the interpretability of survey findings across cultures, new translation methods have been developed and described that may facilitate more valid responses across cultural groups (Erkut, Alacron et al., 1999b).

Another concept implicit in the committee's conceptual approach is the important role of both positive and negative influences on health. If health trajectories are to be modified, then health measurement at a population level needs to clearly account for the presence and effect of influences, their direct and indirect relationship to each other, and to the health outcome of interest. For example, if substance abuse during adolescence is the outcome of interest, a conceptually driven and integrated health measurement strategy would measure and account for the effect of adverse influences on drug use (e.g., peer influences, school performance, lack of adequate parental supervision) as well as protective factors (e.g., mentoring relationships and educational and economic support).

Despite knowledge that adverse health influences often disproportionately fall on some population subgroups more than others, systematic collection of health care data on subpopulations at a local, state, or national level is episodic. Surveys rarely provide enough information to develop a comprehensive picture of the health of young children, or to understand the role of various influences during early childhood, or to assess their receipt of appropriate personal or public health services or the effect of health care on their health. While there has been recent increasing emphasis on the importance of early childhood, as well as considerable focus on adolescence, there has not been the same kind of focus on health influences in the intervening years.

MEASURING BIOLOGICAL INFLUENCES

The range of biological influences on children's health are assessed using "biomarkers," which are indicators signaling events in biological systems or samples (for review, see National Research Council, 1989). There are three categories of biomarkers: biomarkers of exposure, biomarkers of effect, and biomarkers of susceptibility (see Figure 5-1). The markers fall along the time course from exposure (e.g., prenatal exposure to alcohol) to health outcome (e.g.,

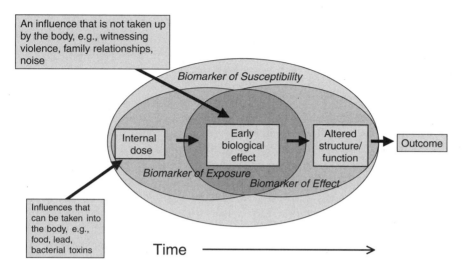

FIGURE 5-1 The three types of biomarkers.
NOTE: The three categories of biomarkers are biomarkers of exposure, biomarkers of effect, and biomarkers of susceptibility. The boxes represent the different steps in the progression from exposures to a health outcome. The solid arrows depict the rate of change from one stage to the next; the time of progression from one stage to the next is highly variable. The nested ovals represent the areas where biomarkers of exposure, effects, and susceptibility may be found and show their overlapping nature (adapted from Committee on Biological Markers of the National Research Council, 1987).

fetal alcohol syndrome). In general, biomarkers of exposure are nearer in time to the exposure (i.e., they are designed to detect exposure rather than the effect of exposure), while biomarkers of effect are generally nearer in time to the outcome (i.e., they are designed to detect the effect of exposure or the effect on health). The time course of moving from exposure to outcome is not continuous. For example, an internal dose can occur quickly after an acute exposure, while a biological effect may take decades (e.g., exposure to radioactive material and the development of thyroid cancer or exposure to asbestos and lung cancer). Biomarkers of susceptibility can mark increased vulnerability at any of the steps between exposure and outcome.

Biological factors that influence health, such as genotypes for functionally important genetic polymorphisms, variations in gene expression, and biochemical measures that reflect body stores or internal doses of environmental exposures, are useful biomarkers. Thus, the concept of biomarkers provides an organizational framework for considering existing indicators and the potential influence of the biological environment. We use this framework in considering current assessments of biological influences, as well as assessment gaps. Identification and selection of particular biomarkers for a specific research or public health purpose would need to include careful consideration of such factors as the ease of collecting a particular biological specimen and the cost of biological analyses.

Biomarkers of Susceptibility

Biomarkers of susceptibility include such factors as biological measures of health and genes. A child's current health as reflected in his or her level of immunity or level of cortisol production may also serve as a valuable indicator of biological susceptibility. Under certain circumstances, age can serve as a proxy for developmental susceptibility, such as the age of risk for sudden infant death syndrome (infants) or testicular cancer (adolescents). The composition of ages in a population, obtainable from the U.S. Census Bureau, can be used as an indirect indicator of susceptibility in the population for specific age-related health conditions. However, most measures of biological susceptibility require some form of biological assay.

As discussed in Chapter 3, polymorphisms (variations from person to person in a gene's molecular structure) in certain genes may impart susceptibility to certain environmental exposures. A biomarker of susceptibility for the individual would be the specific genotype of that gene, while the biomarker of susceptibility for the population would be the frequency of that genotype. An example of an existing database for genes of susceptibility includes newborn screens. Newborn screen testing varies from state to state, but most states include screening for hyperphenylalaninemia (PKU), hypothyroidism, classical galactosemia, and hemoglobinopathies.[1] While congenital hypothyroidism is not always caused by a genetic polymorphism, the screen identifies cases that are genetic in origin. The newborn screen is the only universal population-based database in the United States for children's genetic susceptibilities.

Biomarkers of Exposure

There are several measurement activities for internal dose/body stores/body burdens. Two major programs are being conducted by the Centers for Disease Control and Prevention (CDC): the biomonitoring program and the National Health and Nutrition Examination Survey (NHANES) survey. The process of expanding biomonitoring capability to select state laboratories is currently under way (*Federal Register*, Vol. 68, No. 64/Thursday, April 3, 2003/Notices p. 16287).

---

[1]A listing of the tests done in each state, as well as the summary results of the screening, can be found at the following web site: http://genes-r-us.uthscsa.edu.

Biomonitoring is the direct measurement of environmental chemicals, their primary metabolites, or their reaction products in people—usually in blood or urine specimens. The CDC Division of Laboratory Services has developed methods to measure 200 substances in blood or urine, including but not limited to polychlorinated biphenyls, dioxins, furans, the persistent organic pollutants, DDT and its metabolite DDE, nonpersistent organic pesticides and their metabolites, polyaromatic hydrocarbon metabolites, phthalate metabolites, metals (e.g., lead), volatile organic compounds, and phytoestrogens.[2]

The NHANES survey also includes information about the health and diet of people in the United States. There are both questionnaire and laboratory measurements on a survey of 4,800 children younger than age 19 over a 2-year cycle. Laboratory measurements include iron status, vitamin stores and folate levels, and indicators of specific infections such as viral hepatitis.

Biomarkers of Effects

There are few measurement activities related to biomarkers of effects that are not measurements of health. For example, the NHANES survey measures a few, such as physical growth, biomarkers of inflammation and bone density, and liver, kidney, and respiratory function. NHANES also measures immunization status by measuring antibody levels as a result of immunization. While patterns of changes in gene expression may be a sensitive and specific biomarker of effect, no current population-based measurement activities of gene expression are currently taking place, except in clinical settings for research purposes.

Challenges in Measuring Biological Influences

Several methodological issues are of concern in measuring biological influences. First, obtaining biological samples from fetuses and children is difficult. Samples for biomarkers must be obtained ethically, non-invasively and with a minimum of pain, and be acceptable to both child and parent. Table 5-1 provides examples of types of samples with their advantages and disadvantages. Although it may soon be possible to determine multiple polymorphisms in individuals, the ethical issues in doing so are complex. Guidelines on the ethics of this testing have been proposed (Bakhtiar and Nelson, 2001).

Second, validating a biomarker as a true measure of a biological influence on health is difficult and time-consuming. A number of steps are necessary, includ-

---

[2]The current national status report of population exposure levels (from the CDC's 2002 NHANES) for 116 of these chemicals can be found on the CDC web site: http://www.cdc.gov/exposure report/.

TABLE 5-1 Appropriate Biological Samples in Which to Measure Biomarkers Indicating Fetal/Pediatric/Adult Exposure/Effect

Samples	Advantages	Disadvantages
Adult/Pediatric		
Urine	Large sample size	Requires cooperation, difficult in young children
Hair	May indicate timing of exposure	Requires cooperation, may not be desirable, requires special analytical techniques
Blood	Battery of biomarkers may be used	Invasive, painful, difficult to obtain in young children, amount of blood limited in young children
Breath	Easy to obtain large quantities	Requires special equipment, technology is limited, requires cooperation
Saliva	Easy to obtain	Requires cooperation, sample size limited
Transdermal	Easy to obtain	Requires special equipment, technology is limited, requires cooperation
Nails	Easy to obtain, may indicate timing of exposure	Requires cooperation, may be difficult in young child, sample size limited
Newborn[a]		
Cord blood	Large volume available, discarded sample, battery of biomarkers may be used	Narrow window of opportunity to collect, single time point for measurement
Placenta	Large sample size, discarded sample	Narrow window of opportunity to collect
Umbilical cord	Large sample size, discarded sample	Narrow window of opportunity to collect
Amniotic fluid	Large sample size, discarded sample	Difficult to collect, narrow window of opportunity to collect
Urine	Concentrates metabolites, discarded sample	Difficult to collect
Hair	May indicate timing of exposure	May not be available, may not be acceptable to parent
Breath	Easy to obtain	Requires special equipment, technology is limited
Saliva	Easy to obtain	Small sample
Nails	May indicate timing of exposure	Extremely difficult to obtain, invasive
Transdermal	Easy to obtain	Requires special equipment, technology is limited
Meconium	Easy to obtain, may indicate timing of exposure, discarded sample	None

[a]Obviously, biomarkers measured in newborn samples only indicate fetal exposure retrospectively.

ing (1) developing and validating a biomarker to identify a chemical or biochemical exposure or exposure effect; (2) selecting the biological sample (e.g., blood, breath, or urine) to measure the biomarker; (3) addressing ethical, practical, and cost-related obstacles in actually obtaining the sample; (4) developing a method for analytical quantification of the biomarker in the specific sample (addressing how much biomarker can be recovered from the tissue sample, how much variation exists in recovery of the marker between samples, biomarker stability in the chosen sample, etc.); and (5) ascertaining biomarker sensitivity and specificity to exposure or effect.

Validation of a marker also depends on its expected use. Although biological markers observed well before the onset of disease may have little value for predicting the later occurrence of disease, they may be more useful for identifying exposed populations for long-term follow-up. Examples of biological samples appropriate for biomarker determination are hair, saliva, blood, urine, breath, umbilical cord, umbilical cord blood, placenta, stool (including the first stools passed by a newborn, called meconium), and toenails.

Addressing Gaps in Measuring Biological Influences

The importance of biomarkers has been insufficiently appreciated in assessing children's health and its influences. Biomarkers may be useful even beyond measuring the effect of chemical or environmental agent exposure. For example, biomarkers might be developed that could indicate environmental interactions with the other spheres of influences. This is relevant for all aspects of health measurement, because for any influence to affect physical health or well-being, it must be translated through the child's internal biological environment. Such biological events could potentially be measured. While biomarkers have been associated mainly with toxic events and poor outcomes, biomarkers of positive influences and positive effects could be developed.

When biomarkers of exposure and effect are collected, most often they are collected at the same time in the same person. Yet the effect of a particular exposure often does not occur until later and sometimes a long time after the exposure. Without longitudinal studies, the possibility of understanding the cause-effect linkage is lost, and the effect may be attributed incorrectly. Thus, the opportunity to develop high-impact health policies is lost.

Another methodological gap is the paucity of biomarkers when the exposure does not result in systemic absorption. Two examples are the respiratory system and the skin. While air pollution can be measured and quantified, indicators of dose to the airways or the biologically effective dose have not been developed. The absence of valid indicators may obscure the linkage of exposures to effects on health. Thus, the influence on occurrence of asthma or other important respiratory diseases of some elements in air pollution remains controversial. Development of new biomarkers using breath or nasal secretions may potentially be useful in this area. Where biomarkers have been developed, such as the collection of urinary and salivary samples for cotinine levels, as biomarkers of environmental tobacco smoke, they have been very useful.

Finally, current biomarker methods are based mainly on analyzing one biomarker at a time. For biomarkers for which a battery of tests and an algorithm have been established, sensitivity and specificity improve, thus indicating that systems or arrays of biomarkers may have far more potential than isolated single measurement biomarkers. For gene expression alteration/biomarkers, further application of systems biology approaches with pattern identification/informatics technology are likely to be fruitful. A rapidly developing technology used for complex pattern recognition is the electronic nose. Inspired by the ability of dogs to determine complex patterns of odors, current testing on the device has been done on classifying bacteria or fungi by detecting their odors (such as identifying women with Type II diabetes by urine odor—(Mohamed et al., 2002). It is possible to imagine that this technology might be useful in measuring volatile biomarkers from skin (e.g., those emitted by melanomas and detected by dogs) (Church and Williams, 2001).

Currently, NHANES limits its biomarker assessment to children old enough to tolerate the drawing of blood. Smaller children are subjected to fewer laboratory assessments due to the smaller sizes of their blood samples. Development of more sensitive laboratory techniques using noninvasive biological samples is needed. Biomarkers in exhaled breath, urine, and saliva may prove very useful for this age group. Current examples of the usefulness of these techniques include using breath carbon monoxide levels to predict neonatal jaundice (Smith et al., 1984) and urine toxicology for parental substance use. Similarly, the development of programs, such as the newborn blood screen, could be extended to meconium, cord blood, cord, and placenta, which now are typically discarded. While some measures of infection are currently taken (e.g., rubella, herpes), development of biomarkers for emerging infectious diseases such as West Nile virus, Lyme disease, or hantavirus warrant additional research. Prior research has shown a correlation between the formation of chemical modifications of DNA (DNA-adduct) formation and health effects, yet current measurement activities do not include these genotoxic changes.

MEASURING BEHAVIORAL INFLUENCES

Given the central role of children's behavior on their health, whether by active participation in health promotion or disease intervention efforts or by behaviors that increase the risk for poor health, a systematic strategy for assessing and monitoring such health influences is critical. However, apart from youth, parent, or teacher reports and limited use of urine or hair tests to detect the use of illicit drugs, there are no concrete or fully objective tests for the presence of such behaviors. Moreover, infants and young children pose especially difficult measurement challenges, because they do not have the capacity to report on their moods or cognitions. To fully understand the relationship between children's behaviors and health across regions and populations, optimal measurement strategies in most cases require (1) reliance on multiple informants (single-informant data on youth behavior are usually incomplete and should be used with caution), including reliable observational data about the behaviors of infants and young children; (2) combining measures of behavior across informants and settings; (3) demonstration that the behaviors are not simply normal variations; and (4) demonstration that the behavior is in fact related to adverse health consequences. Multi-informant reports are not always needed, but the validity and adequacy of single-informant data should be scrutinized during the planning and execution of studies of children's behavioral influences. Moreover, because children's behavior is constantly changing, measures must be sufficiently sensitive to detect such changes, as well as able to detect relevant differences in the timing, duration, and intensity of behavior influences on health.

To what extent do studies take into account these factors? Data regarding child and youth risk behaviors are gathered routinely from a number of national surveys (see examples below), some consisting of one-time investigator-initiated (even longitudinal) projects, and others consisting of programmatic efforts to collect such information regularly. However, across the broad range of studies listed in Appendixes A and B, most do not meet the requirements outlined above.

As an example, in the National Health Interview Survey (NHIS), four questions from a single informant (parent-caretaker) are asked about children's risk behaviors. Similar limitations are found in most other national surveys, with the notable exceptions of the Youth Risk Behavior Survey (YRBS) and the current NHANES study, which devote significant time to interviewing children in major behavioral areas related to adverse outcomes (e.g., substance use). In the current NHANES survey, multi-informant interviews are conducted using a well-validated instrument (the Diagnostic Interview Schedule for Children—Shaffer et al., 1996; Jensen et al., 1995). However, for the NHANES study, valid determinations and differences within and across any single geographic policy region (such as a city, county, or state) are not possible, given the sampling frame and sample sizes for this particular survey, rendering the study inadequate for adapting regional policies to variations in regional behavioral influences on health.

The YRBS, which attempts to track 10 high-risk youth behaviors, based on representative samples of entire classrooms within schools within states, has modest promise for policy and planning purposes, although the data are self-reports. While innovative, this methodology is largely dependent on the states' own resources to implement the surveys and, in any given year of the survey, as many as 50 percent of states may not have valid or presumably generalizable data. Moreover, rates of specific high-risk behaviors are solely dependent on youths' self-reports (using a pencil and paper survey measure administered in classroom group settings); are often much higher than those found in more in-depth, methodologically rigorous surveys; and systematically miss school dropouts and youth not at school that day or in alternative placement settings. Publicly available data are reported every 2 years. Under conditions of complete implementation and ideal circumstances, representative classroom data could be obtained from states concerning these high-risk behaviors among high school students. This survey also assesses exercise and positive health behaviors. However, due to the modest levels of funding and lack of centralized control of assessment and sampling procedures, the survey relies on each state to conduct and follow-up the data collection procedures. This produces great unevenness in actual survey execution.

Several other recurring national surveys offer highly relevant information in very specific, targeted areas. For example, the Substance Abuse and Mental Health Services Administration's National Household Survey on Drug Use and Health (NHSDUH) assesses information relevant to the prevalence, patterns, and consequences of drug and alcohol use among individuals age 12 and older, as well as family environment and parenting practices or perceptions that might influence substance use practices among youth. The Monitoring The Future study (funded by the National Institute on Drug Abuse, conducted by the Institute for Social Research at the University of Michigan) assesses substance use, other behaviors, attitudes, and values of 50,000 U.S. secondary school students, college students, and young adults; periodic follow-up questionnaires are mailed to a sample of each graduating class for several years after study entrance.

Another source of behavioral data on younger children is the National Labor Survey on Youth, which continues to follow the children of women in the original cohort. This survey includes the child Behavior Problems Index, but the early rounds of the survey primarily include children born to young mothers.

Data regarding youth behavior and its implications for health are sometimes available from investigator-initiated surveys. For example, the National Longitudinal Survey of Adolescent Health (ADD-Health) began in 1994–1995 with a sample of 7th- through 12th-grade schools. Interviews were attempted with the more than 100,000 students attending these schools, with three follow-up personal interviews conducted with a random one-fifth of these students. Health-related behaviors have been relatively well measured in each survey wave through questionnaire responses.

Absent from current efforts to measure children's behavioral influences is consideration of their attitudes, beliefs, expectations, and cultural factors that shape decisions to seek health care or engage in health promotion or illness prevention activities. For example, "local" instruments have been developed by researchers exploring in a cross-sectional and prospective fashion the relative roles of parents' and peers' perceptions and risk involvement on risk and protective behaviors among adolescents (Stanton, Li, Galbraith et al., 2000; Cottrell, Li, Harris et al., 2003). As noted in Chapter 3, substantial evidence indicates that these factors exert major influences on youths' health behaviors and subsequent health, whether related to their health behavior choices, tobacco/alcohol/

substance use, diet, or exercise or to their compliance with health care interventions. According to findings from the Global Burden of Disease study, these behavioral aspects of health are likely to exert even greater influence in coming decades, as behavioral and life-style-related health conditions (e.g., auto accident injuries, consequences of smoking, depression) become predominant in their overall impact on children's health and illness (Murray and Lopez, 1996).

Another area with significant measurement gaps concerns infant and young children's behavior. Some data are gathered on a recurring basis through the National Household Education Surveys Program to address a wide range of education-related child behaviors, including emerging literacy and numeracy in very young children. These surveys assess, from the perspective of the parent and teacher, aspects of school readiness, children's experiences in early childhood programs, and school adjustment, but they do not generate state or local estimates of differences in behavioral influences on health outcomes. However, other data pertaining to developmental milestones for cognition, behavior or social development are not assessed. An important exception to this rule is the Early Childhood Longitudinal Study—Birth Cohort (ECLS-B), a large-scale (N = 12,500), nationally representative, and longitudinal study that follows a single cohort of children from birth to entry into 1st grade. Because of its longitudinal design, this study will enable researchers to examine children's cognitive, social, behavioral, and emotional growth and to relate their growth and change to their experiences in early child care programs. While this study is likely to yield important findings concerning children's behavioral development, it is time-limited and cannot be used for ongoing monitoring of behavioral influences of U.S. infants and young children. A similar study of the 1998 kindergarten cohort (ECLS-K) also contains rich data on some aspects of behavior in a large cohort over time.

Challenges in Measuring Behavioral Influences

There are many special challenges in assessing children's behavioral, emotional, and cognitive influences on health because information may be highly stigmatizing, raise fears that the child will be "labeled," or may concern illegal activity, such as criminal acts or substance abuse. It has been well established in behavioral research that large variations in observers' reports exist (e.g., see Achenbach, McConaughy, and Howell, 1987; Jensen et al., 1999), sometimes because there are differences in how different persons perceive the same behavior (perhaps as a function of different ethnic or cultural backgrounds), and sometimes because different persons do not always witness the same behavior, since behavior may vary from setting to setting.

For all of these reasons, measurement of behavioral influences calls for obtaining multiple sources of information, ensuring that the measures of behavior do not rely on single items, and including measures of functional impairment with measures of behavior, in order to establish whether the behaviors have clinical significance. Finally, careful attention to gender-related, age-specific, and culture-specific behaviors is essential. Many behaviors must also be assessed in a developmental context. For example, bed-wetting or separation fears at age 4 are normal, but they convey different significance at later years. Similarly, aggression in young children is quite different from such behavior in adolescents, in part because older youth have much greater physical capacity, learned knowledge, and access to other ways to deal with anger. Thus, similar constructs might need to be measured differently across the age spectrum to track the effect of a particular behavioral or emotional construct on later health outcomes.

Addressing Gaps in Measuring Behavioral Influences

Among the influences on children's health, the salience of behavior to long-term health, especially regarding obesity, HIV/AIDS, sexually transmitted diseases, substance or alcohol use and addiction, motor vehicle accidents, teenage pregnancy, school dropout, and homicide and suicide, is generally accepted (Murray and Lopez, 1996).

In addition to stigma, which makes these areas difficult to address a priori, failure to be conceptually clear about which behavioral constructs are being measured also contributes to difficulties in measurement. Thus, one may assess some form of behavioral problem, but whether it is a measure of a *risky behavior* (but not ostensibly a sign of health or illness per se) or a measure of the presence or absence of mental health or illness is not always clear. Many surveys include a few behavioral items, but rarely are there clear conceptual linkages to whether the items are related to a health condition per se (mental health or illness) or only to *influences* on future health (e.g., a risky behavior that may predispose to future adverse health outcomes).

Some of this conceptual confusion may be designed explicitly to avoid the possibility of stigma or stigmatizing a population, especially in surveys conducted by federal agencies of disenfranchised groups that are already prone to stigmatization (e.g., studies of economically depressed groups). As a result, most studies that attempt to assess children's behavior rely on assessments of single behaviors or overall functioning, without reference to the central health conditions that reflect most of the population-attributable risk for adverse outcomes and persisting disability. One illustration of this lack of conceptual clarity is the extent to which surveys may attempt to measure adolescent suicidal ideation—essentially a normative behavior in youth—but fail to consider in the measurement strategy the assessment of major depressive disorder, the single greatest risk factor for completed suicide (Shaffer and Craft, 1999).

Most existing surveys have not devoted sufficient methodological attention to distinguishing sufficiently between behavioral information gathered for diagnostic purposes (e.g., major depressive disorder) and information obtained for purposes of assessing risky behaviors. This difficulty is not the sole problem of survey designers, but it may have to do with how the mental health, education, and medical fields conceptualize mental health or illness and risky behaviors. Many mental health disorders seem to merge with the day-to-day problems experienced by everyone. This results in the absence of clear, critical indicators for mental health and illness that have strong face validity and that are clearly linked to functional impairment and the need for treatment. This reflects a more general failure in behavioral health research.

Another assessment gap is the fact that, among the few studies that attempt to address the problems noted above, few are nationally representative (NHANES, NHIS, National Household Education Survey, and NHSDUH being notable exceptions). Instead, most are samples representative only of a particularly community or region, usually with time-limited funding sources as a part of an investigator-initiated research study. While some regional studies are longitudinal, nationally representative surveys tend to be ad hoc or one-time-only. There is no clear ongoing commitment or funding, or health-monitoring strategy with explicit ties to national policy. Furthermore, no data are currently available meeting these three criteria that can also be used to assess these constructs in policy-relevant localities, such as cities, counties, or states.

In addition to the general methodological inadequacies in assessment of key behavioral characteristics among children, such as failing to obtain behavioral data from multiple informants and failing to distinguish between behavioral risk factors and actual behavioral disorders, most available datasets have not linked the behavioral measures to other influences that may affect behavior, such as family and parenting variables, peer influences, educational functioning, other aspects of physical health, and neighborhood and school resources. A notable exception is the ECLS of the National Center for Educational Statistics.

PHYSICAL ENVIRONMENTS

Our discussion of measurement of influences in the physical environment focuses on chemical exposures and aspects of the built environment to illustrate measurement challenges related to measuring the physical environment. Similarly complex measurement challenges and in most cases a paucity of data exist related to noise and other exposures of concern; home, school, and work settings; and safe environments free of injury.

Chemical Exposures

Environmental pollutants are measured in media, such as water, air, some foods, and soil, as reviewed in two recent Environmental Protection Agency (EPA) reports (U.S. Environmental Protection Agency, 2000a, 2003). However, these measures do not always take into account children's unique exposure patterns and pathways of exposure. In addition, there are few measures of microenvironments in private homes, such as indoor air pollution or noise or indicators of noise. Radon is measured in individual houses, and ultraviolet B radiation (UV-B) is measured in some regions. However, how these measures compare with children's actual exposures is unknown. There are few surveillance systems for monitoring children's exposures, job descriptions, work (including agricultural) at home, or their work-related injuries and illnesses.

Challenges in Measuring Chemical Exposures

Not much is known about specific aspects of the physical environments in which children spend their time, nor are there methods to determine the highly exposed subpopulations of children. The methods generally used are to determine exposure chemical by chemical, without consideration of mixtures of exposures or cumulative effects of exposure. Methods to predict individual exposures accurately from environmental indicators are under development (e.g., U.S. Environmental Protection Agency, 2000, 2003). Measurement of occupational risks to children, especially those in unregulated settings, may conflict with homeowners rights. The Bureau of Labor Statistics of the U.S. Department of Labor and state departments of labor need to develop mechanisms for more efficient data collection of children's occupations and health effects, as well as for better access to datasets that are potentially useful, such as work permit information issued by school boards.

Addressing Gaps in Measuring Chemical Exposures

The health effect of a physical agent to which children are exposed may be unknown. A recent analysis by the EPA discovered that 43 percent of high production volume (HPV) chemicals (the 2,800 or more chemicals released at greater than 1 million pounds per year) have no basic toxicity testing, and only 7 percent have a complete set of basic toxicity tests (U.S. Environmental Protection Agency, 1998; Goldman and Koduru, 2000). Many fewer have any developmental toxicity testing. These chemicals are not monitored in the environment, nor is biomonitoring available for most of them.

Less clear than HVP chemicals are the other chemicals in the environment to which children are exposed. How should the decisions be made about which to monitor? The CDC has come up with a strategy for adding additional chemicals to the NHANES survey, but this strategy has yet to be evaluated.[3] It focuses on chemicals with known toxicity or that are relatively easy to assay, such as heavy metals.

------

[3]See http://www.cdc.gov/nceh/dls/nominations.htm.

The Built Environment

In the United States cities have evolved rapidly toward the pattern known as sprawl, with geographically dispersed metropolitan areas, segregated land uses, heavy reliance on automobiles as the dominant transportation mode, low connectivity, and high neighborhood fragmentation. A majority of children in the United States now grow up in the suburbs. This built environment pattern has major health implications in four areas: air quality, physical activity patterns, injuries related to motor vehicle use, and "sense of community" (Frumkin, 2003). However, in all four cases, knowledge is incomplete, both in terms of understanding and assessing current problems and in terms of designing solutions. Researchers have identified key questions, and active investigations are under way. For instance, using multilevel exposure ascertainment, investigators are able to jointly assess neighborhood-level characteristics, such as collective efficacy and variations in violence, and individual-level characteristics (Sampson, Raudenbush, and Earls, 1997).

To measure physical features of a neighborhood (e.g., the exposure), many parameters of sprawl have been identified (e.g., percentage of the population living in urbanized areas, residential density, accessibility of the street network, proximity of different land uses to each other, pedestrian oriented design) (Frumkin, 2003) and combined into indices. Often these measures are limited by the availability of data; for example, in the relatively complex index proposed by Galster et al. (2000), data were available for only 13 cities. Moreover, when data are available, they can sometimes be mapped only to relatively large geographic units, such as metropolitan areas or counties. Data on smaller units, such as the census tract (geographic areas encompassing 4,000 to 6,000 individuals, with boundaries drawn to approximate neighborhood areas) or even the block, provide more information on individual and family exposures but are more elusive.

In studies of children's health, the preferred measures of "exposure" to sprawl are perhaps best defined by what health outcomes are of interest and what biological mechanisms are hypothesized. For example, in studying the association between sprawl and physical activity, one could measure the proportion of roadway miles with sidewalks, the acreage of parkland per capita in a defined area, the mileage of bike paths, the mean distance of homes to the nearest parks, or the mean trip distance from homes to elementary schools. Such data are available from a variety of sources, including U.S. census data, Department of Transportation road data, marketing databases, and metropolitan planning agency databases.

In addition, direct observation using standardized instruments—analogous to the questionnaires used in epidemiological research—may be applied to the built environment. Such instruments need to be validated prior to use. An example of such a measurement approach is the Built Environment Site Survey Checklist (Weich et al., 2001). Using this instrument, research staff make and record observations about housing type, density, age, space around the buildings, proximity of trees, accessibility of recreational facilities, playgrounds, and gardens, and even signs of vandalism and graffiti. While it is labor-intensive to collect data in this manner, a range of variables can be studied, including many that have great a priori appeal in characterizing the quality of places.

Some studies have assessed exposure by surveying respondents about their perceptions of these conditions. For example, people can be asked to rate the "walkability" of their neighborhoods (Leyden, 2003), the safety of allowing their children to walk to school (Dellinger and Staunton, 2002), or other perceived features of the built environment. In one investigation conducted as part of the Alameda County Study in California, participants were asked to rate the seriousness of six potential neighborhood problems: crime, nighttime lighting, traffic, excessive noise, trash and litter, and access to public transportation (Balfour and Kaplan, 2002). Other areas of concern may relate to the availability of stores that sell tobacco, firearms, and liquor to youth. Such measures carry the problems of many questionnaires, such as variable responses among participants and response bias. Moreover, there may be an element of self-fulfilling prophecy: respondents who rate their neighborhoods as more walkable are likely to walk more, but this may reflect factors other than the physical design of the neighborhood.

To the extent that environmental factors affect people's behavior, that behavior might be considered an early biological effect (see Figure 5-1). An important example is travel behavior—the number of trips per household each day, the mode of travel used, and the distance per trip. A leading source of such information is the National Personal Transportation Survey, renamed in 2001 the National Household Travel Survey.[4] Other features of traffic safety and injuries related to the physical constructions of vehicles and roads are also available. Additional data are gathered in academic and governmental travel studies such as SMARTRAQ.[5] Such information was traditionally collected through surveys, using either retrospective recall or diaries; new techniques, such as personal digital assistants with global positioning system capability, have improved the completeness and accuracy of travel data.

Of note, studies may be conducted that assess the association between an exposure and a biological effect in the sense discussed here. For example, one might hypothesize that certain neighborhood features, such as low density or automobile dependence, are negatively associated with children walking or biking to school. While not extending all the way to a health outcome such as obesity, this association would be an important part of understanding the health implications of the built environment.

---

[4]Available at http://www.fhwa.dot.gov/policy/ohpi/nhts/.

[5]See www.smartraq.net.

Challenges in Measuring the Built Environment

Assessment of physical neighborhood and the built environment is burdened by several problems. First, in Sampson's (2001) words, "the tendency of research on child development has been to focus quickly and narrowly on poverty," especially in high-poverty urban neighborhoods. Moreover, most of the research in this area conceptualizes the neighborhood only as a social construct, using metrics of residential stability, income, education, employment, family structure, and crime, while neglecting physical aspects of the built environment. Finally, most of this research focuses on adolescents, perhaps because they spend more time out of the home and are therefore more exposed to neighborhood factors. This produces large gaps in data collection on other aspects of the built environment and its effects on children's health across the age span.

Addressing Gaps in Measuring the Built Environment

Further research and systematic assessment are necessary to ascertain how the built environment affects sense of community or social capital in ways that shape the development of younger children. In addition, to improve measurement of the built environment, standardized instruments need to be developed, validated, and implemented at geographic levels useful for local planning.

SOCIAL ENVIRONMENTS

As with our discussion of social influences themselves, we organize our measurement discussion into categories of family, community, culture, and discrimination.

Family Environment

The Current Population Survey and the Survey of Income and Program Participation are prime examples of high-quality surveys conducted by the Census Bureau that gather information about many of the components of family demography and process—in particular, family income, family composition, parental schooling, and occupation. These surveys typically contain very few data on children's health. Surveys focused on children's health and its influences often collect some data on the components of family socioeconomic status (SES), but these data are often too crude to serve most analytical purposes. For example, data on family income are sometimes gathered or recoded into such categories as poor, near-poor, or nonpoor, so that it is impossible to estimate social gradients in health at all levels of income.

Vital statistics data contain relatively little information on SES. Birth records contain educational level achieved by the mother but, starting in 1995, do not provide data on the education level of the father. Death records contain data on the decedent's occupation and, beginning only in 2003, educational level. No information regarding parental SES is gathered on death certificates, a serious omission in the case of child deaths.

Other than gross indications of economic status by receipt of public health insurance, clinical data almost never contain any measure of SES, whether about income, education, or occupation of parents. Studies using clinical data or vital statistics sometimes rely on proxy measures of SES obtained by linking addresses to census tract data and attributing to individuals the SES characteristics of their neighborhoods, for example, mean levels of income or of educational achievement in a census tract. Given the heterogeneous nature of families living in a given neighborhood, neighborhood-based measures of family SES contain considerable error (Geronimus, Bound, and Neidert, 1996; Demissie et al., 2000).

When data on neither income nor education are available, race and ethnicity are often used as proxy measures of social class, based on knowledge of the higher frequency of low income among black and other minority groups. The fallacies of doing so are illustrated in data showing the health disadvantage for low-income white people in Appalachia, which is home to predominantly white populations (Centers for Disease Control and Prevention, 1998b). Thus, using race and ethnicity as proxies for social class makes invisible the health problems of low-income white children. Saliently, the risk of dying is higher in low-income groups, even after taking into account health risk behaviors (Lantz et al., 1998).

The National Survey of Early Childhood Health (NSECH) includes detailed assessment of hours and activities spent by parents with children; breast-feeding practices; daily routines including the frequency of playing, singing, and reading to the child; number of children's books in the household; disciplinary practices; parental perceptions of infant temperament; the role of parenting, and their perception of themselves as parents; and pediatric care (including an assessment from the parent's point of view of the usefulness of their provider's health prevention education efforts). The NSECH also assesses family income, medical insurance coverage and adequacy, child care and child care affordability, and receipt of nutritional benefits such as WIC and other low-income benefits.

The Child Well-Being and Welfare module used in two states assesses income, health care coverage, day care utilization and costs, employment, income and job stability, relocation information, reading in the household, and information regarding school and out-of-school extracurricular involvement of the child. Parents are also asked questions about their relationship with and feelings about the child. The National Survey of Children with Special Health Care Needs (NSCSHCN) collected data on children with a wide range of health conditions and included a few questions on the effect on the family, but virtually no data on family structure.

The National Child Abuse and Neglect Data System, a partnership between the U.S. Department of Health and Human Services and the states, collects annual statistics on child maltreatment from state child protective services agencies. The goal is to increase understanding of the magnitude of the problem, the characteristics of those affected, and what type of services are being provided by state and local agencies. Given that the majority of abusers are parents, these data do concern family and family functioning, albeit for a special subsample.

Available surveys also provide family environment information well beyond the traditional demographic variables. For example, the Current Population Survey and especially the Survey of Income and Program Participation augment their efforts with occasional questionnaire supplements to gather limited information regarding health and health insurance coverage, child care, and various other family topics. The NHIS assesses demographics and income, as well as health care seeking for each household member, including children. The U.S. Department of Agriculture's Quality of Continuing Survey of Food Intakes by Individual Survey assesses the adequacy of diet of children ages 2 to 9 years nationwide. Data regarding limited aspects of parenting, nurturing, day care/child care, and school readiness are collected periodically in other surveys.

Challenges in Measuring Family Influences

Decades of methodological research have produced at least rough consensus on how to measure family environment components in surveys. As to SES components, Entwisle and Astone (1994) provide recommendations regarding the measurement of education and occupation, while Hauser and Warren (1997) do the same for occupation and Duncan and Peterson (2001) make recommendations regarding the measurement of income, wealth, and employment. As to family process measures of parenting and the home learning environment, national surveys such the National Longitudinal Surveys of Youth and the Early Childhood Longitudinal Study, Kindergarten Class of 1998–99 provide consensus measurement methods. Thus, one key challenge regarding family environmental measurement in surveys is less how to do it than how much of it should be carried over into surveys focused on health.

With regard to SES, although most health-focused survey data collection provides measures of at least one of the components, clinical data almost never contain any such measures, and there continues to be dispute about the appropriateness of doing so. Ross et al. (2000) summarized the various ways of measuring SES. They argue for the importance of a theoretically based choice, depending on the health measure and the context in which analyses are done. Duncan and Magnuson (2002) argue that estimating the importance of any single component of SES requires measurement of all of them to guard against omitted-variable bias.

Primary challenges to SES measurement are (1) including at least some measure of SES in all data collections and (2) choosing measures that best reflect the theory about the relationship between social disadvantage and the particular measures of health being assessed. Health-focused data collection providing a myriad of health measures should consider collecting information on all of the important components of SES, since it is possible to do so without devoting excessive amounts of interviewing time to it.

A second level of SES challenges is to appreciate and account for their dynamic nature. Family incomes are often highly volatile from one year to the next (Duncan, 1988), and education levels can increase well into adulthood (Magnuson and McGroder, 2002), while occupation and wealth typically change more slowly. Designers of health-focused longitudinal surveys should realize that it may be necessary to include SES-related questions in a number of interviewing waves.

It is more difficult to draw general conclusions about the challenges of measuring the diverse set of other family environmental influences we have considered. With regard to family structure, an important challenge is to gather needed detail on the relationships among the individuals living in the same household. Whether an adult male is the biological father or stepfather to the children is an important distinction for assessing risks to child well-being. By the same token, whether two unmarried adults of the opposite or even same sex are functioning as partners or merely roommates also appears consequential for child well-being. And yet many surveys fail to gather household composition data in a way that captures these distinctions.

Data collection efforts that aspire to understand family environmental influences on children's health should consider including measures of parenting and the home learning and physical environments but, here again, the measures used should match the conceptual orientation of linkages between family process and health outcomes.

Addressing Gaps in Measuring Family Influences

Clinical records pose a special challenge in regard to the assessment of SES influences. Clinical facilities are reluctant to collect information on aspects of SES from patients, believing that this may be interpreted as an attempt to discriminate on the basis of such aspects in providing health care. However, most clinical facilities collect residential address data, if for no other purpose than bill collecting. When geocoded and matched to characteristics of area of residence related to social class, address information can be very useful for population or subpopulation analysis of the relationship between receipt of health services and socioeconomic characteristics (Krieger, 2000).

Methodological advances now enable researchers to estimate multilevel models of the various ecological levels of influence on health. These techniques were developed for use in the social sciences (Blalock, 1984; Di Priete and Forristal, 1994) and have increasingly been used to study the interacting influences on health at both individual and environmental levels in adults, but there are few such studies of children in the United States.

Analysis of the association of SES with health measures would be facilitated by the longitudinal and simultaneous ascertainment of most or all of the important SES components—income, education, occupation, and wealth. Analysis of the effect of income (or wealth) should be mindful of the likely confounding of influences as well as of interactions between SES levels and other influences. For example, Hispanics have better health than the majority population, despite having worse health behaviors and lower average income and education (Hayes-Bautista, 2003; Morales et al., 2002).

Community Environment

Most broad-based neighborhood studies rely on data gathered in the decennial census. Every 10 years, the U.S. Census Bureau provides information that can be used to construct neighborhood-based measures, such as the fraction of individuals who are poor, the fraction of adults with a college degree, and the fraction of adult men without jobs. Such data are available for census tracts as well as larger geographically defined areas. Matching neighborhood-level census information to survey or administrative data requires only a valid street address. The administrative, academic, and commercial value of such matched data has led to the development of a number of efficient address-matching computer programs, as well as a healthy market providing matching and other geography-related commercial services, including geographic information systems. Although such techniques have been useful in managing and analyzing neighborhood data, they are often cumbersome to apply to national datasets.

All in all, apart from privacy and confidentiality issues surrounding the need to gather and store information about the exact addresses of individuals and families, the decennial censuses provide the geographic dimension of demographic and many economic risk factors.

The Census Bureau is developing the American Community Survey (ACS)—a "rolling census" that involves a continuous sample survey of the nation's population. Two noteworthy advantages to such a design are much lower cost and timelier information. The survey is designed to provide geographically specific demographic and economic information more frequently than once a decade (the interval depends on the size of geographic area). However, the fate of the ACS was not certain during the committee's deliberation, as it was not yet funded by the U.S. Congress.

The social organization of neighborhoods' (values and interactions of neighbors) appears influential for children's health (Sampson, Morenoff, and Gannon-Rowley, 2002), but measures of social organization are unlikely to make their way into the decennial census or ACS. Approaches for measuring social organization include surveys and systematic social observation. The Project on Human Development in Chicago Neighborhoods (PHDCN)[6] illustrates both approaches. To gather information on its sample of children in a randomly chosen set of Chicago's neighborhoods, the project conducted a separate survey of a representative sample of adults residing in those neighborhoods. The questionnaire for this second survey included questions on social interactions among neighbors. Mounting an independent survey to gather these kinds of neighborhood level data on social organization would be expensive, although a parsimonious set of observations might be added to existing surveys (such as the NHIS) that require home visits. For example, similar to an approach to measurements of the built environment, a measure described as systematic social observation (Reiss, 1971; Sampson and Raudenbush, 1999) relies on trained observers to systematically record such indicators of social organization as broken windows, vandalism, and evidence of drug use in a well-defined geographic area. Data can be gathered either with direct recording or by systematically coding videotapes taken of the neighborhood areas (Raudenbush and Sampson, 1999). Systematic social observation methods are less expensive than surveys, but they gather different kinds of data about social organization.

Standardized measures of neighborhood institutions and facilities (e.g., parks, the quality of local schools, churches, bus or train service, youth activity centers) are not readily available from any centralized source. Some of these characteristics can be obtained from surveys of the children or parents who are reporting on health outcomes. However, such reports can often identify what families use, but not what is actually present in their neighborhoods. A study by Morland, Wing, Diex Rouz, and Poole (2002) demonstrated that supermarkets are nearly nonexistent in the poorest fifth of the neighborhoods studied.

Investigators have generally considered both childhood victimization (direct exposure) and witnessed violence (indirect exposure) when studying the prevalence and effect of community violence in relation to children's health (Martinez and Richters, 1993; Smith and Martin, 1995). Although most investigators define victimization in a consistent manner (e.g., intentional acts initiated by another person to cause harm), there is much more variability in the definition of witnessed violence. Some authors have referred specifically to eyewitnessed violence, while others have included hearing violent events (e.g., gun shots and screams), and others have included witnessing lesser crimes (e.g., property damage and the viewing of violence on television and in the media). With increasing interest and attention paid to a broader conceptualization of children's exposure to violence (including victimization and witnessed violence) investigators are tending to view children's exposure to violence in terms of levels, rather than direct or indirect exposures (Buka et al., 2001).

---

[6]see http://www.hms.harvard.edu/chase/projects/chicago/about/.

Typically investigators have developed their own questionnaires, used a modified version of the National Institute of Mental Health's Survey of Exposure to Community Violence (Martinez and Richters, 1993), or used a modified version of the instrument used for the National Crime Victimization Survey (Katz, Kling, and Liebman, 2001). Most measures tend to weight violent events equally in spite of the obvious differences in item content (e.g., seeing someone hit versus seeing someone shot). Finally, with a few notable exceptions (Cooley, Turner, and Beidel, 1995; Selner-O'Hagan et al., 1998), the psychometric characteristics of these instruments are largely unknown (Buka et al., 2001). The instruments lack uniformity in their methods of administration, definitions of violent events, and descriptions of where the violence occurs. Importantly, most instruments fail to separate the nature or effect of exposure by setting, despite the acknowledged importance of such distinctions (Selner-O'Hagan et al., 1998).

Data regarding peer interactions and their implications for health are available from several national surveys. From a methodological perspective, the most remarkable is the National Longitudinal Survey of Adolescent Health, described above under behavioral influences. In addition to extensive measures of health and risk behaviors, the questionnaire asked each student to name his or her five best male and female friends. The study's design provides data on direct reports from youth, coupled with limited information from all best friends and extensive information from a random subset of best friends. Peer relations also are assessed in a variety of surveys conducted by the U.S. Department of Education, the National Center for Health Statistics, the Substance Abuse and Mental Health Services Administration, the U.S. Department of Labor, and in surveys such as Monitoring The Future.

Challenges in Measuring Community Influences

As with other influences, the task of securing unbiased estimates of neighborhood effects is fraught with methodological challenges (Manski, 1993; Duncan and Raudenbush, 2001a). One important problem arises from the fact that families are not randomly allocated to their residential neighborhoods, which may lead researchers to mistakenly attribute to a neighborhood effects that are really caused by unmeasured differences in the children's families.

A second challenge is to isolate effects of very high concentrations of certain risks (e.g., poverty, crime) from more general influences of urban neighborhoods (e.g., traffic, noise). Representative population surveys typically draw relatively few families from high-poverty urban neighborhoods. Analysts using these surveys base estimates of neighborhood effects on differences among relatively advantaged, mostly white families and children. If neighborhood conditions matter more for disadvantaged than advantaged children, then studies of neighborhood effects based on broad population samples may miss an important part of the story.

One solution to interpreting the effect of this bias is to analyze what neighborhood they moved into. The Department of Housing and Urban Development is conducting precisely such a study. The Moving To Opportunity experiment randomly assigned housing project residents in five of the nation's largest cities to one of three groups: (1) a group receiving housing subsidies to move into low-poverty neighborhoods; (2) a comparison group receiving conventional Section 8 housing assistance but not constrained in their locations; and (3) a second comparison group receiving no special assistance. Orr et al. (2003) detail program effects 4–7 years after families were randomly assigned to these three groups. The evaluation showed significant improvements in neighborhood conditions and adult mental health but mixed results for children, with mental health improving for girls but behavior problems increasing for boys. A 10-year follow-up is planned as well.

Assessing the effect of violence on children is also challenging. First, investigators must measure simultaneously multiple facets of community violence. Measures of violence in the home (domestic violence) and violence in different community contexts (in the home, near home, in school and near schools) must be quantified so that the independent contributions of each exposure can be assessed. Second, few measures are available that distinguish among different forms and severity of violence. The adverse health consequences of exposure to extreme and acute violence (e.g., kidnapping, mass shooting) are likely to affect children differently than chronic exposure to community violence. Third, given the wide range of age and developmental diversity in children exposed to violence, multiple measures taken from children, parents, and other primary caregivers are needed. Moreover, the degree to which young children can reliably report exposure is an important concern. Also, sole reliance on parental reports of child exposure to violence are likely to underestimate children's actual exposures (Martinez and Richters, 1993; Taylor et al., 1994). And compounding these above-noted difficulties, research evidence suggests that it is difficult to determine the relative effects of different types of violence exposure, because study subjects reporting to have witnessed violent events are also likely to have directly experienced lesser types of violence (Buka, Stichick, Birdthistle, and Earls, 2001).

Addressing Gaps in Measuring Community Influences

The decennial census and, if fully implemented, the ACS provide abundant and fairly timely demographic and economic information on the nation's neighborhoods, cities and towns, counties, and states. Indeed, the United States gathers and releases much more of this kind of information than most other developed countries. However, the census questionnaire lacks comprehensive measures of health and health risk behaviors, and the linking of these data to other information sources is somewhat difficult.

Measures of most other important aspects of the community context (social organization, amenities such as parks and public transportation, and safety) as well as media exposure currently can be gathered from administrative sources or special surveys, but at considerable expense and often not consistently from one geographic unit to the next and, hence, they do not permit generalizable interpretations.

Although there are routine sources of information on youth perpetration of violence, none exists to monitor youth exposure to community violence. Routine population surveys are needed to identify regional and secular trends. Such efforts would provide the foundation for attempts to collect data and design important intervention and support programs for the most affected communities. For example, there is a paucity of data on children's exposure to community violence in nonurban settings (Buka et al., 2001; Smith and Martin, 1995).

At present only a few longitudinal multilevel studies of children's exposure to community violence exists. Longitudinal studies, such as the PHDCN (Earls and Buka, 1997), hold the promise of allowing for a more comprehensive evaluation of the complexities of the types of exposure to violence, the context of exposure, and the contribution of potential risk and protective factors in determining child risk.

In addition to the major lack of systematic data collection, several important methodological issues confront future studies of the effects of violence on youth. These include the need to (1) develop consistent definitions of community violence; (2) develop violence exposure measures of proven validity and reliability; (3) determine how best to measure exposure to community violence in young children, including comparisons of child versus parent report and assessment of levels of violence witnessed; and (4) evaluate effects of acute and chronic violence separately.

In addition, research in this area would be facilitated by allowances that distinguish consistently between different forms and severity of violence. More attention should be paid to evaluating the extent to which the effects of children's exposure to community violence are mediated by family and community response to community violence; for example, the family conditions that reduce the likelihood and consequences of exposure to community violence. Similarly, future research can improve understanding of the role that community violence plays in family violence. At least one team of investigators has noted a strong positive relation between exposure to community violence and the incidence of family violence (Osofsky et al., 1993). This challenge is further complicated by the issues and limitations in confidentiality and mandated reporting regulations under such circumstances, especially when a child's health is in danger and the perpetrator is one of the child's caregivers.

Many surveys include one or a few questions assessing aspects of peer relationships throughout childhood. Lacking in most are robust measures of peer relationships with strong psychometric properties that provide a cohesive story across the developmental stages. Thus, there is a need for at least some surveys to gather in-depth information about peer relations, which was last done for middle and high school students in the National Longitudinal Survey of Adolescent Health in the middle 1990s. As youth approach adolescence, peer group acceptance becomes of even greater importance and conformity to perceived norms assumes an important role in the adolescent's life; surveys assessing health and well-being should include a greater focus on these domains. Numerous surveys document involvement in risk behaviors, but few assess these aspects in any depth, and most rely on secondhand reports of peers by parents or the youth themselves.

Cultural Influences

Current national and regional efforts to assess population health collect data from population subgroups with different cultural backgrounds. Although the role of culture has been invoked as a contributor to observed health disparities (e.g., Hayes-Bautista, 2003), surveys typically gather few data that would help assess how culture contributes to health disparities.

One problem is that population samples include too few members of important population subgroups. Techniques for oversampling such subgroups can be used to draw large enough samples to support reliable statistical inference, particularly when subgroup members live in close geographic proximity to one another.

Another problem in most current measurement activities is the use of pan-ethnic labels that obscures cultural differences among groups. Pan-ethnic classifications, such as Hispanic, black, and Asian, reflect a classification system that neglects national origins and reflects membership in minority groups in the United States only in relation to the white Caucasian frame of reference (Portes and Rumbaut, 2001). The use of these convenient group definitions obscures important differences between the national groups in terms of migration, original culture, and social and cultural capital, all of which can have important consequences for children's health.

For example, using the Hispanic Health and Nutrition Examination Survey, (conducted in 1982–1984) that oversampled Mexican Americans, Cubans, and Puerto Ricans, investigators have shown very different rates of asthma, lead levels, and health care utilization (Mendoza, Takata, and Martorell, 1994). Similarly, Becerra and colleagues (1991) have shown differences among these groups in infant mortality and low birthweight, including data to support the finding that recent immigrant women from Mexico have the best birth outcomes among Hispanic subgroups, despite their relatively low SES and poor acculturation to the dominant culture. Additional research to improve understanding of this "immigrant paradox" is warranted.

Another problem is that racial and ethnic information has been gathered in different ways in different surveys. For example, national health surveys and the official decennial census and survey data are not comparable in their use of ethnic/racial labels and the definition of such labels. In some instances, for example, the African American and black labels can be used interchangeably, while in other cases the label black might include West Indians or Africans who don't consider themselves to be African Americans. These distinctions are important. The Office of Management and Budget (OMB) provides useful standards for gathering such information in both administrative records and surveys. The standards capture country of origin for those reporting Hispanic ethnicity and allow respondents to select more than one race. The 2000 census allowed Hispanics to designate multiple races independent of their ethnicity for the first time in U.S. history. The option of selecting more than one race reflects increasing recognition of interracial marriages and unions and the rejection of the "one drop rule" as historically defined (a person was automatically considered black if any close or distant relative was black). This option is likely to be used by increasing proportions of the population.

Surveys such as the Current Population Survey (CPS) have adopted the OMB standard related to racial and ethnic data and provide a timely and reliable method for capturing data on immigration. The CPS asks for the birth countries of the respondent, the respondent's father, and the respondent's mother. This allows children to be identified by generation and country of origin of self and parents. Health and access to insurance vary substantially across both immigrant generation and ethnicity.

Acculturation level has also been associated with health outcomes (Hayes-Bautista, 2003). Questions related to language(s) spoken at home, how long a child and his or her parents have been in the United States if not native born, and whether born a citizen, all included in the census, can serve as proxies for acculturation. Questions related to language may be the most useful. Children who speak a language other than English at home often have parents with limited labor market opportunities, which affects their employment, job benefits, and access to public services.

Challenges in Measuring Cultural Influences

There are many challenges to measuring the effect of culture on health. One is the definition and operationalization of culture. Assessing the effect of culture on health and its interactive relation with other influences requires standard definitions and measures of cultural processes. As discussed in Chapter 3, culture can refer to values, perceptions, and interpretations as well as behaviors that constitute daily routines and responses to environmental challenges that reflect such cultural views. There is little consensus on what is important and measurable.

Aside from the lack of standard definitions and measures, differences in cultural background in this country are highly confounded with socioeconomic and minority status, making it difficult to isolate the effect of one from the other or their interactions. When this is done, in some instances, cultural differences disappear when education is controlled for (Laosa, 1980; Solis et al., 1990), and sometimes they remain (Gutierrez, Sameroff, and Karrer, 1988; Harwood, 1992; Ogbu, 2003).

These findings support the stance of some investigators that health outcomes are a function of the compounding effects of many characteristics that are, in reality, difficult to isolate (Boykin and Toms, 1985; García Coll et al., 1996). It might be more efficient to measure and delineate their interactive effects over time than to try to isolate them. In this view, cultural differences are most important when they are compounded by oppression, poverty, and discrimination. Although some health outcomes are still adverse as a function of cultural background in high socioeconomic groups (Steele, 1997; Ogbu, 2003), the expectation would be that cultural differences in the context of relative oppression, poverty, and discrimination would need most attention from the standpoint of health policy and health care delivery.

In addition, cultural differences may also be very important when demographic variables (i.e., poverty, lack of English proficiency) predict negative health outcomes but these adverse outcomes are not observed (Hayes-Bautista, 2003; Fuligni, 1997; Portes and Rumbaut, 2001). Measuring how cultural processes lead to resilience in health outcomes is an area in which knowledge is particularly lacking.

Given how little is known about the way in which culture directly influences health, or the extent to which it is confounded with other influences (such as social class), a research agenda to develop validated and standardized measures is warranted.

Addressing Gaps in Measuring Cultural Influences

In order to make data compatible for aggregation and analysis, collection of data on cultural group membership should be systematized and standardized across all levels of local, regional, and national data collection. Following the most recent OMB guidelines might be the way to work toward standardization, with the recognition that categories change over time and need to be clearly defined to ensure comparability of data over time. Specifically, the OMB standard related to capturing data on ethnicity, country of origin for self-identified Hispanic populations, and multiple races should be used in all health data-gathering efforts at the local, regional, and national levels.

Beyond this information, to help understand the established relationship between generation and health outcomes, it would be very beneficial to identify children by immigrant generation using questions about birth country for children and their parents and, if born elsewhere, how long they have been in the country. Ideally, this information should be obtained regardless of whether the parent lives in the household. Similarly, given the relationship been acculturation and health outcomes for some populations, if an acculturation measure cannot be used, questions related to languages spoken in the home should be incorporated in studies.

Work toward standardizing the assessment of cultural group membership should also be done with the recognition that such membership alone does not capture cultural processes. Ethnic identification, place of birth, recency and pattern of migration, and language proficiency and choice are only proxies for cultural processes. Adding these items to extant or planned surveys or to any intake or identifier data will provide information on factors that have been found to correlate with health habits, practices, and outcomes (Portes and Rumbaut, 2001), but will not address the underlying mechanisms.

For example, there is a growing and consistent literature that points out the existence of health disparities along ethnic, racial, and cultural lines; however, the processes that underlie these differences, including the likely confounding effect of social class, are hardly understood. In order to address this knowledge gap, it is necessary to oversample subpopulations that are important because of their current or projected demographic growth or their overrepresentation in high-risk or resilient groups. In addition, future efforts should engage in the measurement of actual practices and daily routines that reflect in part cultural adaptation to present demands (e.g., Gallimore, Weisner, Bernheimer, Guthrie, and Nihira, 1993; National Research Council, 1984; Rogoff, 1990; Weisner, 1997, 2002).

Furthermore, not all members of an ethnic/racial group will be similar in their adherence to particular cultural values and practices. The role of acculturation—the adoption or rejection of new ways of being as a function of contact with a different culture—has been identified as a very significant source of variability among members of the same cultural group. Members of the same group can differ in how assimilated, resistant, or bicultural they can be; yet most surveys fail to use available methods for ascertaining these differences. Several scales have been developed for certain populations and could be further developed as a standard way to measure acculturation for inclusion in local, regional, and national surveys.

It is important to promote the development of measures that are psychometrically valid and reliable across all cultural groups being measured. Standardization on one group or on a national representative sample does not guarantee cross-cultural validity and reliability. Measures must also be linguistically accessible and valid. Translations and back translations, although a standard way of translating measures, do not guarantee cultural equivalence (e.g., How does one translate "nervous breakdown," or "feeling down," or "eating regularly?"). Other methods should be used to ensure linguistic accessibility and psychometric validity and reliability (see for example, the dual focus approach, Erkut et al., 1999a).

In general, measures and ways of administration need to be culturally sensitive (e.g., what is considered private information may vary according to age, gender, and cultural background of the interviewer and the interviewee). This requires extensive pilot testing of all assessments across all groups under study and in-depth training of survey personnel on administration methods that will lead to reliable and valid data across cultural groups.

Discrimination

Studies have shown disparities in treatment and outcome between minority- and majority-culture children after controlling for other social indicators, such as SES. Discrimination is sometimes mentioned as possibly having a causative role in these disparities, but its contribution has rarely been studied directly. There are many possible reasons for this, including a lack of understanding of the multiple mechanisms by which discrimination may affect health; a lack of an a priori conceptualizing of discrimination as a potential influence separate from other social stratification mechanisms, such as race, ethnicity, and socioeconomic status; and difficulty in operationalizing and measuring discrimination.

As noted in Chapter 3, there is a sparse but growing literature on the effect of discrimination and racism on health. Most of the studies concern adults. Not surprisingly, these studies use instruments and questionnaires that measure discrimination (and perceptions of discrimination) in largely adult contexts and as such are not directly applicable to children. Instruments are lacking that are explicitly developed to measure experiences and perceptions of discrimination in child-specific contexts, sensitive to the particular conceptual and measurement issues regarding children of different developmental ages and from different ethnic groups. Thus, a concerted effort to develop measures is warranted.

Questions specifically pertaining to discrimination should be validated and then included in research related to minority child health and development. One example is provided by Erkut, Alarcon, García Coll, and colleagues, who developed questions pertaining to discrimination for their studies of the physical and psychological health of Puerto Rican children and adolescents in the greater Boston area (Erkut, Alarcón, and García Coll et al., 1999b; Alarcón, 2000). These questions are good examples of how researchers need to take into account developmental age (e.g., the wording and complexity of the questions for the 1st to 3rd graders compared with young adolescents) when constructing appropriate questions, and how to incorporate age-appropriate contexts into the questions. These questions have not been psychometrically validated; although they may service as a basis for further testing, they have some limitations, as noted below.

Challenges in Measuring Discrimination

One of the major challenges in studying the effects of discrimination, prejudice, and racism on children's health and development is finding ways of disaggregating the effects of this particular social stratification mechanism from other interrelated variables, such as social class, ethnicity, and minority status. These variables need to be clearly defined and operationalized and then placed into models for the study of the determinants of children's health. Once such model has been proposed for the study of developmental outcomes in minority children (García Coll et al., 1996); similar models need to be constructed for the study of sociocultural disparities in children's health.

Another challenge is that the effects of discrimination on children's health are likely to be interrelated, that is, discrimination suffered by the child, the parent, the family, as well as neighborhood level-discrimination (e.g., segregation, with its effects on housing stock, neighborhood safety, social capital, and even differential exposure to environmental pollutants) may affect children's health. An integrative, ecological approach is needed, one that is able to measure and tease out the complex interactions among institutional and personal discrimination at multiple levels and their unique and cumulative effects on children's health.

The measurement of discrimination directed to and perceived by children poses unique methodological challenges. A child's perception and understanding of the causes of a negative social interaction will depend in large part on his or her age and developmental level. An understanding of child developmental theory is necessary in order to create instruments and measures that are valid for children at different ages and stages. Children (as well as adults) will sometimes not attribute a negative social encounter to racial discrimination. The challenge for the researcher is to find methods to delve beneath the surface to see if racial or ethnic discrimination may be part of the child's explanatory model, but to do it in a way that is not leading. Methods used in the cognitive social sciences (card sorts, ratings, triadic comparisons, and sentence frame formats; see Weller and Romney, 1988) may be helpful.

Since the dimensions of discrimination will be different for different minority groups, another challenge is to create instruments that tap into the unique aspects of discrimination in each group but can also be used comparatively in studies of multiple groups. Perceived discrimination may be based on such factors as language or accent, skin color, food preferences, family or household structure, or customs. Salient factors for one group may not be the same as for another group. Creating measures that have salience within a particular group (which anthropologists call *emic*) while also allowing for intergroup comparisons (i.e., *etic*) is a methodological and measurement challenge.

Researchers also differ on whether racial discrimination is best measured by experimental or experiential methods. Each method has its own advantages and disadvantages. The experiential survey approach takes into account the real-life social contexts in which discrimination is experienced, drawing on actual instances of discrimination encountered or perceived by the respondent. Because of this nonabstract approach, experiential surveys may be more developmentally appropriate for younger children. One benefit of the experimental approach is that setting and stimulus are controlled for. However, experimental techniques could lead to an underestimation of negative situations as being attributed to discrimination (see Szalacha et al., 2003).

Concerns and worries over *potential* discrimination, and not *actual* experiences of discrimination, may also have effects on the health and well-being of minority children. In the study of Puerto Rican children discussed above, 47 percent of the sample indicated that they worried about possible discrimination, and this discrimination anxiety was significantly related to low self-esteem (global self-worth) (Erkut et al., 2000). Studies regarding stereotype threat in black college students (Steele and Aronson, 1995) also reflect the consequences of perceptions and worries that minorities face on a regular basis and may be applicable to encounters with the health care system.

Discrimination based on race and ethnicity is an indisputable fact of life for many members of racial and ethnic minority groups. Its effects on physical and mental health in adults have been documented, and it is beginning to be studied in children. Perhaps the most crucial question that can be asked is what accounts for the variation among individuals in both the perceptions of discrimination and more importantly in its effects on health and well-being? Why do two individuals who are exposed to the same stressful stimulus have different responses to that stimulus? What are the social and psychological milieus that allow one child to thrive under such circumstances while another child becomes emotionally, educationally, or physically distressed? Focusing on the variability of responses to discrimination will help guard against viewing minority children's health disparities from a purely deficit model. It will allow for an analysis of health disparities that balances risk with resilience, perhaps explaining differences as being a function of protective and adaptive responses to a particular social context (LeVine, 1977).

Addressing Gaps in Measuring Discrimination

Discrimination is a social stratification mechanism that warrants further consideration as one of many mediators of health outcomes in minority children, including the multiple levels and mechanisms through which discrimination may have either direct or indirect effects on their health. These include both institutional and personal discrimination and discrimination not only directed to the child but also directed at other family members and caregivers, as well as neighborhood-level processes. It also includes actual experiences of discrimination as well as worries about being discriminated against. Since the relationships among discrimination, other social position variables, and children's health are complex, analytic strategies that are robust and can account for the effects of indirectly measured (latent) constructs should be used. Health researchers need to become familiar with techniques, such as structural equation modeling, which can be used to determine the direct and indirect effects of latent constructs, such as discrimination, racism, self-esteem, locus of control, cultural identity, and racial socialization.

Instruments need to be developed that can adequately measure perceptions of racism and discrimination in different age groups (from young children to adults) and different ethnicities. Such instruments should be tested for conceptual and measurement equivalency across ethnic and age groups within each group. Ultimately, large-scale national surveys such as the Health Interview Survey, NHANES, and National Longitudinal Survey of Youth should incorporate measures of racism and discrimination, whether limited to a single question or full instruments. One approach may be to create instruments that have a core set of generic items or subscales that are appropriate to measure racial discrimination among all minority groups, as well as additional items or questions salient to each particular ethnic minority group to ensure emic validity. Such instruments could potentially be used in comparative studies of the effects of discrimination among different groups as well in studies addressing the specific dimensions of discrimination salient within each group.

The development of such instruments is likely to require the use of both qualitative and quantitative methodologies, from ethnography and focus groups to confirmatory factor analysis and Rasch modeling. The utilization of multidisciplinary research teams, which include representation from such fields as public health, clinical health research, pediatrics, child development, education, anthropology, sociology, and psychometrics, would help to create instruments that are theoretically driven, conceptually valid, and psychometrically sound. Although not specific to children or to health, a recent National Research Council report (2004) outlines a series of recommendations related to measurement of discrimination.

SERVICES

Evaluating the effect of services on children's health is an important consideration both in terms of understanding the relative role of various influences on health and in relation to public policy decisions regarding services expenditures. In 2000, federal spending on children under age 18 was estimated to be $25 billion on Medicaid and the State Child Health Insurance Program (SCHIP) and approximately $123 billion on a wide range of other services, including food stamps, nutrition programs, social services, and other health and human development programs (http://www.cbo.gov/showdoc.cfm?index=2300&sequence=0). These federal expenditures do not include additional spending by state and local governments directed at promoting the health of children or improving their neighborhoods, or expenditures by their parents, families, or their parent's employers. From the standpoint of federal, state, and local policy, decision makers need to know whether expenditures on services result in improved children's health. Measurement systems can monitor trends in services and provide information to help target research on the effectiveness of specific services.

Given that the data systems and approaches to quality measurement are more advanced for health services than other services, the majority of the discussion that follows focuses on health services. The federal government has developed several different data collection mechanisms to monitor the delivery of health services and, more recently, the costs of these services. Existing surveys monitor the patterns of health service use and disease, but they lack the detail required to assess the appropriateness and effectiveness of the care provided. Nor do they provide a more nuanced assessment of health care access based on need. For example, evidence from health services research indicates that certain aspects of the regular source of care are associated with better outcomes at lower cost, but existing surveys, for the most part, do not adequately obtain information on such aspects of care as continuous person-focused care over time, comprehensiveness of care, and coordination of services.

Most approaches to assessing the quality of care focus on individual physician-patient encounters rather than on quality of the system that delivers care. With the exception of selected health services delivery systems, no existing data sources deals with the adequacy of the place where people receive their regular source of care as measured against well-accepted criteria of primary care. It is estimated that as much as 30 percent of U.S. health care costs are a result of inappropriate interventions (Schuster, McGlynn, and Brook, 1998); despite this, most quality measures focus exclusively on underprovision of services rather than overprovision of services.

Several recently designed surveys, including the NSCSHCN, the National Survey of Children's Health, and the NSECH attempt to improve measurement of the performance of health services, including disparities and gradients in health service provision. For example, the NSCSHCN included several measures about the acceptability of care for this subset of children, including whether or not the care provided to a family is "family-centered," meets their expectations, and provides a high standard of interpersonal quality. It also includes components of services that allow the measurement of some aspects of the system, in terms of operationalizing whether or not the children have a medical home. The NSECH provided information about perceived accessibility, continuity, the appropriateness of the content of care, as well as the acceptability of the care to parents. The NSECH also collected information about parental childrearing behaviors and assessed missed opportunities to provide specific components of well-child care that parents expressed an interest in receiving. It also collected information about parents' reported discipline practices, inquired into whether their regular provider had discussed discipline issues with them, and, if not, whether or not parents would have found such a discussion useful, thus providing a measure of unmet need for health services and missed opportunities to provide a service perceived by parents as useful (Regaldo, Sareen, Inkelas, Wissow, and Halfon, 2004).

While improving the quality of health care for both adults and children is recognized as a national imperative, there has been relatively slow progress in developing quality of care measures for children's health. The Institute of Medicine's (IOM) report *Crossing the Quality Chasm* (Institute of Medicine, 2001a), adapting and modifying a model proposed by the Foundation for Accountability, suggested that the focus of services should be on staying healthy, getting better, living with illness, and coping with the end of life. While these represent appropriate foci for adult health services, they omit the important role of development in the context of children's health. Moreover, coping with the end of life—an important issue for the small proportion of children who have life-threatening or terminal illnesses—is a relatively rare occurrence in childhood. The "staying healthy" rubric misses the importance of promoting optimal health and development. In addition, it is important to consider how health services delivered by both the personal medical care system and population health services perform and affect health outcomes in children. *Crossing the Quality Chasm* outlines several domains to measure the quality of services provided. These include medical services that are safe, effective, patient- and family-centered, timely, efficient, equitable, and coordinated.

The Foundation for Accountability, through its Child and Adolescent Health Measurement Initiative, has developed consumer surveys that can be administered to parents by health plans, Medicaid programs, and medical practices in order to assess the content and quality of the services that are being provided. The Young Adult Health Care Survey assesses perceptions of the content and quality of care for adolescents (Bethell, Klein, and Peck, 2001a); the Children with Special Health Care Needs Module for the Consumer Assessment of Health Plans Survey assesses the quality of services provided to children with chronic conditions (http://www.faact.org/faact/site/CAHMI/CAHMI/home?action=ViewGuidedTour Section&id=80); and the Promoting Healthy Development Survey assesses the content and quality of developmental services to children from birth to age 3 (Bethell, Peck, and Schor, 2001b; Bethell, Reuland, Halfon, and Schor, 2004). Although these mailed surveys provide information on quality as perceived by individual responding consumers, they are used primarily in populations already receiving health services in certain types of facilities rather than in the population in general. Thus, they systematically exclude the populations that are most deprived of needed services.

At present the major system that is used to measure the quality of personal health care provided by large health care organizations in the United States is the Health Employer Data Information System (HEDIS), operated by the National Committee on Quality Assurance (NCQA). HEDIS also assesses enrollees in health plans and contains very few indicators of the quality of children's health care or measures of the quality of care they receive. For example, the only measures of well-child care—which constitutes a major aspect of primary health care services for children—are the number of doctor visits children received and whether or not they have been immunized or screened for previously undetected health conditions (e.g., anemia) These are arguably important and necessary measures, but clearly not sufficient to determine if children have had their developmental risks assessed in a timely or appropriate fashion, whether their behavioral and emotional problems have been recognized and dealt with, or whether they have been followed to ensure resolution or improvement of their problems. They also assess only children in participating insurance plans (Kuhlthau, Walker et al., 1998; Perrin, Kuhlthau et al., 1997; Newacheck, Stein et al., 1996). Moreover, HEDIS has no comparable data collection on those without insurance, the underinsured, or those not enrolled in a health services organization that provides data to NCQA.

There has been progress over the last several years in measuring the quality of health services provided to children and the potential effect of different kinds of health services on their health. However, such measurements are not being collected as part of routine monitoring of quality and are not being collected at all on the most deprived segments of the population. Moreover, since the data collection mechanisms (even within HEDIS) are voluntary, some health maintenance organizations have decided not to monitor the health of children. Here, as in many other instances, the efforts are directed principally at the health of adults. Moreover, they are family-based and not a community of population-based assessments and give no clues either about averages or distributions in the population.

Challenges in Measuring Services

Although the United States has relatively good statistics on overall access to and use of health services, primarily through its national surveys, the data are notably inadequate for assessing access to and use of different levels of health services (including primary care and specialty care) and the effectiveness of those services. In current data, the concept of "access" is often confused with use of services, despite the fact that access facilitates care but does not reflect services sought or provided. Health surveys usually address the issue of access to and use of "a regular source of care," which may or may not be a primary care source. Modifications of survey questions sometimes inquire whether the source is the same for both preventive and illness care (with increased likelihood that the source is primary care if both are the same), but there is still no direct data on the extent and distribution of primary care at any geographic level in the United States or on the actual services provided.

Although some effort has been directed at improving measurement of personal health care services, far less has focused on assessing the performance of the community health infrastructure on which many parents rely (Fawcett, Pain, Francisco, and Vliet, 1993). The community service system includes a range of child development, behavioral, and mental health services and centers; programs to address the needs of children with learning disabilities and behavioral problems; health education programs provided through public health departments; educational services; nutritional services; and other programs provided by public health systems and communities (Halfon, Inkelas, Wood, and Schuster, 2001). At present, there is no systematic measurement of the effectiveness and efficiency of these community service systems or their capacity to meet the service needs of their communities and provide services acceptable to parents.

There are also major gaps in understanding the delivery of health services and the potential effect of these services on special populations. For example, although the number of children in foster care has increased dramatically over the past two decades and the high prevalence of mental health conditions in this population is solidly documented, there has been little focus on the accessibility and appropriateness of health services provided to children in foster care. It is not known whether health care providers and local health care systems are capable of providing mental health and developmental services to this high-risk group of children, the degree of continuity in the services provided, or whether the services are actually effective in addressing each child's particular needs (Rubin et al., 2004; Simms, Dubowitz, and Szilagyi, 2000; Horwitz, Simms, and Farrington, 1994; Takayama, Bergman, and Connell, 1994; Halfon, Berkowitz, and Klee, 1992; Halfon and Klee, 1987). Such measures would not only be helpful in specifying the burden of illness in this high-risk group of children, but in better understanding whether local and state authorities responsible for ensuring the well-being of children in foster care are actually meeting their legal and morel responsibilities.

A similar case can be made for a number of other special populations. For example, while the *Report of the Surgeon General's Conference on Children's Mental Health* (U.S. Public Health Service, 2000) documented the increase in mental health needs and the widening gaps in unmet needs for services, there is very little information at the federal, state, or local level on the affect of preventive, treatment, or rehabilitation services on children with mental health problems or on monitoring of the extent to which gaps are being closed.

It is also important to consider how services may be arranged and delivered based on population health needs. In keeping with the concept of health that was adopted for this report, we consider the services not only to prevent and treat diseases, conditions, and impairments, but also to prevent the effect of adverse influences and promote optimal health. The latter factors are especially important for children with serious ongoing health conditions. While only a minority of children have such conditions, they use a disproportionate amount of personal health care services and their medical expenses account for a substantial portion of health care expenditures (Ireys and Perry, 1999).

Addressing Gaps in Measuring Services

Better questions about access to and use of services are required to obtain more adequate information about types of care needed and received. This requires an understanding of the relative importance of primary care and specialty care, to improve the quality of decisions on personnel training, resource distribution, and financing and organization of services.

A continuing imperative is to improve methods and measures for all services. Clinical measures of quality that are based on evidence from various types of research studies are developing at a relatively rapid pace, but efforts to develop measures of health services performance are not. Recent research has demonstrated that the quality of systems for delivering primary care for children can be assessed using criteria that are widely accepted as constituting good primary care. These are based on characteristics including accessibility for first-contact care, person-focused care over time, comprehensiveness of care, and coordination of care when people have to be seen elsewhere (Cassady et al., 2000; Starfield et al., 1998). However, there has been little movement to incorporate primary care measures into existing data collection efforts. Moreover, there has been no effort to develop ways of conceptualizing and assessing the adequacy of specialty care services. Recent research is showing the variable nature of need for specialty services, including the need for advice and guidance, confirmation of initial opinion, and need for definitive interventions that can be provided only at the specialty level (Forrest, Glade, Baker, Bocian, Kang, and Starfield, 1999; Forrest, Rebok, Riley, Starfield, Green, Robertson, and Tambor, 2001) Both national and international data indicate great variability in referral rates from primary care to specialists and from one cultural context to another (Forrest, Majeed, Weiner, Carroll, and Bindman, 2002a). Although much of this variability can be attributed to age and case-mix differences, considerable variability remains even after controlling for these characteristics. Moreover, there is consistent and robust evidence of gaps in coordination of care, even though better coordination has been demonstrated to improve at least some aspects of the results of care (Forrest, Glade, Baker, von Schrader, and Starfield, 2000). Thus, for policy-related measures to be available and adequate, policy makers need to encourage and support efforts to develop criteria for referral and then to develop evidence-based guidelines to monitor rates of referral in different areas and in different population subgroups to ensure the most effective and equitable use of health services personnel and resources.

To capture the performance of both the personal health care system and the public health system, allow systematic assessment across the range of different performance attributes, and consider disparities in the distribution of services across various populations, an integrated measurement system should adopt a broad set of performance categories. As illustrated in Table 5-2, these categories include the effectiveness, efficiency, availability, appropriateness, capability, safety, continuity, acceptability, coordination, and equity of services. Such an approach would build on work in other countries, for example Australia, where broader measures are used to assess population effects as well as individual effects.

The table suggests how each attribute might be operationalized using a specific health service—developmental assessments—as an example. Although data would come from health service encounters and parents' perception regarding services, the committee has not laid out the specific data collection necessary. These same attributes and a similar kind of matrix could be constructed to assess the performance of other services, including other health care services, such as prenatal care, primary services to children, and specialty services.

A growing body of scientific evidence highlights the importance of the early years and experiences, developmental supports, and services that children receive. National and local research studies have highlighted gaps in the availability and quality of existing early childhood health services (Bethell, Peck, and Schor, 2001b; Bethell, Reuland, Halfon, and Schor, 2004). The federal Maternal and Child Health Bureau (MCHB) has launched a State Early Childhood Comprehensive Systems Initiative. Through this initiative, specific states are starting to improve the availability of health, early intervention, education, and family support services. There is very little information on the performance of these emerging early childhood service delivery systems and their effect on children's health.

Measurement of the effect of services on children also plays an important role in the context of other influences, especially when identifying the most effective and efficient intervention points along the pathway to health. Depending on the performance of a service, it may act to improve or modify health and reduce disparities that are due to social and economic differences or to environmental exposures. Understanding the potential effect of a service on populations requires understanding the variation in the performance of the service (e.g., effectiveness, efficiency, availability, and appropriateness) across populations, and the impact on variation in health. Performance is affected by factors intrinsic to the services delivery system and the context in which they operate. It is important to understand how its performance is affected by factors intrinsic to the service delivery system, geographic variations in the delivery of services, and a range of other potentially interacting factors. Accurate measurement of services and evaluation of their effect on children is important in order to partition the effects of the availability and delivery of services and their unique contribution to health outcomes in relation to the other influences on health.

POLICY

There are relatively few efforts to assess the effect of policy changes on health, particularly children's health. In rare cases (e.g., welfare reform, residential mobility programs, health insurance), random assignment evaluation studies have been mounted. Occasionally, rigorous longitudinal designs have been imple-

TABLE 5-2 An Integrated Service System Performance Approach
(Population-Level Developmental Assessment Example[a])

Performance Attributes	Construct
Effectiveness	Care/service intervention or action achieves desired results at individual, family, and community levels
Efficiency	Achieving desired results with most cost-effective use of resources
Availability	Ability of clients/patients to obtain care/service at the right place and right time, based on needs and is equitable
Appropriateness	Care/service provided is relevant to client/patient needs and based on established standards
Capability	Self-assessment of skill to conduct appropriate risk assessment
Safety	Potential risks of an intervention or the environment are avoided or minimized
Continuity	Ability to provide uninterrupted care/service across programs, practitioners, organizations, and levels of care/service over time
Acceptability	Care/service provided meets expectations of client, community, providers, and paying organizations
Coordination	Different aspects of care are connected seamlessly
Equity	Absence of systematic differences across population subgroups

[a]At national level, if we want to measure how care of children can impact development.

mented to assess the effect of specific policies. For the most part, laws are passed
and regulations written without specification of the aspects of health that are
likely to be affected, the mechanisms by which that is likely to occur, or funding
for rigorous evaluations. As a general rule, evaluations of the effect of new policies
on children's health, including not only health policies, but also most environmental, education, welfare, and other social policy, come from academic research
studies conducted after the policy is implemented.

The kinds of data systems that are the focus of the committee's report can be
used to provide a limited assessment of certain policies. In general, however, there
is little activity in the United States to measure the effect of policies on children's
health. The United Kingdom, Canada, and Australia have gone several steps further by developing approaches that attempt to assess policy effects more systematically and comprehensively.

Data collection by agencies such as the National Center for Health Statistics
and ongoing surveys by the MCHB and the Agency for Healthcare Research and

Measurement Strategies	Example Measures
Providers are using appropriate screening/ surveillance measures to detect problems	Rates of children receiving indicated assessments with appropriate instruments
Estimating costs of interventions	Average expenditure per child identified
Parents report services are available and they can have problem assessed	Rates of children actually reaching indicated services
Rates of services based on American Academy of Pediatrics guidelines	Proportion of children appropriately identified
1. Routine periodic survey of provider about knowledge, skill, and tracking needs	1. Self-assessment of skill to conduct appropriate risk assessment
2. Community health service—asset mapping of developmental services in community	2. Adequate referral services
Monitoring of avoidance of unsafe or unwarranted interventions	Rates of initiation of inappropriate modes of therapy
Same provider/practice conducting assessment	Rates of children with regular person conducting assessment
Assess parent satisfaction with assessment and its results	Satisfaction with care by ethnicity, income, and practice type
Spectrum of care provided without conflict in advice and/or management	Rates of conflicting advice or incompatible management strategies (e.g., drug incompatibilities)
Population-based monitoring of all aspects of health system performance	No differences in access to or receipt of individual services

Quality have unexplored potential for assessing the effects of policy changes on children's health outcomes. For example, state trends in health insurance coverage using the Census Bureau's CPS could be expanded to assess the effect of Medicaid or SCHIP policy changes on enrollment. Available national surveys such as the NHIS and the Medical Expenditure Panel Surveys could potentially provide insight into effects on access and utilization. They do not provide the state-level estimates necessary to monitor such programs as Medicaid and SCHIP, which are under state jurisdiction. National data systems provide very few data to assess whether policy changes designed to affect enrollment, access, or utilization of health care services actually result in changes in children's health outcomes. The best attempts that have been made to examine the effect of changes in Medicaid on children's health have been done using very long time frames and very gross and narrow measures of health outcomes, such as infant mortality (Currie and Gruber, 1996b).

Many health and other social policies are focused on reducing disparities in access, utilization, and health outcomes based on such social factors as differences in income, race, ethnicity, and gender. Even when relatively good data can be collected on the outcome of interest—such as infant mortality—and overall trends in that outcome accurately measured, existing data systems do not include sufficient other variables to test what accounts for the observed trends. Moreover, existing data also may not be able to differentiate between overall and subgroup trends. For instance, even though infant mortality rates have decreased for all ethnic and racial groups, disparities between whites and blacks have actually increased. This indicates that the influence on the absolute trends is likely to be different from the influence on the disparities trend (Wise, 2003). Because one of the two goals of *Healthy People 2010* is to eliminate disparities, it is important to develop data systems that can measure the effect of policies on health outcome disparities.

A success story in assessing the effect of a major health policy is the national Back to Sleep campaign (Wise, 2003). Because the outcome of interest is infant mortality and because there is a specific long-standing data collection system for this outcome, it has been possible to monitor the effect on sudden infant death syndrome (SIDS) specifically from the time that this national Back to Sleep campaign was introduced (American Academy of Pediatrics Task Force on Infant Position and SIDS, 1992; Pollack and Frohna, 2002; Lesko, Corwin, Vezina, Hunt, Mandel et al., 1998). Using infant mortality data, which contain some information on social class, it was shown that the Back to Sleep educational initiative dramatically reduced mortality rates due to SIDS, but also increased social disparities (Wise, 2003). Research studies were required to demonstrate that the effect of this new information and educational program has a bigger uptake and adoption by wealthier and more educated families. This was an important source of information for national, state, and local policy makers and programs interested in making midcourse corrections in their Back to Sleep campaign.

Measurement of the effect of policies related to the physical environment can be done at several different levels, including the monitoring of air, water and food quality, biomonitoring, and health effects. However, for environmental policy changes, the use of multiple indicators, as shown in Figure 5-1, allows rapid assessment of changes in influences by measuring environmental indices and biomarkers of exposure. These can then be correlated over time with changes in biomarkers of early and late effects, and finally with indicators of health. If a "significant risk" rather than an "actual harm" standard prevails in environmental policy (as it did for leaded gasoline), then biomarkers of exposure, while an indirect measure of children's health, could be used to document significant risk. The presence of an environmental influence for which there is evidence of likely harm, as measured using biomarkers, can then be used to guide environmental policy decisions.

While *Healthy People 2010* provides a possible framework for evaluating the effect of some influences on health, including policy changes, its structure does not permit examination of changes (improvements or decrements) in children's health from a dynamic perspective, as conceptualized in this report. *Healthy People 2010* provides a large number of indicators that reflect particular aspects of health—for example, behaviors influencing health, mental health, injuries, and vaccination status—but it does not offer a model for assessing the interaction or accumulation of these indicators in children or groups of children. There has been little work on how indicators of health can be combined to form a composite of health at the individual or population level or to profile health and changes in health at the population level across the group of indicators. Similarly, developmental concepts (e.g., rates of change in health potential over time) are not incorporated in the 2010 goals or objectives. The effects of policy changes cannot be adequately assessed without tracking the way these changes and their consequences affect children's developmental trajectories.

A number of other countries are ahead of the United States in monitoring both health overall and children's health in particular. In England, Canada, and Australia, major efforts have been undertaken to monitor the health of children over time. Although health was conceptualized in conventional ways using such indicators as mortality and morbidity, rather than in a dynamic manner, a recent effort carried out in the Canadian province of Manitoba (Manitoba Centre for Health Policy, 2002) provides lessons for future U.S. efforts. Data were organized by regions of the province, with each region characterized by an overall measure of health—premature mortality—and the areas ranked from high to low. These rankings were similar to the areas' ranking by socioeconomic status measures, reflecting worse health in more socially deprived areas. Areas were also ranked on the basis of mortality rates, adolescent reproductive health, acute and chronic conditions, and injury rates and these rankings were compared against the overall rankings. In this way, areas that performed better or worse than expected given their overall health status (i.e., premature mortality) were identified, making it possible to link particular policies (including those relating to health services) in different areas to level of performance on various health indicators. This is an important example of using ongoing data collection for monitoring children's health. It represents public commitment to children and demonstrates the feasibility of implementing such an effort on a large scale.

In Vancouver, British Columbia, Canada, a major initiative has been launched to measure and link measurement of children's health, development, and educational achievement for all school-age children to all existing programs and policies that affect these outcomes. Through the nationally sponsored Canadian Human Early Learning Partnership, this pilot project in Vancouver has mapped differences in children's health and social outcomes at the neighborhood level and related those differences to the availability and delivery of different health education and social service programs (Hertzman, McLean, Kohen et al., 2002). While representing a step toward a more extensive, ongoing, and integrated data system to measure and monitor the longitudinal health and educational trajectories of children, this initial effort aggregates health, human services, and neighborhood data and links them at the level of the individual child and neighborhood. The framework used in Vancouver to collect and report data on children provides an opportunity to monitor continuously the effects of a range of policy changes.[7]

Challenges in Measuring Policy

Measuring the effect of policies on children poses extraordinary challenges, given the many other influences that concurrently affect children's lives. Few attempts have been successfully mounted in this regard, particularly in areas in which the policy is not explicitly targeted toward children. As discussed previously, use of ongoing data collection for this purpose is exceptionally rare, but are noteworthy for the quality and effect of the information they provide.

One of the major challenges has to do with the frequently changing nature of the policy environment. Policies put in place during one administration may be accompanied by attempts to evaluate its effect, only to have that program changed or eliminated by the next administration.

The most convincing studies of policy effects involve random assignment to an experimental and control group. This is not only expensive and at times difficult to implement, but it can also be difficult to justify ethically, especially when a given policy is enacted with the purpose of benefiting children. Nonetheless, without such studies, the best intentions of policy makers can have untoward effects.

Promising alternative strategies rely on the natural experiments provided by changes in national or state policies over time (e.g., Currie and Gruber, 1996a) and ongoing data collection. In this case, sharp policy changes from one administration to the next or from one state to another aid evaluators, since they can then look for health care and health changes surrounding the policy changes. These evaluation studies require consistent and representative measurement of children's health and other demographic as well as policy conditions before and after the changes of interest. Studies based on trends in state-specific policies benefit greatly from consistent information across states and time regarding exactly what state policies have been implemented.

Assessments of policy effects—indeed, the design of policies themselves—are limited by conceptualizations of what constitutes health for children. Current policy perspectives continue to focus largely on diseases and illnesses and health services relevant to those diagnoses rather than on facilitating healthy development. To embrace a more dynamic view of children's health, policy approaches need to consider health in a developmental context, focusing on facilitating well-

---

[7]For additional information, see http://www.earlylearning.ubc.ca/CHILD/.

ness and health potential. This broader conceptualization will require consideration of not only biological factors, but also the range of behavioral, family, neighborhood, community, and system influences on children's health. A good example is the Sampson, Raudenbush, and Earls (1997) analysis of the importance of a community's "collective efficacy," discussed in Chapter 3. Understanding the factors that enhance collective efficacy would allow a community to develop policies intended to improve it, thereby improving the healthy development of its children.

Evidence about the importance of particular influences on health usually comes from studies of the relative risk of particular influences on a specific health outcome. The information provides a numerical estimate of the extent to which exposure to an influence increases the likelihood that a particular health outcome will occur, compared with the situation when the influence is not present. Clinical decision makers usually rely heavily on such evidence to justify interventions to reduce exposure to such influences in individuals.

In contrast, policy makers concerned with population health are more appropriately interested in attributable risk, that is, the extent to which different influences contribute to health outcomes. This is important for making policy decisions about which influences are most likely to improve health outcomes in the population. Such evaluations have much more potential to contribute to rational decisions about the most effective strategies to improve health. The challenge for such evaluations, however, is to include multiple types of influences as well as their interactions, in order to avoid attributing more benefit to certain types than to others. For example, McGinnis and Foege (1993) reviewed studies of the effect of certain behaviors on subsequent death and concluded that the combined behaviors accounted for 50 percent of deaths. The study was relatively unusual in examining attributable risk and an important model for needed studies, although it did not include a full range of influences. Moreover, it did not assess the interactions among the various types of influences, thus raising the likely possibility that behavioral factors were a result of, confounded by, or interacted with other types of influences that were not studied. Their report, for example, explicitly recognized the importance of appropriate health services (in the form of primary care) and socioeconomic characteristics, but it did not consider the effect of these services on the prevalence of the behaviors.

Where there is evidence that certain exposures are likely to cause ill effects, the wise course of action is to avoid such exposures, especially for children. Ill effects experienced during childhood alter future health. Policies that limit the release of noxious chemicals or other agents and the building of safe schools, houses, roadways, and cities can be expected to maximize the potential for good health, both of children and the adults they become.

Addressing Challenges in Measuring Policy

Monitoring policy effects on child health has not been a national priority. While existing laws require that environmental impact statements be developed when new roads, bridges, or dams are built, there is no such requirement to monitor the effect of labor, health, housing, energy, or transportation policies on children's health. Yet as noted earlier, such policies can exert important yet unintended and unanticipated effects on children's health, sometimes positive and sometimes negative. Given strong evidence that children's health sets the stage for life-long health, assessing the effects of policy on children's health should be given much more attention.

Existing ongoing data systems have several limitations as a tool for assessing policy effects, including their limited focus on particular diseases, the relative lack of longitudinal data, and the inability to link data across systems. Given the latitude afforded to states to implement policy, there is also a need for better tracking of state-specific policy implementation from one year to the next. Approaches being undertaken in Canada, England, and Australia provide valuable models for the United States. These models should be considered as new approaches to measuring children's health are developed.

CONCLUSION

Additional well-designed research and evaluation that address the challenges articulated throughout this chapter are needed to fully understand the range of influences and the interactions between them. The conceptual basis of many studies of children's health would be improved by the simultaneous study of at least one factor from each important category of influences known to be associated with health—an exception is the assessment of social class. In this way, studies can avoid the most egregious biases from failing to include variables that influence health and that interact in powerful ways with variables that have been included. A prototype of such a study is that of Lantz et al. (1998), which included both behavioral as well as social factors in the analysis of a national dataset. This was a study of adults; similar studies are warranted for children.

No single survey collects data on all influences on children's health in a comprehensive manner; it would be both financially and methodologically onerous to do so. Ensuring that the portfolio of surveys collects at least some data on multiple salient influences and improving the comprehensiveness of individual surveys drawing on the content of existing surveys should be priorities as research continues to elucidate the dynamism of health and its influences. Surveys focused on child outcomes other than health would profit from paying more attention to health outcomes and influences. For example, education-focused datasets often provide rich information on the child's readiness for literacy, family access to resources, and school quality but lack data on the child's biomedical markers and family health care seeking and health care access. Similarly, surveys focused on health outcomes have comparatively little information on such influences as family and communities variables.

Over time, a comprehensive continuous measurement system should be informed and evolve based on knowledge gained from continued research and expanded data collection in existing surveys.

6

Developing State and Local Data Systems

Existing state and local data constitute an underutilized resource for monitoring children's health and its influences. Effective use of existing data could serve many diverse functions, for example:

• a data system could provide a state or local health department with data on a range of health indicators to monitor children's health over time and inform policy decisions;
• a user-friendly web site could enable community groups to compare child health and environmental risk factors in their own communities with those in neighboring communities and with state and national averages;
• an integrated data system could enable public health professionals to identify geographic clusters of birth defects diagnosed months or years after birth, to link these birth defects with the prenatal histories of the mothers and to the newborn screens, and to determine whether environmental toxins are identified in the cluster areas;
• a data system could enable a pediatrician to determine whether a child being seen for the first time has received a full course of immunizations or enable the coordination of care among multiple providers serving the same child.

All of these information needs could be addressed by combining existing data from such sources as vital records, birth defects registries, Medicaid records, immunizations registries, the decennial census, and education records. But doing so requires attention to privacy concerns, standardization of data, political will, and financial resources. While there are challenges to creating an integrated data system, the opportunities far outweigh the challenges. In addition to an ethical mandate to know what is happening to children (e.g., when they are at risk, whether their health is changing for the better or worse), a solid data foundation to monitor risks and changes in health is crucial to evidence-based policy making and accountability, particularly in an environment in which states are being given more decision-making responsibilities. There is also a clear need to better understand and act on disparities in health to ensure the long-term productivity of the nation and the health of its citizens.

The chapter begins with definitions and then provides descriptions of data systems, including examples of state and local efforts to build children's health data systems and federal efforts to encourage such systems. It then outlines the needed steps that would facilitate all states and communities using available data to monitor their children's health and the influences on it.

DATA DEFINITIONS

For purposes of this report, data are tools to measure health, influences, and their indicators. A *data element* is a specific component of data with a clear, standardized definition to ensure that the numbers collected accurately represent the component. Age, birthweight, income, source of insurance, educational level completed, and race are examples of data elements. A *dataset* refers to observations and measurements collected through a single mechanism, effort, or type of scientific investigation. For example, data from a range of questions asked by a survey, such as the census or the National Health Interview Survey, is a dataset. Other examples of datasets are law enforcement records (e.g., incidence of domestic violence, juvenile arrests, and homicides), vital records (e.g., birth, death, marriage, and divorce records), immunization registries, newborn metabolic screening results, program encounter data, results of school readiness assessments, reports of childhood abuse, and health data for children in foster care. A *data system* is an integrated system of multiple datasets, including the combination of software and hardware that makes possible the manipulation or interpretation of data and datasets.

Data integration refers to the combination of data from more than one dataset into a data system. Data integration facilitates maximal use of data and improves surveillance of children's health and the factors that affect it. Single datasets allow an assessment of only a narrow set of aspects of health. Data integration can involve either aggregation of data from multiple datasets or linkage of multiple datasets at the individual level.

VALUE OF DATA SYSTEMS

Good integrated data systems increase knowledge that can be used by states, communities, and policy makers who design policies and fund interventions that affect children's health. Data systems can also be used to communicate knowledge about children's health to the public. Integrated data systems provide early information to identify areas of vulnerability, monitor health disparities, and detect manifestations of adverse effects on children's health across time, across domains of health, or for a variety of subpopulations defined by geography, ethnicity, or other characteristics.

Integrated data systems with data linked at the individual level also allow individual children or groups of children to be followed longitudinally across datasets to better understand why a characteristic or problem develops in some children but not others, and they support epidemiological studies of the potential effects of certain health influences. Linked datasets from multiple service systems, such as public health, education, human services, child welfare, juvenile justice, and health care, enable particularly useful longitudinal analyses. Based on guidelines to protect privacy and confidentiality, there should be limited access to linked data systems for a range of purposes. For example, policy makers can forecast and monitor the effect of their policies on children; researchers can determine best practices for health, social, and education services; the particular impact of multiple health influences on children can be determined; and management of patient care can be improved.

A community can be empowered when it has information specific to its children. States and some communities collect a wealth of data about children and their health. If data at the state or community level are scattered among several agencies or departments, it is difficult for community groups to compile them. Community groups and local policy makers are much more likely to use data systems that combine administrative datasets from multiple state and community sources (without identifiers) and are easily accessible to the public. Making children's data systems accessible on the Internet can enhance distribution and use by individuals outside government and the research community. The responsibility for providing much of these data is the public health department at the state and local levels. Since one of the three core functions of public health is assessment, data collection and dissemination is a major activity. The Institute of Medicine recommended in 1996 that the state health department be responsible for the provision of data. More specifically, within the public health department, the Title V maternal and child health program is mandated by federal law to be the lead on maternal and child health issues.

Advances in the systematic collection, analysis, and reporting of data have been made in recent years. Standardizing data definitions and collection methods is an important step in improving the value of data elements, datasets, and data systems and has been a priority of the National Center for Health Statistics (NCHS). Federal, state, and community programs have been encouraged to adhere to guidelines established by NCHS in order to improve the comparability of data. Without standardization, even sophisticated, integrated data systems cannot provide good information.

In addition, advances in technology and architecture for linking data systems allow for the integration or linkage of a large number of datasets on different platforms. Information technology systems in the future will increasingly separate the data elements from the business rules for combining the data elements; this will allow for more uses of the data elements and less recoding or reliance on one or more software packages.

DATA SYSTEMS

Both aggregation and linkage can serve a range of state and local purposes. While both strategies can be utilized for the same datasets, aggregation alone is most common because it offers fewer challenges; the technology, expertise, confidentiality, and security issues are relatively simple. There is increasing interest in linked datasets given the expanded analyses they enable, but for some jurisdictions the expense, privacy obstacles, or other implementation issues make this an unreasonable short-term objective.

Aggregated Data Systems

The oldest and easiest method is to aggregate data from multiple datasets of counted events, problems, or traits for a population group defined by residence in a geographic area or some other factor. Population subgroups may be further defined according to age, race, gender, or other data elements included in the datasets. For example, each of several datasets collected by the federal, state, and local government could be aggregated to the same geographic level to provide a more detailed picture of the health of the entire population of children or a subpopulation. Individual identifiers are typically removed before data are shared for aggregation. Many data-holding agencies (e.g., state or local departments of education) are prohibited by state privacy laws from sharing data unless personal identifiers are removed.

Policy and program decisions about children's health and environments can be enhanced when aggregated data are provided on the web in a user-friendly manner. Massachusetts and Missouri are two examples of states with web-based systems that provide children's health data from a variety of sources at several levels of geography. Aggregated data can be used to compare a multitude of health characteristics or influences on health for children in one community or across communities. Local and state programs use data such as these to better plan for services and improve programs and policies as well as evaluate programs over time; several states have systems that make aggregate data available on a regular basis. Consistent with the expectation that collection and provision of data are core functions of public health (Institute of Medicine, 1988, 1996, 2001a), public health departments are responsible for the provision of these aggregate-level data on a timely basis.

Aggregated data cannot be used to track individual children or groups of children over time, so they cannot be used to fully understand the significance of particular health factors or influences. Surveillance efforts that count events or conditions are useful for determining when there is an unusual incidence or cluster of a disease or condition that deserves closer scrutiny or identifying problems, such as high levels of substance abuse or injury, but they do not usually provide data that would help in determining why the condition has occurred.

Although states and communities may be organized differently, all have similar departments or divisions providing services to families and children: Medicaid and the State Children's Health Insurance Program, public health departments that provide such services as maternal and child health (Title V), family planning, and communicable disease services, child welfare, public assistance, education, mental health, housing, developmental disabilities, and juvenile justice. States are required to aggregate data for some federal reports, such as the one associated with the Maternal and Child Health Block Grant (Title V), but many states and several large cities have gone beyond mandated requirements to improve their health assessment and planning capabilities for children.

Making Public Health Data Available on the Internet

There is wide variation among states and communities on the number of datasets they aggregate and the accessibility of this information to communities and the public. The final report on the Evaluation of State-Based Integrated Health Information Systems commissioned by the Centers for Disease Control and Prevention (CDC) attests to the variation among states in the distribution of health data on the Internet (ORC Macro, 2000). The report summarizes an inventory of 53 state and local public health department web sites. Data were found on 51 of these 53 web sites. Key findings were:

• The most common datasets contained population data on death, birth, and low birthweight.

• Few sites provided data on health care or hospital utilization, social programs, or behavioral risk factors, such as smoking, alcohol use, obesity, and seat belt use, despite the fact that half of the sites contained other behavioral risk factor survey data.

• Only 10 of the 51 web sites were designed to allow users to formulate their own queries of the data system in addition to the graphs, charts, and tables created and provided by the states.

• About half the sites disaggregated data for geographic units—typically by county.

• Some web sites were geared for public use, others for use by researchers.

• The assistance provided for use of the web sites varied according to the complexity of the site, including whether the site could be queried and users could create both tables and graphs.

The study was limited to an evaluation of web-based efforts since a key purpose was to evaluate the accessibility of health data. The study of web sites also discussed some of the difficulties facing a state that donates nonproprietary software to help another state develop its health data system. The donating state often lacked the training and technical resources to assist the recipient state in getting the system operational. At the same time, states often were reluctant to purchase proprietary systems due to the initial and ongoing costs involved.

Many more states and communities are aggregating health data that were not included in this study, but they have not yet fully utilized the web to make aggregate, queriable data publicly available. In the committee's view there is great value in federal government efforts to partner with states to develop web-based data systems that, at a minimum, make aggregate data available in a form that can be queried for various geographic levels and for different measures over time. For many states, such a system would be a significant advance over current single dataset analyses.

Aggregating Children's Datasets Across Department Lines

Some states and communities have aggregated children's data without individual identifiers from datasets in two or more governmental departments or agencies. Over the past decade, several larger cities and counties have developed children's data systems to assist with policy development, service planning, and program accountability. While states may aggregate data by county or city, communities often need to analyze data for smaller, neighborhood-based units, typically a census tract. This is important for identifying areas with the greatest problems and the highest priority for resources. Some critical children's data are often more accessible to cities than to states. For example, a police department can contribute data regarding arrests for juveniles by geographic location, age, race, and reason for arrest. Education data can include absentee rates, suspensions, expulsions, number of special education students, number taking medications for chronic conditions, and proficiency scores by school. In contrast, education data in many states are not standardized, computerized, or in a central database, so collecting this information may require contacting each school. If a community has concerns about a particular area or group of the population and wants additional information, it may develop or use existing tools to collect these data.

Many communities have developed efforts to monitor and track the health and well-being of children in their communities and develop strategic priorities. Los Angeles County has one of the more comprehensive children's data systems and, through the Los Angeles Planning Council, produces a Children's ScoreCard every 2 years with data by services planning area. This data system contains aggregated, geographically coded data on children from health, education, social services, juvenile justice, and law enforcement agencies at the county, city, and state levels. However, Los Angeles goes beyond integrating the existing administrative datasets collected by government agencies and designs its own survey to capture data elements needed for planning children's health services. For the 1999–2000 health survey done by the Department of Health, 6,000 interviews of parents with children under age 18 were completed in a county with 1.3 million families with children. The sampling for this survey was designed to provide estimates for the service planning areas of the county. While only large communities like Los Angeles may have the resources for such a data system, they also must deal with such challenges as collecting data from many agencies, schools, and municipalities, as well as with geocoding data according to service planning areas or the equivalent (see Box 6-1).

The MassCHIP system in Massachusetts provides data on the web that can be queried at various substate levels. The data come from multiple state agencies as well as some sources external to government. Data include expanded Behavioral Risk Factor Surveillance System data on children and families that can be aggregated at various substate levels. MassCHIP also produces reports on the Kids Count indicators and the Maternal and Child Health *Healthy People 2010* objective for each city, town, and region of the state (see Box 6-2).

Many states or communities produce periodic reports, sometimes referred to as "report cards," modeled on the types of indicators identified by the Federal Interagency Task Force on Child and Family Statistics or the KIDS COUNT initiative. In some cases, these reports are produced by government agencies and in other cases by community groups. For example, Philadelphia Safe and Sound is an organization dedicated to improving the lives of Philadelphia's children through "a committed public-private collaborative" and publication of *Report Card: The Well-Being of Children and Youth in Philadelphia*, which monitors key indicators of childhood health, safety, and development (Philadelphia Safe and Sound, 2001).

Linked Data Systems

There is a growing interest in building data systems that are more sophisticated and have greater potential for policy and research purposes by linking individual-level data from two or more datasets. Linking datasets using consistent individual identifiers significantly increases the benefits of a system, even if personal identifiers are removed after the linkage. For example, linking would allow determination of whether conditions or behaviors co-occur, in what proportion of children, and in which areas of the state or locality. The advantage of this model is that it offers an opportunity to identify clusters of children who have specific characteristics, traits, behaviors, and health conditions and to follow individual children in a population longitudinally. This type of data system, if it provided valid and reliable data on a large and diverse population of children, could allow all the functionalities (surveillance, monitoring, forecasting, indicators to be used for accountability or quality improvement, and research) envi-

BOX 6-1
Community Report Cards on Children's Health

Local efforts to monitor and track the health and well-being of children through community report cards demonstrate a vital interest on behalf of communities to understand how children are faring. More importantly, these report cards—also referred to as "score cards," "profiles," or "data books"—help communities develop strategic priorities for action that can improve children's health.

The development of community report cards is often initiated by local health departments, local government agencies, colleges and universities, nonprofit organizations, and foundations. They sometimes involve community residents and stakeholders, require a significant investment of time and resources, and have a range of target audiences, including policy makers, professionals, media, and community groups.

Community report cards not only track health conditions, but also focus on broader indicators of child health and its influences, including social and emotional well-being, safety and crime, education and workforce readiness, and economic well-being. Some report cards disaggregate their data by geographic areas, ethnic groups, or socioeconomic status; track data over time; and offer policy and programmatic recommendations.

An example is the Los Angeles Children's ScoreCard, developed and published by the Los Angeles County Children's Planning Council, a public-private partnership organization created by county government. The ScoreCard tracks a set of indicators across five outcomes of child well-being—good health, social and emotional well-being, safety and survival, economic well-being, and education/workforce readiness. The indicators to be collected are determined by key stakeholders, including community representatives; tracked over time; and disaggregated by the eight regions of the county. The report also captures how communities are translating the data into action, by highlighting the work of nine regional children's councils whose efforts are aligned with the five outcomes and indicators that are of most concern to that region.

Los Angeles County has used the ScoreCard to guide community action on children's health issues. Concerned that only 75 percent of children had health insurance, in 1997 the county—in partnership with the community—established as a goal enrolling 100,000 more children into MediCal. By the end of that year, 124,000 children had been enrolled. By 1999, the number of children with health insurance increased to 80 percent. The numbers of children immunized also increased by 15 percent between 1997 and 1999.

The ScoreCard is published every 2 years and is the primary source of data on children's health and well-being in Los Angeles County.

BOX 6-2
MassCHIP

MassCHIP, the Massachusetts Community Health Information Profile, is a dynamic, user-friendly information service that provides free, online access to sociodemographic, health, and social indicators. Using MassCHIP, one may query, pose questions, and retrieve information on a variety of health and related topics concerning children, youth, and families for a range of geographic areas in order to assess health needs, monitor health status, and evaluate health programs. MassCHIP includes data that reflect a broad view of population and public health.

MassCHIP currently contains over 28 major datasets from health, education, and human service agencies. For example, it currently contains data from the Office for Child Care Services; the departments of Education, Social Services, and Transitional Assistance; the divisions of Employment and Training, Health Care Finance and Policy, and Medicaid; the Board of Registration in Medicine; and the Bureau of the Census, in addition to the Department of Public Health.

Developed originally with grants from MCHB/HRSA and CDC, MassCHIP has a number of easily accessible (via the web) reports on 23 specific topics. Included among the options are specific "instant reports" on adolescents, children with special health care needs, perinatal indicators, *Healthy People 2010* maternal and child health objectives, and the KIDS COUNT indicators for all levels of geography, including census tract, city and town, county, region of state, school district, etc.

In addition to "instant topic" reports, users can generate their own reports across datasets and time periods for different geographic areas. To execute the most flexible queries, users must download the application onto their computer and access MassCHIP data servers through the Internet. MassCHIP returns counts of events and a wide variety of statistical measures, including percentages, age-specific and age-adjusted rates, and standardized incidence ratios. The system provides charting and mapping options and results may be exported.

MassCHIP is currently in transition onto the web with enhanced functionality and appearance. The first phase is complete with Instant Topic reports on the web; in the next phases, the user-friendly custom report functions will also be available on the web. It was awarded the Massachusetts Investing in Information Award for improving the state's health information infrastructure by the Massachusetts Health Data Consortium in 1998.

For additional information, see http://masschip.state.ma.us/.

sioned by the committee as desirable for a data system of the future. The disadvantage of linking datasets is that more concerns are raised about confidentiality and privacy, discussed later in this chapter.

A linked data system must adhere to state and federal rules and regulations regarding the collection and dissemination of confidential data; the Health Insurance Portability and Accountability Act and similar state laws provide the context for how data systems can be developed and used in the future. All states have procedures for how to obtain access to confidential information; these rules are followed internally within health departments for linking data between key surveillance systems. Unique identifiers that allow data for the same individual to be linked without that person's identity revealed are often used when data are shared.

Two decades ago, the University of Miami undertook one of the earliest efforts to link data at the state level with financing from the Florida departments of education and health (personal communication, Fredia Wadley with Keith Scoot and Rachel Spanjer, 2003). The Florida Department of Education initiated the linking of datasets because it would help elucidate the problems of future cohorts of students and support better policies and planning to meet student needs. However, Florida is still one of the few states in which the education department shares its data with individual identifiers with another state agency (see Box 6-3).

Tennessee has been developing a data system on children over the past 5 years. The first phase aggregated datasets across five state-level departments serving children. The second phase linked the datasets with individual identifiers to allow case managers in the various state departments to access information on the Internet for their clients.[1] Initially the information provided by each program was limited. Case managers could find out what other state services were being provided and whether other case managers were assigned to the same child, but they had to contact other relevant programs to gain more information. The final phase is being developed and is to contain a record of all state services and health care information for children in foster care.

Health providers who have been approved to access the system for their foster care patients will be able to view records for their clients and input specific diagnostic, treatment, and referral information. Although there are only approximately 10,000 children in state custody at any time in Tennessee and a total of 15,000 in an average year, these children present an enormous challenge to state and to health providers. Locating and making available social, education, and health records to those service and health providers attempting to make adequate assessments and plans for these vulnerable children has been a long-standing problem. A second challenge has been tracking these children as they receive multiple services and therapies and sometimes relocate to other regions of the state. The type of system being developed would not only help in resolving these two problems common among states but would also serve as a prototype for broader children's health data systems (Urbano, 2001).

The Robert Wood Johnson Foundation All Kids Count initiative has a recommended approach to creating an integrated data system for the early years that grew out of efforts to develop and implement immunization registries. Rhode

---

[1]Internet access by the general public was not allowed.

BOX 6-3
Florida's Children's Registry and Information System

The Florida Department of Education and the University of Miami's Child Services and Policy Research (CSPR) Center have worked together for 20 years on various research and service programs. As part of these cooperative efforts CSPR has created a linked database with data from education, birth records, nutritional programs, and the public defender's office. These data are used to assess risk factors for poor school outcome, to evaluate program effectiveness, and to contribute to instructional improvement, cognitive test development, and screening. CSPR, as an agent of the Florida Department of Education, is able to access school data and not violate the requirements of the Federal Education Right to Privacy Act. CSPR has been successful in responding to the needs of the Department of Education that could not be addressed without a linked database for longitudinal studies.

Florida is fortunate to have a statewide school database that receives data from the 69 county school systems. While the county systems have more detailed information than the statewide database, placement, achievement, attendance, and disciplinary actions are available in the statewide database.

CSPR manages the Children's Registry and Information System (CHRIS) for the Florida Department of Educations' Florida Diagnostic and Learning Resources System (FDLRS), which is the state's child find agency. Each regional FDLRS center has a CHRIS database that tracks the services and placements of children from birth to age 5 (although the FDLRS emphasis is from birth to age 3). The CHRIS databases are then combined into a statewide database maintained at the University of Miami and also linked to other CSPR databases.

Florida also has a program for following children after completion of their secondary school education. The Florida postschool follow-up program tracks individuals to assess their attainment by linking data from a variety of sources (employment, corrections, and postsecondary education).

Island is one of the states that have linked their immunization registry with other state datasets. Rhode Island's children's data system, KIDSNET, links nine datasets from programs that serve children in the state health department. While other state health departments have integrated many of their datasets, Rhode Island is unique in that it has concentrated on integrating the data available on children. Data from KIDSNET is made available in both aggregated and linked form, depending on the user (see Box 6-4).

Other examples include the systems in Missouri (MOHSAIC), Oregon (FamilyNet), and Utah (CHARM). The Maternal and Child Health Bureau and the CDC have over the years funded various states to develop integrated child health data systems. The technology available today can produce linked data systems. The challenges stem from a lack of awareness about the potential benefits, a need for strong commitment and leadership at all levels of government among the various data owners, the reality of government budget crises, and increasing concerns about confidentiality and privacy. Even if these challenges are overcome, it will take time and resources to build linked systems.

BOX 6-4
KIDSNET in Rhode Island

KIDSNET is an integrated information management and tracking system for new-born metabolic screening, newborn developmental risk assessment, newborn hearing loss, childhood blood lead screening, childhood immunizations, the Special Supplemental Nutrition Program for Woman, Infants, and Children, early intervention, maternal and child health home visiting, vital statistics, and other preventive pediatric health initiatives. KIDSNET is primarily a tool to ensure timely delivery of preventive services to all Rhode Island families with children born after January 1, 1997. In addition, it serves as a resource and link to ensure coordinated access to community-based family support services for providers of childhood immunizations to these infants and toddlers.

A KIDSNET goal is to continue enrolling significant additional providers so that over 90 percent of KIDSNET records contain immunization information, the only data component of KIDSNET that cannot be supplied by existing program data systems and that requires reports from providers. The 150 primary care provider offices participating in the state health department's Immunization Programs Universal Vaccine Purchasing and Distribution Program (which makes vaccine for children's antigens available for free to all children receiving care in the state) are eligible to be KIDSNET providers. They are equipped, trained, and supported by health department staff to use KIDSNET and are then able to get practice-based rates and reports on how well they are screening for lead poisoning, immunizing, and related goals.

In addition to supporting primary care providers in their efforts to provide a "medical home" for their patients, KIDSNET has had the secondary function of supporting public-private partnership efforts to ensure the completeness of childhood lead screening to an entire population, regardless of their type of insurance. This collaborative quality improvement strategy has been recognized by the secretary of the U.S. Department of Health and Human Services as a model effort. Driving population-based quality improvement activities using shared data will soon test the completeness and accuracy of the immunization data in KIDSNET.

A third use of KIDSNET is system performance evaluation. Under the state health department's authority as the Title V agency for Rhode Island, indicators of a medical home are being developed to reflect the values of continuity, comprehensiveness, and coordinated care. Using linked data at the individual child level, these indicators will be used by a multidisciplinary team to develop quality improvement activities that will attempt to ensure a medical home for all preschool children in Rhode Island.

ISSUES RELEVANT TO DEVELOPING DATA SYSTEMS

Addressing Ethical Concerns

Ethics pervades discussions of the collection and use of data. It is accepted that certain types of health data serve a public good and are in the interest of the community so can and should be collected. For example, certain vital statistics are required to be reported in all jurisdictions. Similarly, reporting of some conditions is mandatory. In the case of children, this includes birth defects (in some jurisdictions), newborn metabolic screening, newborn hearing screening (in some jurisdictions), certain infectious diseases, all cancers, and suspected abuse and neglect. The exact list of reportable conditions is further guided by state law. There is also general consensus that it is appropriate to track the rates of some potentially sensitive population characteristics using aggregated data (e.g., suicide rates, adolescent pregnancy). Much of the information that is collected in national and state surveys is also reported as aggregated data. However, reporting of data also raises issues of privacy and confidentiality.

Privacy and Confidentiality

Virtually all of the datasets used to obtain aggregated data include detailed information on individuals or in some cases on all the individuals in a family or household. This provides the mechanism for review and analysis of data pertaining to individuals and the cross-tabulation of data to assess how two or more characteristics are associated. For example, one could determine the proportion of white males in rural areas who are immunized. In order to examine such relationships, identifiers are routinely removed to preserve anonymity.

Although the agency that collected the data could theoretically identify the individual, and in some cases does go back to collect additional information (as for example in a follow-back or longitudinal study), the information that could be used for identification is stripped from the file before the data are analyzed. This protects the individual who provided the information, but at the same time allows analysts to query the data so that multiple pieces of information can be combined to assess the relationships between elements in the dataset.

Numerous data are available in public use datasets that can be analyzed both by public health officials and by investigators in research institutions. This mechanism has provided a great deal of current information about children's health. The removal of individual identifiers protects the individual's privacy while advancing the public interest to learn more about children's health. Furthermore, there are requirements to ensure that individuals with rare conditions are not identifiable by prohibiting the reporting of units of analysis (such as geographic sites) that would allow the person to be traced.

Data anonymity is now possible with current technologies, even for linking individual data across time within a survey or agency and also across surveys and agencies. In such cases, individual identifiers are removed from the data and are known only to the persons who have access to the linking process. The data stripped of identifiers can be used for a wide range of purposes, while still allowing for the protection of individual interests. Again, standards would be needed to ensure that individuals with particular profiles of rare occurrence could not be identified.

Private Lives and Public Policies, a National Research Council and Social Science Research Council report of the Panel on Confidentiality and Data Access, made recommendations designed to aid federal statistical agencies in their stewardship of data for policy decisions and research (National Research Council and Social Science Research Council, 1993). Recognizing the tension between individuals' rights for privacy and the public's need to know certain information for the good of society, the panel stated that "Sharing of identifiable data for statistical purposes can have many potential benefits, including the enrichment of cross-sectional and longitudinal datasets, evaluation and improvement of the quality of census and survey data, improvement of the timeliness and consistency of statistical reporting, development of more complete sampling frames, and improvement of comparability between data developed by different statistical agencies" (p. 40). The panel also posed questions to consider before linking records:

1. Will the linkage process conform to all statutory confidentiality standards of the agencies involved?
2. Will the linkage conform to pledges made to data providers concerning the use of their information?
3. Is linkage of data the only feasible way to develop the desired statistical products?
4. Are the uses of the data sufficiently important to justify introducing additional risks of disclosure?
5. Should resources and costs be considered in obtaining the desired data by other means?
6. Who will have access to the data? Who should decide?

These questions form a good basis for making decisions affecting the development and maintenance of data systems at all government levels. Since federal and state laws vary according to the data elements and datasets involved, general statements cannot be made to fit all federal and national efforts to develop systems of data. However, some overriding issues must be addressed at the federal level before states can move forward.

The first question of the Panel on Confidentiality and Data Access related to barriers to agencies sharing data. The Federal Education Right to Privacy Act presents some legal concerns for sharing education data on individual students. An exception provides that schools can share individual data on students if they are used to improve instruction (National Education Goals Panel, 1997). Nevertheless, it is unlikely that state education departments will participate in linking their datasets with those in other departments as long as they are unsure of the interpretation of the law and this exception. Sharing of education data and health data collected in schools (e.g., school-based health centers, school nurses) could be facilitated with an amendment to clarify that student data can be used for research and planning when they (1) benefit the health and well-being of students and (2) confidentiality is protected.

Some state Medicaid programs also cite Section 1092 (a) (7) of the Social Security Act as limiting the sharing of Medicaid data with individual identifiers. This section limits the use of individually identifiable Medicaid data to purposes directly connected with the administration of Medicaid. Some Medicaid programs believe that linking data helps in meeting the needs of their participants and improving programs and do not see this as a barrier, while others take a more restrictive view.

The Health Insurance Portability and Accountability Act of 1996 (HIPAA) also raised concerns about sharing individual data. The final rule required health plans, health care clearinghouses, and health care providers who conduct certain financial and administrative transactions electronically to disclose how they will (1) use, store, and share health information; (2) ensure patient accessibility to their medical records; and (3) obtain patient consent before releasing patient information (U.S. Department of Health and Human Services, 2003). The act establishes mandatory procedures for the linkage of data sets. Although HIPPA is explicit about covered health entitities under the law, very little reference was made to uncovered entitites, especially those in public health departments. All state public health mandated data systems, such as registries and communicable disease reporting systems, must include all relevant cases in the dataset.

Informed Consent

Linkages that do not remove identifiers can be desirable for purposes of care management. In these situations, the goal of linking the data is to allow relevant service providers to know what other service sectors are involved in an individual's care. In these situations, the balance of individual interests with public interests (for example, to save money, avoid duplication of services) may become more complex. These issues are sometimes handled by suggesting that consent be obtained for such linkages.

In order for consent to be informed, parents must be told and must understand who will have access to the data, how they will be used, and any risks associated with their child's data being in the system. Parents must also be assured that no negative action will occur if they refuse consent. Consent forms can be designed to have a list of data elements that can be shared and those that are not to be released. A critical question is whether a parent can consent for a child, especially if, as is often the case, the ultimate uses or potential uses of the data are not known at the time that the permission is obtained. In addition, new knowledge might make parents want existing data elements to be kept confidential. State laws and regulations differ on this point, though generally uses of data are restricted to what was included in the original consent. Federal guidance on this point will be increasingly important as new technologies push the current boundaries of research and make possible previously unforeseen analyses.

Data Security

With any collection of data containing personal identifiers or a potential for breach of confidentiality, there will be questions about who has access to the data and who makes access decisions. Advisory groups consisting of data experts, data providers, and data users, frequently used by state health departments to guide data system development, can be created to provide guidance consistent with federal, state, and local laws and policies for dealing with issues of access, privacy, and ethics. Advisory groups can decide which data elements should be excluded in the data system, or should be accessible only after the identifiers have been removed, or should be shared only after a unique identifier has been assigned. This same advisory committee could also develop protocols on what data could be available to researchers or other groups and under what conditions. Policies and procedures should be developed before proceeding with the development of the data system. Guided by state laws regarding confidential data, state health departments have such procedures and policies in place for health department data.

Even data that are a matter of public record have the potential to stigmatize counties. Many states distributing data for HIV/AIDS cases do not report a number for a county until the total number of cases reaches a specified level. The concern is that if only a couple of cases of HIV/AIDS are reported in a small community, certain individuals might be labeled, correctly or incorrectly, as having AIDS due to their sexual preference or life-style. Communities have also expressed concern about reporting certain youth characteristics (e.g., a high percentage of sexually active adolescents or a high incidence of sexually transmitted diseases). Schools have refused to participate in surveys designed to determine risk behaviors of students if the results were to be made known by school or community, fearing that characteristics perceived as negative can stigmatize the school and create problems for the school with community leaders. Many state public health departments have developed their own rules about suppression of small numbers of cases. HIPAA also includes data suppression and reporting rules. Additional federal standards on this issue could facilitate a consistent approach across states.

Some security concerns relate to the technological design and maintenance of a system. Over the past few years, several widely publicized breaches of network security and global viruses have elevated concerns about the security of online data. Most of these incidents have not involved health-related data, but they have fostered the perception that any online data poses a security threat (Eng, 2001). Today's technology allows databases to be designed to provide security against direct query of certain attributes. Any specific user can be given restricted access to specific parts of a database. Such a multilevel database stores data according to different security classifications and allows users access to data only if their security level is greater than or equal to the security classification of the data (National Research Council, 1993).

Another concern is what Lunt and collegues (1990) call an inference channel. An inference channel is said to exist in a multilevel database when a user can infer information classified at a high level for which he or she does not have access based on repeated queries of information classified at a lower level to which the user does have access. Techniques (e.g., query restriction, response modification) exist to limit the potential for such inferences, and consideration should be given to these approaches in designing data systems. Extensive security protocols in place for public health bioterrorism systems also provide possible models.

The Census Bureau has implemented an approach that makes sensitive individual-level data available to researchers in seven data centers across the country (see Box 6-5). This approach demonstrates that there are viable strategies for making individual data available without compromising confidentiality, representing an initial step toward improving access to data. However, accessibility under this model is limited, the relatively small number of centers makes the process somewhat cumbersome, and it can require significant expense by researchers who are not located near a center. Additional and expanded approaches should be developed to continue to make Census Bureau and other datasets, such as those available through the NCHS, more accessible. Although NCHS has a mechanism in place to make sensitive data available at their headquarters, the process is more cumbersome than the Census Bureau's approach and currently does not meet the needs of data analysts outside the center.

Emerging Issues

Another set of complex ethical issues arises from the relatively new ability to collect and store biological specimens for long periods of time. For example, all states collect drops of blood from newborn infants on special absorbent cards. These are used for mandatory newborn screens for inborn errors of metabolism and other congenital conditions. There is inconsistency in the screening procedures used across states and in the procedures used to handle such specimens after collection. However, it is technically possible to take anonymous fragments of these specimens to look at population exposures to infectious diseases (such as to determine rates of HIV transmission) or noxious chemicals (e.g., pesticides or

---

BOX 6-5
The Census Bureau's Research Data Centers Program

The Research Data Centers (RDC) program of the U.S. Census Bureau's Center for Economic Studies is one promising model for enabling knowledgeable researchers working outside a data collection agency to access otherwise confidential respondent-level information. This increases the research value of data that has already been collected and provides feedback from the research community to the bureau about its data products.

There are currently seven regional centers: in Ann Arbor, Michigan; Boston, Massachusetts; Berkeley, California; Chicago, Illinois; Durham, North Carolina; Los Angeles, California; and Pittsburgh, Pennsylvania. Access to the data is strictly limited to researchers and staff authorized by the Census Bureau. The computers in the RDCs are not linked to the outside world. Researchers must conduct all of their analyses within the RDC, may not remove confidential data from the RDC office, and must submit output to Census Bureau personnel for disclosure review prior to removal from the RDC. In establishing these centers, university-based researchers, sometimes in collaboration with other local-area research groups, submit detailed proposals for setting up a secure computing facility that meets strict Census Bureau requirements. Researchers interested in using the centers submit proposals that must be approved by both the RDC and the Census Bureau and are required to obtain special sworn status from the Census Bureau. Approved researchers are subject to the same legal penalties as regular Census Bureau employees for disclosure of confidential information.

For additional information, see http://www.ces.census.gov/ces.php/rdc.

---

persistent organic pollutants—Burse, DeGuzman, Korver, Najam, Williams, Hannon, and Therrell, 1997).

In addition, it would be possible for an investigator to approach families several years after a baby's birth to obtain permission to use identified samples to conduct a retrospective study of a toxic agent to assess the body burden at the time of birth. In this case, presumably the family could make an informed decision about the merits of the study and the risks to the child, if any, of making this determination. It is likely that interest in conducting such retrospective analyses will grow with the further sophistication in understanding of biological mechanisms of gene-environmental interaction.

What is much less clear is whether it is ethical to ask parents for consent to use their baby's biological samples for open-ended purposes at the time of the infant's birth, since it is not clear what the implications are for future risk to the child of information that might be obtained at a later point. For example, if genes are identified that are associated with increased risks for antisocial behavior, might a child's genetic profile be used to exclude him or her from some activities, or if a child is found to have a genetic predisposition for an illness, might he or she be charged a higher premium for life insurance? Many would argue that the parents could not anticipate the potential consequences of the permission they were granting.

These examples illustrate some of the complexity of the ethical issues involving the use of different methods for monitoring children's health and its influences. Because of this complexity, the committee recommends that special attention be given to these issues. In the committee's view, linkage of currently available data, using existing and emerging technologies, can advance understanding of disparities in health and ways to address them. Not utilizing these capacities also raises ethical concerns, because it means that information within our grasp is not used to improve children's health.

Standardization of Data Elements

Standardizing data elements and the methodology for their collection is vital to having reliable analyses. Various agencies of the federal government have taken the lead in this area, and there is good rationale for strengthening the coordination and collaboration of all the federal agencies providing funds and guidelines for the many programs that require collection of administrative data on children's health or health influences. States must also be partners in the process, since they not only collect data for the federal programs but also for state programs. States are most likely to adopt standardization guidelines if they are developed by the federal government in collaboration with the states. Standardization would produce comparable data across states and reduce the time and resources needed for individual states.

Medicaid and education programs represent a large part of government budgets at all levels. There are federal requirements for both programs to collect a significant amount of data, but it is not specified or mandated that states collect all data elements in a standardized way. For example, Medicaid requires a comprehensive physical (including behavioral) examination and developmental assessment on children receiving an Early, Periodic Screening, Diagnosis and Treatment (EPSDT) examination. The federal Medicaid guidelines do not require the use of standardized tools for these assessments, or that there be a reduction in the reimbursement if all sections of the EPSDT exam are not completed. As a result, documentation for these assessments may be absent. Even when they are present, there is no way to aggregate these data in any meaningful way, since the tools and documentation vary so greatly.

A similar problem exists for education data. States and school districts do not always require their schools to use the same tools and methodology for collecting data. While all schools are now required by the No Child Left Behind Act of 2001 to conduct annual assessments at specific grade levels, it is left to the

---

BOX 6-6
Vancouver, British Columbia

In Vancouver, the Canadian Early Learning Network has begun an important and ambitious data integration and mapping project designed to provide an integrated view of children's health and development at the neighborhood level. Using the geocoded results of a school readiness assessment that is now provided to all children at kindergarten entry, they have linked school readiness measures at a school or neighborhood level to a range of other indicators of health, educational achievement, and availability and receipt of services. For example, at a neighborhood level, data are provided about the relationship of low school readiness scores (overall or in a particular domain) with availability of child care, libraries, use of health services, etc. Because it is being done at the school or neighborhood level, it mitigates some of the confidentiality issues, since data are not analyzed at the individual level. Moreover, this school or neighborhood analysis strategy also lends itself to population-based approaches to finding ways of addressing disparities and gradients in health and developmental outcomes, not just those that focus on a particular child. This is important if the type of population health approaches that a community seeks is to shift the curve in a positive direction for the entire population.

---

states, and often the school systems within a state, to determine which tools will be used for assessment. Similarly, *Readiness for School: A Survey of State Policies and Definitions* documented in fall 2000 that only 13 states conducted statewide screenings or assessments when children enter kindergarten; 5 states required the screenings or assessments but local school districts decided how to do them; and 26 states did not mandate any readiness assessments. The National Education Goals Panel (1997) has made recommendations for defining and assessing school readiness, but educators have not been able to reach consensus on if, what, or how this should be done (Saluja, Scott-Little, and Clifford, 2000). Standardized data on school readiness and performance in grades 4 and 8 could advance efforts to identify practices most effective in helping children perform at the same level of their peers even though they are behind when they start kindergarten (see Box 6-6 for an approach in Vancouver using school readiness data).

Infrastructure Needs

Technical Issues

In developing a data system, it is important to follow a logical cycle from planning to development to implementation and to involve relevant program and community leaders in developing system specifications. Such a system should be developed with a clear set of requirements based on the various processes or outcomes desired. When system needs are well defined, technical solutions can be purchased to meet specified requirements. Although building or purchasing a system is likely to be feasible, doing so will require resources. Federal programs such as the Title V program should consider a dedicated funding stream for the design and implementation of well-developed data systems to guide policy development and aid program monitoring.

However, states and communities that are developing information systems on children are struggling to develop or purchase software as well as obtain necessary hardware. Building the infrastructure for such a system may require steps as simple as having enough computers for field staff in the various children's services agencies who will be putting data into the system. Another challenge is acquiring the hardware and processes necessary to address access and security concerns. Proprietary systems that come with support services may be too expensive for a state or community to purchase. States willing to donate their system to another state may not have the manpower resources to help in the training and implementation phase of the project, even in the absence of patent or copyright protection. Obtaining software can therefore be a major barrier for a state or community trying to develop a data system on children.

In addition, data system developers must grapple with datasets that sometimes contain incomplete and inaccurate data. Standardization of data elements will help to reduce inaccuracies. Involvement of the people and programs responsible for providing relevant data in the development of system specifications will also help address these issues, particularly if the system is designed to provide useful information to the people responsible for providing the data.

Personnel

Personnel time and expertise are necessary to identify and integrate datasets, to create and maintain data at the substate level (e.g., county, city, or census tracts), to make the data available for others to disaggregate at these levels, and to create web sites with tutorials on how to use the data. A greater level of manpower and expertise is needed to create linked data systems and protect the data in those systems than for aggregated systems. Hiring adequate staff to develop and maintain such data systems is a barrier for many states and communities. However, every Maternal and Child Health (MCH) Title V program has one or more personnel trained in data analysis and applications, and there is a national network of state MCH data contacts. CDC and HRSA have helped to develop and train data expertise in each state; CDC has fostered the development of a network of maternal and child health epidemiologists.

The National Action Alliance started in 1997 as the national action agenda for building data capacity for maternal and child health. The initial leadership group, which consisted of the Association of Maternal and Child Health Programs, CityMatCH, HRSA, and CDC, has now expanded to include other state affiliates (the Council for State and Territorial Epidemiologists, the National Association of Public Health Statistics and Information Systems), the National Association of County and City Health Officials, the Association of State and Territorial Health Officers, the Association of Schools of Public Health, and the Association of Teachers of Maternal and Child Health. The National Action Alliance has advocated for better maternal and child health data and information systems, increased opportunities for field-based capacity building, sufficient well-trained people in the field, as well as increased communication and opportunities for research and evidence-based practice.

Concerns About Data Linkage: Territoriality and Competing Sectors

Data linkage raises concerns as more information becomes available about specific individuals. Parents may be reluctant to have their children's data in a linked system. Government agencies, health providers, health insurers, and even legislators may oppose data linkage because of the accountability issues it raises. Data are very important for ensuring accountability, but not everyone welcomes accountability with the same enthusiasm. Competing private entities may have concerns about how data will be collected, analyzed, utilized, and reported and may fear that negative data could be presented in a manner that threatens the stability and future of a facility, organization, company, or community.

Geographically Coded and Valid Data for Smaller Geographic Units

Geographically coded data can help communities understand children's health and its influences in their communities. They provide communities with an efficient method for determining *what* or *where* their problems are and allow them to compare their community with other similar communities. Most data now are geographically coded at the state and county level, and some public health data, such as cancer data, includes geocodes. However, few communities have data other than decennial census data available at smaller geographic levels, such as the census tract level. In some cases, administrative data sets that incorporate geocodes do not retain multiple geocodes, which negates geographic tracking over time.

Geocoded data can also assist states and communities in their efforts to target limited resources to meet the greatest need, forcing communities to recognize problems that they might not acknowledge without data to apply to them. For example, although a state may recognize that it has a higher incidence of youth alcohol and drug use or juvenile arrests than surrounding states or the nation, communities can deny that the problem relates to them if there are no data specific for their community. Rural communities may be surprised at their incidence of specific social and health problems because they have associated these problems with urban areas (e.g., drug abuse). Middle and upper income communities may also underestimate the risk behaviors of their children and youth without data that are specific to them.

Most national and state surveys are not designed to produce valid data at the community level, whether that is a county, city, or census tract. While the expense of producing tract-level survey data may be prohibitive, county, city, or town-specific data are often feasible and enable meaningful geographic analyses within a state. Some states have invested in expanding both the Behavioral Risk Factor Surveillance System and the Youth Behavioral Risk Factor Survey, funded by the Department of Health and Human Services and designed to produce state-level estimates, in order to have county-specific data. Expanding these surveys (and others) to obtain census-tract-specific data is also an option for communities. Many states are using this approach to develop substate estimates as well as stable estimates for ethnic and minority groups. States should ensure that data are captured at substate levels that make sense for the geographic characteristics of their state. Additional federal resources to states and communities targeted to data and analysis would advance efforts to make substate data available and ultimately improve efforts to target resources to needs.

MOVING FORWARD IN BUILDING DATA SYSTEMS

As the technology is available to build systems of data providing benefits for children, how does the nation move forward? Some states and large cities have had success in building children's health data systems; these systems need to be expanded to other areas.

Federal-Level Vision and Leadership

The federal government has a key role to play in establishing data standards, providing resources to states to develop data systems, providing guidance on data system development, and facilitating the availability of state or local-level data. The vision for what these data systems can produce to improve children's health should be shared by the multiple federal agencies serving children and communicated to the leadership of all states and to the public to generate commitment. The federal government should take the lead in convening and determining the elements and standards for a children's data system for use at the national, state, and local levels. Several federal efforts have supported or could facilitate state and local-level data systems, but increased efforts are needed.

As mentioned in Chapter 4, the MCHB and CDC have led government efforts to collect and report state-level health indicators for children. The MCHB has played an important role designing a unique set of performance standards. Created in partnership with the Association of Maternal and Child Health Programs, all states receiving federal maternal and child health block grant dollars are required to collect and submit certain data elements that are used to create profiles for states and the nation. These data, however, are largely anonymous and cross-sectional. As such, they do not allow assessment of change over time except for individual elements at the population level.

The Division of Services for Children with Special Health Needs of the MCHB recently began a new effort to develop comprehensive, community-based systems of care for children with special health care needs. As states develop systems of care, they are being asked to measure and monitor their progress in meeting specific goals and to build state capacity for data-based decision making. The MCHB has developed a standard definition for children with special health care needs and supported research used to develop a screening tool to identify them. The screener has been used in a survey using the State and Local Area Integrated Telephone Survey (SLAITS) platform and by the Consumer Assessment of Health Plans Survey used by Medicaid and commercial managed care organizations. This is a good example of the federal leadership required to establish standardized data collection protocols for states.

CDC has been the leader in defining standard definitions for key data registries and systems used to monitor health outcomes in states; these include definitions for HIV/AIDS, sexually transmitted diseases, birth defects, and cancers. CDC has also developed the National Electronic Disease Surveillance System (NEDSS), originally piloted in Nebraska and Tennessee, which establishes standardized data elements and can link with state systems to use state data to get national totals for specific indicators. However, data are retained and analyzed at the state level. NEDSS is important because the system is using a set of data and technology standards based on the Public Health Information Network to collect basic data from a variety of settings rather than requiring reports using standard software or hardware across states. While this makes it difficult to pool data at the national level, it provides advantages for states and anyone reporting data to the state. There are great expectations for NEDSS as a prototype to facilitate better aggregated and linked data in the future at the state and national levels. Although its design is intended for surveillance of infectious diseases, the approach could be readily used for assessment of children's health over time and across groups as defined by the committee. Some states currently building child health tracking systems (e.g., Utah, Massachusetts, Tennessee, Washington) are using the NEDSS approach and standards.

The National Committee on Vital and Health Statistics, which advises the secretary of health and human services on national health information policy, presented the report of its Workgroup on the National Health Information Infrastructure (NHII) in November 2001 (U.S. Department of Health and Human Services, 2001a). The report, *Information for Health: A Strategy for Building the National Health Information Infrastructure*, envisions a process for building a 21st-century health information system, emphasizing the importance of an effective, comprehensive health information infrastructure that links all health decision makers, including the public. The heart of the plan is sharing information and knowledge appropriately so that they are available to people when they are needed to make the best possible health decisions. It seeks to serve all individuals and communities equitably. The plan does not include a large centralized data warehouse with information on individuals stored at one site. Instead, it is to be a system with a set of technologies, standards, applications, systems, values, and rules that allow access to specific data only on an approved and a "need to know" basis. Personal health, health care providers, and population health are the three key dimensions. These dimensions provide a means for conceptualizing the capture, storage, communication, processing, and presentation of information for each group of information users.

While the NHII would offer opportunities for standardization and linkage of datasets, it is not currently designed to be an information system to monitor children's health. As proposed, it provides a framework for integrating data on health services and population health. To be used for children's health, it would have to be expanded to reflect a board definition of children's health and to include specific child health variables, and standard definitions for additional child health variables would need to be developed. This might be done through a partnership of the HHS agencies that collect data on children's health and could provide a valuable tool for states designing data systems.

Although linking existing data systems will be an important first step in monitoring children's health at the state and local levels, additional data may also be required. The SLAITS platform developed by the NCHS in CDC provides a valuable mechanism for states to collect additional data. When collecting additional data, states would be well served to use existing survey questions and mechanisms developed at the federal level to allow comparisons with national standards and avoid investing resources to develop instruments that are already in place. The federal government could play a lead role in guiding states in such efforts.

The Institute of Medicine's report *Fostering Rapid Advances in Health Care* also provides recommendations on health data systems (Institute of Medicine, 2002a). It proposed federal funding of 8 to 10 demonstration projects to establish computerized clinical information systems and Internet-based communication in the health field. These proposals have concentrated on designing a national information infrastructure for health services and if implemented should explicitly include child health measures as a core component of the infrastructure.

The MCHB and CDC have funded some states to develop integrated child tracking systems that combine datasets, such as vital statistics data on births, newborn screening, and early childhood programs. Funding for continued and expanded demonstration projects to create and share children's health data systems can greatly facilitate the process of building information systems for children. To facilitate analysis of the costs and benefits of these data systems, an area about which there are very few data, demonstration projects could be required to collect relevant data. Multiple variables will affect the cost of these data systems, including the method for integration, the software used, the number of datasets included, and the existing technological NCHS infrastructure. The benefits will also vary depending on whether aggregated or linked data systems are developed, how the data are used, who has access to the data, and how many critical datasets are included. Expanded model demonstration projects would offer continued opportunities to develop comprehensive data systems and to estimate costs and benefits based on the types of data system and their intended uses.

The federal government could also advance the development of data systems by convening relevant federal, state, and community stakeholders to explore the range of privacy and confidentiality issues, including the sharing of individual data (with identifiers) among departments of government and to develop clear guidance related to privacy and confidentiality.

State and Community Vision and Leadership

Several governors and mayors have recognized the value of appointing a Children's Cabinet, a public health agency, or similar entity to coordinate and improve services influencing children's health across multiple state departments and agencies. This same type of leadership and political will is needed to create data systems across departmental lines and to resolve funding and data sharing issues. States and localities will need the vision to see that these data systems have the potential to increase the effectiveness and efficiency of their services to children, provide data for accountability, and empower communities to act (see Box 6-7 for one state example). But this vision has to spread across the many departments and agencies that are involved in providing relevant services. A financial investment will be required for the development of any data system, and states and localities without an adequate infrastructure will require a greater investment. States might take a graduated approach. An initial first step is the enhancement of state public health web sites with aggregated health data. The next objective could be aggregated children's data available on the Internet followed by the linkage of many of the state's datasets on children for government and private research purposes. These three steps are well within the reach of all states within the next few years.

It is equally important for communities within states to evaluate child health. While it may not be feasible to collect every relevant data element at the census tract level or even the city or county level, states and communities should improve efforts to work together and share the financing of data collection efforts. Just as it can be more economical for states to enhance national surveys to get valid data for the county level, the same is true for communities that might want to expand either a national or state survey to meet their own needs. This could involve increasing the sample size to obtain data valid for a smaller geographic unit or adding new questions to an existing survey, as some communities do now using the Behavior Risk Factor Survey or the Youth Risk Behavior Survey.

State-level aggregated data that are available to the public on the Internet will

BOX 6-7
Maine Marks

Maine Marks, a statewide initiative originally funded by the U.S. Department of Health and Human Services, is a partnership led by senior staff of the governor of Maine's Children's Cabinet.

The four goals established by the Children's Cabinet are:
- to develop, implement, and report on a set of indicators to measure progress on the child and family well-being outcomes of the governor's Children's Cabinet;
- to develop and maintain a set of partnerships in support of the Maine Marks program;
- to provide education and training on the function of and use of social indicators in policy making and program management;
- to maintain and enhance the use of Maine Marks for all Maine citizens.

The decision-making criteria for the Maine Marks indicators:
- have enduring importance to child health and well-being in Maine;
- have implications for policy or action;
- are outcome-oriented not just process measures;
- are relevant to policy makers, state agency managers, community leaders, citizens, and youth;
- are readily and uniformly understandable and meaningful;
- are goal-driven, i.e., "What should we be tracking?" not "What can we easily track?"
- are consistent with existing measurement and reporting standards from other sources;
- are representative of the larger population, not just one group;
- have a consistent data source, one in which the indicator was measured in the same way over multiple observations;
- reflect a balance between traditional and promotional indicators.

There are three types of indicators developed by the Maine Marks initiative:
- the fully developed indicators (number = 40) with at least three years of historical data;
- the partially developed indicators (number = 28) with a year of data but not enough history to ascertain a trend;
- to be developed indicators (number = 12) with no data yet but for which future information will be developed.

The information collected by the Maine Marks initiative is made available for smaller geographic areas within the state.

be most accessible to communities for planning and monitoring the health of their children. In addition to making the data available, states should provide the tutorials and explanations that can promote utilization of the data by the public, interested organizations and researchers. While accessibility via the Internet is very important, states will often need to provide technical assistance to communities in understanding and utilizing their data. This is especially true for small, rural communities with very limited resources. Similarly, one of the most important steps that a community can take is to ensure that there is a designated agency or entity responsible for reviewing available data on children and making a report to the community on an annual basis. Knowledge is empowering, and a community empowered with data is more likely to develop necessary interventions to improve their children's health.

A logical point of accountability for data collection and provision and in some cases leadership is the state maternal and child health agency, which is directed by statute to ensure the health and well-being of all mothers, children, and youth. This includes making data readily available; in recent years this includes reporting consistent data to the federal government as part of the block grant. In collaboration with the federal MCHB, states are also working to improve state data capacity. The state maternal and child health office may be a logical locus for leadership on state data systems; at a minimum, state efforts should attempt to build on this existing capacity.

CONCLUSION

Many steps have already been taken to develop data systems that can better evaluate and monitor the health of children at the federal, state, and community levels. The technology and some models are available to direct the next steps leading to better data systems and improved children's health that can result from use of these systems. Vision, leadership, political will, and investments will be needed to meet this challenging but attainable goal.

7

Conclusions and Recommendations

The health of children is a product of complex, dynamic processes produced by the interaction of external influences, such as children's family, social, and physical environments, and their genes, biology, and behaviors. Because children are rapidly changing and developing in response to these interactions, the developmental process plays an important role in shaping and determining their health. Nonetheless, the routine approaches to defining and measuring health in many national, state, and local data collection and measurement efforts are adult-based and capture neither the developmental essence of nor the multiple influences on children's health.

In the committee's view, healthy development is both a component of children's health and a manifestation of it. It is often the case that existing health measurement strategies and systems neither account for the developmental variability of children's health nor include components specific to children. This leads to incomplete measurement of health characteristics, capacities, and influences and a diminished capacity to effectively characterize and adequately monitor the health of children.

Recent rapid increases in scientific information about the development of health, the role of prenatal and early childhood health on adult health outcomes, and the importance of predisease pathways that begin in childhood provide powerful evidence about what is likely to be learned from more detailed, systematic, and longitudinal efforts to measure the multidimensionality of children's health. This growing body of empirical evidence also suggests that as more is understood about how different internal and external influences program the development of biopsychosocial pathways, more effective and appropriate prevention and intervention strategies can be designed, targeted, and implemented.

As reiterated throughout this report, the committee contends that it is in the national interest to place a higher priority on children's health. In the short term, this will result in children whose health and quality of life is improved and who are more ready and able to learn. Children have important value in their own right and are worthy of this type of societal commitment. It is also in the national interest to optimize children's health for two reasons that have longer term implications.

First, the continuing viability of society depends on a citizenry and a workforce that are properly equipped to be productive and committed to serving the nation. Second, failure to improve children's health will have substantial long-term consequences for the health of the adult population, especially in terms of the incidence, timing of onset, and severity of chronic conditions. Events in early childhood can contribute to the physical and mental health morbidity that is often evident and only measurable later on. Thus, society has a choice between addressing that morbidity early in children's lives or dealing with its future consequences. In the committee's view, investing now is the better alternative for all the reasons above and because it is the right thing to do.

DATA AND INFORMATION

Important improvements in children's health will require new data to inform policy and practice. Filling data gaps requires knowledge about the gaps that exist, understanding which gaps are important and how they can be filled, and appreciating what new research and methodologies must be developed to accomplish this. This report has provided a framework for national, state, and local policy makers to identify and fill data gaps and thus secure information needed for consistent, focused, responsive, and effective policy.

The committee also assessed what is currently in place to measure children's health at the national level, as well as approaches that facilitate use of data by states and localities. Over the past century, the United States has instituted important health monitoring and surveillance activities that increased the number of measures of personal and public health delivery systems and initiated important research strategies to better understand the influence of various factors on health outcomes. However, much of this new capacity has been created without adequate attention to the measurement and monitoring of children's health and to the factors that influence it. Inadequate and incomplete measurement obscures the ability to identify important influences on and changes in children's health, including influences that may adversely affect immediate and long-term health outcomes. The lack of information on children's health and its influences can allow harmful exposures (e.g., environmental toxins, damaging social conditions) to go undetected, resulting in missed opportunities to improve prevention, health promotion, and treatment interventions.

Building on what has already been achieved, the committee puts forward an ambitious but attainable vision for the goals of a measurement system for children's health that would need to develop and evolve over the next decade. Such a system would be able to:

• Measure and monitor important trends in children's health and its influences. These measures would span the stages of childhood in order to capture appropriate developmental trajectories. They would also measure trends and influences within important subgroups defined by ethnicity, income, geographic region, and special needs.

• Provide a surveillance and early warning capacity for the detection of significant changes in health, the effect of changing influences on children's health, and identify the need for specific services, interventions, policies, and more detailed evaluations of services and interventions.

• Improve understanding of the mechanisms of children's development and guide evaluations of how changes in behavior, new health practices, and new policy interventions affect children's health.

• Provide indicators of the performance of the personal medical care system, the community health service system, and the broader public health system and how they each operate and interact to influence children's health. Such activities would not only measure the quality of services in the health care systems, but also encourage the integration and coordination of personal, community, and public health services.

Achieving the envisioned comprehensive children's health measurement system will take a gradual, concerted effort over many years. The remainder of this chapter outlines the committee's conclusions and recommendations to begin to move the nation toward this ultimate goal, beginning with establishment of a new definition and framework for understanding children's health and its influences and strengthened national leadership on children's health measurement. We then outline several specific recommendations to address gaps in current children's health measurement efforts and improve state and local use of existing data. We conclude by identifying specific research needs.

A NEW DEFINITION AND FRAMEWORK

Recommendation 1: Children's health should be defined as the extent to which individual children or groups of children are able or enabled to (a) develop and realize their potential, (b) satisfy their needs, and (c) develop the capacities that allow them to interact successfully with their biological, physical, and social environments.

The committee's review of prevailing definitions of health produced few child-based definitions that could incorporate the growing consensus of health as a developmental capacity of the individual child. Existing definitions do not capture the dynamic mechanisms that underlie children's health. The report's conceptual framework builds on the following principles:

- the rate and course of development are fundamental to children's health;
- a broad range of biological, behavioral, and environmental factors affect children's health;
- these influences have cumulative and interactive effects and become embedded in children's developing biological pathways that further affect developing biological systems and predisease pathways, with both immediate and long-term consequences;
- the relative effect of different influences shifts across a child's life span, which calls for attention to the timing of experiences and exposures in understanding children's health, particularly in relation to critical and sensitive periods of development; and
- children's health has a fundamental impact on the course of adult life.

Recognizing that the measurement of health depends on its definition and the first principles about how different factors affect health, the committee sought to develop and adopt a definition of children's health that was compelling and scientifically appropriate.

We began with the definition of health that was adopted as part of the 1986 Ottawa Charter, because of its utility in guiding population health measurement efforts and because it not only encompasses diseases and functional deficits and disabilities, but also accounts for those positive attributes, capacities, and reserves that determine how well an individual or population is able to respond to the challenges that life presents. The committee modified the Ottawa definition in light of what research says about developmental processes that influence health, especially for children. The committee also proposes a set of principles that encompass the processes and pathways that result in different domains of children's health, including health conditions, functioning, and health potential.

In considering the growing literature on factors that affect health, the committee recognized that a comprehensive range of influences interact dynamically with each other. Therefore the committee sought to classify influences in a comprehensive way, encompassing biological, behavioral, and environmental factors. Environment is broadly defined to include community demography and organization, family process, physical environment, and culture. Furthermore, the committee sought to acknowledge the relationships and interactions among influences, as well as how the larger service environments and policies structure those influences.

While much has been learned about children's development and how specific factors affect it and are embedded in biopsychosocial pathways, increased understanding of how these pathways develop is critical, if cost-effective service and policy interventions are to be developed, targeted, and implemented to improve the healthy development of all children. Many have recognized the importance of creating measurement mechanisms that do a better job of capturing these influences and closing the gap between understanding of the influences on health and actions that mediate and modify those influences, in order to improve children's health.

The committee began its work with the general model of the multiple determinants of health adopted by the *Healthy People 2010* report. We moved from this generic model of the determinants of health to a more interactive and developmentally appropriate model that captures the interaction of multiple influences and acknowledges changes in the relative weight of those influences in relation to developmental stage.

This common framework of children's health should be adopted by the diverse group of federal, state, and local agencies with some purview over children's health (e.g., delivery, assessment, assurance, and policy development functions). Each agency should be responsible for developing plans to address relevant health influences within its purview.

A NATIONAL PRIORITY

Recommendation 2: The secretary of the U.S. Department of Health and Human Services (HHS) should designate a specific HHS unit with a focus on children to address development, coordination, standardization, and validation of data across the multiple HHS data collection agencies, to support state-level use of data, and to facilitate coordination across federal agencies. The designated agency's long-term mission should be to

- **monitor each of the domains of children's health (i.e., health conditions, functioning, and health potential) and its influences over time;**
- **develop the means to track children's health and identify patterns (e.g., trajectories) in it over time, both for individual children and for populations and subpopulations of children; and**
- **understand the interaction and relative effects of multiple influences on children's health over time.**

The responsible federal agency should (1) translate recommendations on domains, subdomains, and dimensions of children's health and its influences into improved data collection strategies; (2) identify duplication and gaps in data collection and data display strategies and make data collection efforts more economical and standardized; (3) ensure that all data collection activities are accompanied by data validation; (4) ensure that as many data collection activities as possible are usable at the state and local levels and facilitate state- and local-level use of data; (5) ensure that thoroughly documented data are released on as timely a basis as possible; (6) develop a process for assessing the potential effect of key policy changes on children's health; and (7) facilitate continued research on children's health and its influences.

It is necessary for a single federal agency to take responsibility for the measurement of children's health. The majority of relevant data is collected by HHS, the lead federal agency on health issues. The secretary of HHS should designate and empower a specific unit of HHS and a senior staff person to take steps to make measurement of children's health, broadly defined, a national priority. Several agencies within HHS have children's health or data collection within their purview, including the Maternal and Child Health Bureau (MCHB) in the Health Resources and Services Administration, the National Center for Health Statistics (NCHS) and other offices in the Centers for Disease Control and Prevention (CDC), the Agency for Healthcare Research and Quality (AHRQ), the Office of Disease Prevention and Health Promotion and the Office of the Assistant Secretary for Planning and Evaluation in the Office of the Secretary, the National Institute for Child Health and Human Development and other units in the National Institutes of Health, and the Administration for Children and Families. The committee has not identified a preferred agency but stresses the importance of the designated agency having monitoring and promotion of children's health as a core component of its mandate and having an established leadership role on children's health in the department and with state and local partners.

The designated agency should be charged with better integration of the existing portfolio of health surveys so that the identified gaps, particularly related to measures of functioning and health potential, can be addressed in a strategic and systematic fashion. Strategies to integrate measures and to compare and contrast data from existing surveys should be developed. Steps are needed to improve the health measures in surveys that do not have a primary health focus, but for which current collection of information about health influences could be substantially augmented by adding a parsimonious set of health measures. Many other federal agencies also fund services or research that affect children's health, including the departments of Agriculture, Education, Transportation, Housing and Urban Development, Commerce, Labor, and Justice as well as the Environmental Protection Agency. Many of them also collect data on children's health or its influences. Coordination among these agencies is essential to minimize duplication, improve standardization of data, increase efficiency, and ensure that data collection focuses on the most important variables. The existing Interagency Forum for Child and Family Statistics, if extended beyond its current authorization expiration date of 2007, provides a possible mechanism for this coordination. A lead agency for the multiple relevant HHS agencies will help to facilitate this coordination. Coordination and measurement would also be advanced if the forum adopted a broad conceptualization of health that mandates development of new measures rather than relying solely on existing data.

The committee's definition and model of health have several important implications, most notably how measures of health are conceptualized, operationally defined, developed, applied, and implemented. The committee's analyses of indicators of population health clearly point to the importance not only of measuring diseases, impairments, and functioning, but also of accounting for those positive attributes and capacities that are important determinants of an individual's or population's ability to respond to different experiences, challenges, and exposures.

Similarly the committee reviewed how both negative and positive influences on health develop, aggregate, and interact to produce different levels of vulnerability or bestow greater health capacity and resilience. The committee also concluded that, since prevention and health promotion should be key goals of the health care system, better specification of the relative effect of positive and negative influences, and their origin and timing, would provide important information for improved targeting of prevention and health promotion strategies to optimize the healthy development of all children.

In considering the current status of children's health measurement, the committee recognized the need to articulate a compelling vision for what a children's health measurement system should include; how it would function at the federal, state, and local levels; how it could be used to monitor and assess trends and changes in health, health influences, and health disparities; and how it can serve the important national policy goals of optimizing the healthy development of all children and the adults they will become. Given these compelling policy goals, the measurement of children's health should serve as a sensitive surveillance and early warning system for potential threats to children's health and development, as well as provide information for evaluating policies, services, and interventions in the personal, community, and public health systems. To meet these needs, the measurement system should attempt to provide comparable measures of health and health influences across time and at federal, state, and local levels.

In articulating the importance of a broad, developmentally responsive, multifunctional health measurement system, the committee specified that measures and measurement approaches should be capable of capturing changes in individual and population health trajectories and specifying the importance and time-sensitive effects and interactive influences of different factors on health development pathways. This means that measures of a health characteristic or influence must be consistent and appropriate across developmental stages, and that greater attempts should be made to collect longitudinal information with the greatest likelihood of yielding information about causal relationships and differential trajectories.

The committee reviewed evidence demonstrating that multiple factors, including community demography and organization, family process, physical environment, culture, health services, and policy, make a difference to children's health. The effects of these various factors are known to accumulate over time. It is also known that early childhood conditions matter for adult health. Less is known about the relative power of these influences, their interaction over time, and their precise effect on health.

IMPROVING CHILDREN'S HEALTH MEASUREMENT

Recommendation 3: National surveys of health and health influences, such as the National Health Interview Survey, the National Health and Nutrition Examination Survey, the Early Childhood Longitudinal Studies, and the National Children's Study initiative, should address gaps in what is now collected and reported to reflect a more comprehensive, developmentally oriented conceptualization of children's health and its influences. Particular attention should be paid to adding data on functioning and health potential.

Many surveys in the United States collect periodic health information about children, while many more irregularly collect at least some health-related information. The committee is encouraged that many such efforts are under way. At the same time, it is clear that a number of important gaps remain between the data collected and the committee's definition and model of children's health and its influences, including gaps related to the domains of health, developmental stages, the range of influences, and subpopulations. The lack of data on developmentally appropriate functioning and health potential, two of the three domains of health articulated in this report, is particularly notable. Adding measures that capture data on these domains to the most comprehensive of current surveys would be a significant step in moving toward a comprehensive approach to children's health measurement and should be a priority for new data collections. Existing data on the domain of health conditions should be analyzed in such a way as to provide information that relates to person and populations rather than to individual diseases.

There is a vital need for health survey designs that capture health in more detail during different stages of development. At a minimum, this involves distinguishing the special developmental issues of infants and toddlers (ages 0–3 years), preschool children (4–5), elementary school-age children (6–11), early adolescents (12–14), and older adolescents (15–17). Data on toddlerhood through adolescence are especially lacking.

Understanding of the constellation of both social (e.g., family, peer, neighborhood) and physical (e.g., toxins, violence) environmental influences on children's health has grown rapidly in recent years, as has research on valid and reliable methods for gathering data on many types of influences in surveys. Since environmental influences can affect health in developmentally specific and interactive ways, the committee sees great value in surveys that attempt to measure multiple environmental influences. Thus, surveys directed at understanding children's health should be strategically constructed and organized to capture as many influences as possible, with particular attention paid to measures that cut across domains and are consistent across developmental stages. Similarly, analysts should adopt methods that examine the interactions among various levels and types of influences. For example, comprehensive surveys could include data on family process and neighborhood characteristics, through systematic social observation and parent report, as well as biological markers of health status, and environmental samples.

Individual groups defined by race, ethnicity, low socioeconomic status, or special needs (e.g., children with a chronic physical or mental health problem, those in foster care) constitute a relatively small share of the total population. Consequently, a survey drawing its sample of respondents from the general population will have small numbers of respondents in these groups. It is straightforward to oversample respondents from these subgroups so that sufficient numbers will be included in the surveys. The committee attaches substantial value to these efforts.

Most instruments and measures for assessing children's health are standardized on a particular (usually white, middle-class) population, so it is often unclear how valid and reliable they are for other racial, ethnic, and class subpopulations. It is important that surveys attend to possible cultural biases by using measures of health and health influences that have proven to be reliable for subgroups whose health disadvantages are of interest. As new surveys or measures are developed, instruments and administration methods should be tested on groups that represent major population subgroups to assess validity and reliability.

Regular and periodic surveys could greatly increase understanding of the role played by contextual as well as individual characteristics in overall health. In addition to funding new and independent longitudinal studies of children's health, existing data collection vehicles, such as the National Health Interview Survey, can be used to conduct follow-back studies that provide useful repeated cross-sectional information.

Longitudinal surveys of health and health influences should have high priority in research, since they alone are able to characterize and incorporate temporal and developmental dimensions of health and provide the data needed to construct developmental health trajectories. Ideally, such surveys would be conducted recurrently to enable assessments over time.

The committee's review of the importance of a wide variety of influences on health outcomes demonstrates a need for greater understanding of the effect, distribution, and changing character of different influences on children's health. The committee reviewed many existing surveys and data collection efforts and found that many of the most salient and important influences on children's health are often collected by surveys that were originally designed to measures changes in family life, income dynamics, or educational attainment. The committee determined that, with little additional response burden, health measures could be added to many of these existing surveys (e.g., the Early Childhood Longitudinal Studies), providing powerful additional information at marginal increases in costs. If these health measures were the same as those included in existing health surveys, findings across surveys could be usefully compared.

Piecemeal additions to existing surveys will help advance understanding of the nature of children's health and its influences, but they do not substitute for truly comprehensive data collection projects. Over the longer term, approaches need to be developed that incorporate the following elements: oversampling of disadvantaged groups; tracking of children early in life, collecting prenatal information; frequent interviews and assessments with these children throughout childhood and into adulthood; measurement of assets as well as deficits; comprehensive measurement of multiple contexts that affect children's health, including the biological, demographic, and socioeconomic, at both the family and neighborhood levels, and services and policy environments; measurement of gene-behavior-environment and other developmentally specific contextual interactions; and charting of health and disease trajectories and the relative contribution of various influences on health outcomes.

The National Children's Study being considered by HHS and the Environmental Protection Agency is a possible vehicle for not only collecting data on the functioning and health potential domains, but also implementing a comprehensive, longitudinal assessment of children's health and its influences as envisioned here. Such an approach could contribute greatly to understanding of the dynamics of children's health and its influences.

Monitoring Health Disparities

Recommendation 4: National and state surveys and records-based sources of data on children's health and its influences should gather systematic, standardized data on racial, ethnic, immigration, and socioeconomic classifications in order to measure the origins, distribution, and development of disparities in children's health and facilitate linkage and analysis across multiple datasets.

Although in the committee's view policy makers should pay special attention to the needs of all children, subgroups of children, including those defined by race, ethnicity, and socioeconomic status, experience poorer health outcomes and poorer access to services in ways that affect their future potential for healthy, productive adulthood. Many of the factors leading to the development of health disparities and the gradients in these disparities across populations are poorly understood.

The committee recognizes that reducing population health disparities in children and adults is an important national health policy goal. Research on the origins and development of population health disparities in children demonstrates that many disparities result from prenatal influences or have their origins early in life. Disparities can continue to develop in a linear fashion, or their effects can be compounded as a function of a child's age and developmental process. A key priority is to improve measures that focus on the origins, development, and compounding effects of health disparities.

The growing body of research also demonstrates that most health disparities between populations defined by specific characteristics (e.g., race, income, geography, institutional home, disease state) are the result of differential influences that cut across the population characteristics of interest. Rather than existing as dichotomous measures, many disparities are the result of a gradient of continuous influences across a range of social, economic, ethnic, cultural, and geographic factors. In the committee's view, over the longer term, measures should not be limited to ethnicity and income differentials but must also account for disparities in health outcomes for other vulnerable child populations. This includes those with special medical needs due to genetic defects, injury, abuse and neglect, residential turbulence (including foster care placement and homelessness), and to a range of other factors that lead to systematic differences in health.

The committee identified the need to develop better information and more conclusive evidence to target interventions that have the greatest likelihood of decreasing population health disparities and in order to design effective policies to ameliorate these disparities. Differences in how various cultural and ethnic groups consider health and disease affect the interpretation of inquiries about health and services utilization patterns and therefore should be considered when evaluating the effectiveness of policies and interventions.

To promote a more systematic understanding of the effects of culture, it is important to measure minority and socioeconomic status and acculturation in surveys and in health records and to ensure that measurements be consistent across measurement systems. In the case of race and ethnicity data, this can be accomplished by conforming to current guidelines of the Office of Management and Budget. In the case of immigration data, the committee recommends using such questions as those included in the most current waves of the Current Population Survey.

Despite a large body of research on health disparities across subgroups defined by socioeconomic status, no standards have been established for how socioeconomic status ought to be characterized in surveys and administrative records. However, ample methodological research has led to thoughtful recommendations regarding how surveys and administrative records could gather reliable measures of the education, household income, or occupational dimensions of socioeconomic status. Such recommendations should be considered in the design of surveys and collection of administrative data.

Geographic Information

Recommendation 5: Federal agencies and departments, particularly the Environmental Protection Agency and the U.S. Department of Health and Human Services, should promote the systematic collection, dissemination, and linkage of data on children's exposure to toxins, air pollution, and other environmental conditions, as well as data on policies likely to affect children's health. The Census Bureau should continue to collect and distribute local-area data and facilitate efforts to match these data to existing sources of information on children's health and its influences.

Recommendation 6: Government and private agencies and academic organizations that conduct health-related surveys or compile administrative data should geocode addresses (i.e., provide geographic identifiers) in ways that facilitate linkages to census-based and other neighborhood, community, city, and state data on environmental conditions. With adequate protections to ensure the confidentiality and security of individual data, they should also make geocoded data as accessible as possible to the research and planning communities.

An emerging body of evidence demonstrates a clear association between geographic location and children's health. Suggestive associations have been established for such environmental conditions as neighborhood, socioeconomic conditions, crime, community cohesion, ambient noise, traffic flow, and air quality.

Efforts to monitor and understand environmental influences on children's health are facilitated by the systematic collection of regional, neighborhood, and community-level information. Most importantly, demographic and economic information about neighborhoods (census tracts), communities, cities, and states has been collected and made available to planners and researchers every 10 years as part of the decennial census. Continued collection of most of this information is threatened by congressional plans to eliminate the long-form questionnaire from the 2010 census. The emerging American Community Survey (ACS) has been proposed as the vehicle for collection of long-form data. The committee supports the continued collection of these vital neighborhood data. Information at the census tract level on the demographic and economic characteristics of neighborhoods should continue to be collected at least once every 10 years and preferably more often, through the ACS, the decennial census, or in some other way.

Other local and regional environmental data, such as neighborhood and community-wide crime rates, regional air quality, and doctor availability in a health services planning area, also hold great value for health planners and researchers. Such data can help specify gradients in the effect of different influences, in order to specify thresholds of concern and to better target prevention, intervention, and health promotion activities. Improving the availability of data at the neighborhood, community, or regional level can improve the ability of a local community to target their own efforts and institute community-specific interventions.

Environmental data are valuable in and of themselves, but they also enhance the value of survey and records information. For example, survey-based reports of poor children's health can be related to neighborhood socioeconomic conditions, or crime, or local or state policies regarding health care or welfare reform. Records-based data on substantiated reports of child abuse can be examined to see if cases cluster in certain neighborhood "hot spots." But the geographic dimension can be exploited only if subjects' locations (e.g., homes, schools, workplace addresses) have been coded with geographic identifiers. With proper safeguards, data collectors should make efforts to make these geocodes, which facilitate geographic linkages or the linked data themselves, more available to the planning and research communities.

Balancing Confidentiality with Public Health Needs

Recommendation 7: Administrators of survey and records-based sources of health information should take all necessary legal, ethical, and technical steps to ensure respondent or subject confidentiality while also promoting the availability of needed data to the research and planning communities.

The committee recognizes the importance of maintaining the confidentiality and privacy of data, perhaps especially for children: data can follow them through various programs and systems and be perceived as potentially affecting the provision of benefits and services, and facilitating geographic analysis threatens subject anonymity. Administrative data can be integrated in a manner that prohibits the identification of specific children. Safeguards include obtaining appropriate parental consent for the collection and sharing of data, limiting access to integrated data, ensuring that data security protocols are in place, and in some instances reporting only aggregated data. The committee is encouraged by the many surveys and records systems that have developed geographic identifiers that both safeguard data and make them available to the research and planning communities. However, much more needs to be done to make data, such as that collected by the NCHS, readily accessible to the research and planning communities.

Facilitating State and Local Use of Data

Recommendation 8: The U.S. Department of Health and Human Services should formulate strategies to improve the capacity of state and local communities to monitor children's health and its influences, including fund-

ing state or local demonstration projects, standardization of data elements, and technical assistance.

Both federal and state governments should assist local efforts to measure trends in children's health and development and to address disparities in children's health, health influences, and access to and use of health services. Of greatest use to health planners are the collection and public distribution of data on health and health influences at neighborhood, community, county, and state levels. State web sites with aggregated data hold particular promise as ways of disseminating information inexpensively to large numbers of users without breaching confidentiality. Web sites designed for use by the public as well as public and private researchers with more sophisticated skills have greater usefulness.

Because there are likely to be common technical, methodological, and measurement challenges at the state and local levels, the federal government has an obvious role in convening and supporting efforts to reengineer state and local health information systems. Collaborative strategies to identify and implement promising data system reform strategies should be supported by the federal agencies.

Federal agencies—including but not limited to the CDC, the NCHS, the MCHB, and the AHRQ, operating under the auspices of the newly designated lead HHS agency—should assist states in their effort to improve and create more systematic approaches to measure children's health. They should provide preferential funds for model demonstrations that use standardized data collection methods, aggregate data by local geographic units, and disseminate aggregated data on web sites designed with two to three levels of complexity to meet the needs of the public and researchers while simultaneously protecting confidentiality. Federal guidance and assistance are necessary but not sufficient for states and localities to realize the potential of records data to inform health policy and research. States and communities should establish a process for using the data on children in the allocation of limited resources, policy development, and the evaluation of strategies.

Several areas of children's health measurement are ripe for efforts to integrate data across age ranges, child service sectors, and geographic levels. Several of these areas would build on or be responsive to important and emerging children's health issues that are supported under a range of different federal and state initiatives.

In building and improving the function of data collection systems, it is also useful to institute data integration strategies that capture aspects of health across developmental stages. For example, a possible measure of health potential is profiles of school readiness that can be measured at school entry. Measures of school readiness usually capture several aspects of functioning, such as physical, social, emotional, cognitive, and language functions. Currently, some states and communities are instituting school readiness measures that can be linked to other measures of specific influences, in order to describe the effect of services, service availability, and other factors that impact school readiness profiles. Measures of school readiness in comparable dimensions can be collected at ages 2, 3, 4, and 5 to establish school readiness trajectories for individual children and populations of children. Use of integrated data to produce school readiness trajectories could provide communities with powerful information to improve the delivery of various services and target prevention and promotion activities.

It is also important to consider linking data across different service sectors (health, education, nutrition, child welfare). Such integration strategies using common identifiers can allow communities to understand questions such as whether 10 children are receiving one service each or whether one child is receiving 10 services. Improved integration of data across sectors would provide information to enable different service sectors to align their policies and programs to produce more effective and efficient outcomes.

STATE AND LOCAL LEADERSHIP AND USE OF DATA

Recommendation 9: Governors, mayors, and county executives should designate a central coordinating agency responsible for measurement and monitoring of children's health across agencies, as well as an individual responsible for reporting on progress toward integrating data on children's health. The state coordinating agency should facilitate use of standardized data at the local level.

States and communities must also coordinate the efforts of multiple entities serving children and their families. It is necessary to have a single agency at the state and local levels responsible for evaluating children's health and reporting the results to policy makers and the public. In many states and communities, this single entity would probably be the state or local health department, particularly the maternal and child health agency. However, some states and communities have empowered other structures or entities for this role.

Some state governors have formed children's cabinets that include the director or commissioner of each agency with services for children. A lead state agency may be appointed to coordinate efforts and report to the governor, or a senior official in the governor's office may be given this responsibility. Some mayors have established offices of children's services, children's caucuses, and cabinets that report to the mayor to provide leadership on all issues relating to children. The benefit of having a lead state and community agency responsible for coordinating data efforts related to children is that the responsibility can be institutionalized and continue even with a change in administrations. How the elected official for the state or community achieves leadership for this effort on behalf of children will depend on how the governmental entity is organized and the expertise available within his or her administration. The most important role of the governor, mayor, or county executive is communicating and demonstrating to the administration and the established leadership team that promoting and evaluating children's health are priorities.

The federal government can facilitate the development of state data systems by promoting standardization of data collection methodologies and coordinating data collection efforts among the many federal departments and agencies. Federal data also provide a benchmark against which states can compare their own performance and, if collected for all states, a standard to which states can compare one another.

Recommendation 10: The designated state and local coordinating agencies should advance strategies for standardizing and integrating records, including available administrative records and survey data, to maximize their potential for monitoring children's health and understanding its influences.

Despite increased efforts to collect state- or local-level data through such programs as the maternal and child health block grants and an increase in the number of communities that produce report cards that include or are specific to children, comprehensive state and local-level measurement of children's health is still relatively uncommon.

Substantial administrative data, collected primarily at the state level, could serve as the foundation for efforts to analyze children's health in a community and the factors that might explain health problems. Although improved data integration is not in itself sufficient to answer all questions related to children's health, enhanced efforts to use existing data could advance children's health in many places. Several states and localities have implemented efforts to integrate administrative data that have helped to inform policy and resulted in changes that benefited children. The strategy for a national health information infrastructure developed by the National Committee on Vital and Health Statistics and the National Electronic Disease Surveillance System discussed in Chapter 6 provide a partial framework for these efforts.

As with surveys, record-based data sources on children's health and its influences are most useful if they gather health data on multiple developmental stages, identify subgroups prone to poor health, collect and make available information on the geographic location and environmental conditions of subjects, and at the same time ensure the confidentiality of subjects.

Key to maximizing the utility of records-based sources of information is standardizing given types of data and facilitating the linkage of different types of data. Data standardization would be facilitated through the development and use of national guidelines.

The committee found value in aggregating all administrative data relative to children by multiple geographic units, including, if feasible and relevant to local circumstances, at the census tract level. In cases in which administrative records are not sufficient to provide the needed data for policy development or planning of interventions, states and communities should consider conducting targeted surveys. Of most value would be surveys that model national surveys, thus allowing comparisons with a national standard, or state- or local-level application of national surveys, such as the Behavioral Risk Factor Surveillance Survey. When feasible, strategies to link data at the individual level and then aggregate to community levels should be a goal.

PROMOTING RESEARCH

Recommendation 11: The U.S. Department of Health and Human Services and the Environmental Protection Agency should prioritize research and training on emerging methods for characterizing children's health and understanding influences on it, including research on:

- **creation of improved measures of functioning and health potential;**
- **the relative importance of and interactions among the range of influences;**
- **biopsychosocial pathways of development;**
- **assessment of children's exposures to environmental toxins and other environmental health hazards;**
- **reasons and remedies for health disparities;**
- **longitudinal methods that can identify causal relationships between developmental and functional levels and the health status of children;**
- **development of profiles and integrative measures of children's health; and**
- **construction of trajectories for each domain of children's health.**

Great strides have been made in conceptualizing the dynamic process by which many external influences interact with individuals' biology and behaviors over the course of childhood to determine health. However, empirical studies of the nature and importance of these processes are suggestive but far from definitive.

The research literature provides strong empirical evidence that children's health results from developmental processes involving continuously changing and iterative time frames with differentially sensitive and critical periods of development for prevention and health promotion. At each developmental phase, children experience multiple influences, and their experiences in a given phase will in turn shape their response to influences in later stages of development. Yet current measures of children's health capture neither the iterative nature of these factors nor their interdependence. Furthermore, the measures are generally not robust across different developmental stages, so that health characteristics can be assessed across stages of development in a dimensionally consistent manner.

An earlier section of this chapter delineated the elements of ambitious new surveys that would promote research efforts in this regard. The committee also highlighted important technical and methodological gaps in the ability to measure specific dimensions of health across developmental stages in a consistent and continuous fashion. Some of these gaps require more research on appropriate measures and measurement strategies.

As basic science continues to elaborate the biological, behavioral, and environmental pathways of healthy development, new measures will become available based on how these pathways function. As more is learned about sensitivity genes, and genomic testing becomes more widespread, the value of biomarker assessment is likely to increase considerably. At the same time, the technologies for gathering biomarker data in routine surveys using noninvasive procedures are advancing rapidly. The current and future use of such biomarkers in isolation or in conjunction with other health or health influence (including genetic) measures demands increased research attention. Furthermore, given the complex interaction between genetic and multiple environmental factors, these assessment and predictive efforts should be integrated with measures of other influences and indicators of health to enable the development of composite measures of health.

Given the large number of new chemicals introduced into the environment each year, and the lack of information about their effect on human function and health, particularly their potential effect on children, there is a growing need to measure the exposures of children to these agents more systematically and to understand better their potential effect on children's development. In addition, the levels of agents currently in the environment known to pose an appreciable risk to children need to be monitored and child populations at greater risk of environmental exposures identified.

The committee determined that, despite general awareness of the scope and nature of children's health disparities across population subgroups, the reasons for such disparities are barely understood. A growing body of empirical literature indicates that many disparities begin early in life and increase or are compounded as a child grows. Much is to be learned from longitudinal research on the processes that lead to health disparities among specific subgroups and on the development of measures of health and health influences that are valid across population subgroups. Longitudinal studies that examine cultural processes—acculturation, daily routines, values and attitudes toward childrearing, and the effects of actual or perceived discrimination on health disparities—are needed. In addition, traditional methods for measuring health and social influences are not equally valid across subgroups. Efforts to develop reliable measures to assess the influence of culture and discrimination on children's health need to be supported.

Newly developed statistical strategies, such as growth curve analysis, provide promising ways to test dynamic models of health and health influences using longitudinal data. Here the needs are twofold: (1) to support efforts to develop these models so that they can be applied to conceptual advances in understanding influences on children's health and (2) to support efforts to train new and existing cohorts of researchers in these methods.

Finally, there is a great need for research that can translate what are potentially effective measures used primarily for research purposes into wider application for population health measurement and policy development. At present there is an enormous gap between what can be measured in controlled research environments and what is currently applicable for population and more general health measurement uses. Bridging this gap requires research that can address conceptual, methodological, and technical hurdles, many of which the committee has identified. These hurdles are eminently addressable but require dedicated resources, attention, commitment, and collaboration among researchers and public officials and agencies that could benefit from a more comprehensive and integrated measurement system and resources.

CONCLUSION

Much progress has been made over the past century in understanding the special attributes of children and the importance of their healthy development to the health of the population as a whole. Nevertheless, in the United States, the current failure to adequately consider, define, conceptualize, and measure the dynamic and multidimensional aspects of children's health has profound implications for the entire population, with potentially compromising effects on the nation's health. It is time—arguably overdue—to repurpose efforts at the federal, state, and local levels to focus on the nation's most valuable national resource—children. The reasons for and the steps involved in this establishment of children and their health as a national priority have been described in this report; in short, it is time to develop ways of looking at and assessing children that will demand that the nation nurture and develop their inherent richness and potential across the multitude of geographic, racial, cultural, socioeconomic, and developmental spectrums. This effort requires a shared vision from local communities through the highest levels of national government and should be treated as an urgent national priority.

References

Abel, E.L., and Sokol, R.J. (1987). Incidence of fetal alcohol syndrome and economic impact of FAS-related anomalies. *Drug and Alcohol Dependence, 19*(1), 51–70.

Abel, E.L., and Sokol, R.J. (1991). A revised estimate of the economic impact of fetal alcohol syndrome. *Recent Developments in Alcoholism, 9,* 117–125.

Ablon, J. (1982). The parents' auxiliary of Little People of America: A self-help model of social support for families of short-stature children. *Preventive Human Services, 1*(3), 31–46.

Ablon, J. (1990). Ambiguity and difference: Families with dwarf children. *Social Science and Medicine, 30*(8), 879–887.

Achenbach, T.M., McConaughy, S.H., and Howell, C.T. (1987). Child/adolescent behavioral and emotional problems: Implications of cross-informant correlations for situational specificity. *Psychology Bulletin, 101*(2), 213–232.

Acheson, D. (1998). Inequalities in health: Report on inequalities in health did give priority for steps to be tackled. *British Medical Journal, 317*(7173), 1659.

Agency for Toxic Substance and Disease Registry. (1993). *Case studies in environmental medicine: Reproductive and developmental hazards.* Atlanta: U.S. Department of Health and Human Services.

Aidoo, M., Terlouw, D.J., Kolczak, M.S., McElroy, P.D., TerKuile, F.O., Kariuki, S., Nahlen, B.L., Lal, A.A., and Udhayakumar, V. (2002). Protective effects of the sickle cell gene against malaria morbidity and mortality. *Lancet, 359*(9314), 1311–1312.

Ajzen, I. (1991). The theory of planned behavior. *Organizational Behavior and Human Decision Processes, 50,* 179–211.

Alaimo, K., Olson, C.M., and Frongillo, E. (2001). Food insufficiency and American school-aged children's cognitive, academic and psychosocial development. *Pediatrics, 108,* 44–53.

Alarcon, O. (2000). *Social Context of Puerto Rican Child Health and Growth Study—Final Report.* Submitted to the Maternal and Child Health Bureau, U.S. Department of Health and Human Services.

Alfred, J. (2000). Tuning in to perfect pitch. *Nature Reviews Genetics, 1*(1), 3.

Allen, M., D'Alessio, D., and Brezgel, K. (1995a). A meta-analysis summarizing the effects of pornography II: Aggression after exposure. *Human Communication Research, 22,* 258–283.

Allen, M., Emmers, T., Gebhardt, L., and Giery, M.A. (1995b). Exposure to pornography and acceptance of rape myths. *Journal of Communication, 45*(1), 5–26.

Amato, P.R., and Keith, B. (1991). Parental divorce and the well-being of children: A meta-analysis. *Psychological Bulletin, 110,* 26–46.

American Academy of Pediatrics. (1987). Asbestos exposure in schools. Committee on Environmental Hazards. *Pediatrics, 79*(2), 301–305.

American Academy of Pediatrics. (1997). Noise: A hazard for the fetus and newborn. Committee on Environmental Health. *Pediatrics, 100,* 724.

American Academy of Pediatrics. (1998). Risk of ionizing radiation exposure to children: A subject review. Committee on Environmental Health. *Pediatrics, 101*(4 Pt 1), 717–719.

American Academy of Pediatrics. (1999a). *Handbook of pediatric environmental health.* R.A. Etzel and S.J. Balk (Eds). Elk Grove Village, IL: Author.

American Academy of Pediatrics. (1999b). Media education. Committee on Public Education. *Pediatrics, 104*(2), 341–343.

American Academy of Pediatrics. (2002). The medical home. Medical Home Initiatives for Children with Special Needs Project Advisory Committee. *Pediatrics, 110*(1), 184–186.

American Academy of Pediatrics. (2003). *Handbook of pediatric environmental health.* Committee on Environmental Health. Elk Grove Village, IL: Author.

American Academy of Pediatrics Task Force on Infant Positioning and SIDS. (1992). Positioning and SIDS. *Pediatrics, 89*(6), 1120–1126

Anand, S., and Hanson, K. (1997). Disability-adjusted life years: A critical review. *Journal of Health Economics, 16*(6), 685–702.

Andersen M.R., Leroux, B.G., Bricker, J.B., Rajan, K.B., and Peterson, A.V. (2004). Antismoking parenting practices are associated with reduced rates of adolescent smoking. *Archives of Pediatrics and Adolescent Medicine, 158*(4), 348–352.

Anderson, C.A., and Bushman, B.J. (2001). Effects of violent video games on aggressive behavior, aggressive cognition, aggressive affect, physiological arousal, and prosocial behavior: A meta-analytic review of the scientific literature. *Psychological Science, 12,* 353–359.

Anderson, D.R., Huston, A.C., Schmitt, K.L., Linebarger, D.L., and Wright, J.C. (2001). Early childhood television viewing and adolescent behavior. *Monographs of the Society for Research in Child Development, 66*(1).

Anderson, R.N., and Smith, B.L. (2003). Deaths: Leading causes for 2001. National Center for Health Statistics. *National Vital Statistics Reports, 52*(9).

Association of State and Territorial Health Officials. (2003). *Issue Report: Integrating Information Systems to Improve MCH.* Washington, DC: Author.

Atkinson, A.J., Daniels, C., Dedrick, R., Grudzinskas, C., and Markey, S. (2001). *Principles of clinical pharmacology.* San Diego: Academic Press.

Babarain, O.A. (1996). The IRS: Multidimensional measurement of institutional racism. In R. Jones (Ed.), *Handbook of tests and measurements for black populations.* Hampton, VA: Cobb and Henry Publishers.

Bakhtiar, R., and Nelson, R.W. (2001). Mass spectrometry of the proteome. *Molecular Neuropharmacology, 60,* 405–415.

Balfour, J., and Kaplan, G.A. (2002). Neighborhood environment and loss of physical function in older adults: Evidence from the Alameda County Study. *American Journal of Epidemiology, 155*(6), 507–515.

Ball, S., and Bogatz, G.A. (1970). *The first year of Sesame Street: An evaluation.* Princeton, NJ: Educational Testing Service.

Baltes, P. (1997). On the incomplete architecture of human ontogeny. *American Psychologist, 52,* 366–380.

Bandura, A. (1994). Social cognitive theory and exercise of control over HIV infection. In R.J. DiClemente and J.L. Peterson (Eds.), *Preventing AIDS: Theories and methods of behavioral interventions* (pp. 25–59). New York: Plenum.

Barker, D. (1998). *Mothers, babies, and health in later life.* Edinburgh: Churchill Livingstone.

Barnard, K.E., and Kelly, J.F. (1990). Assessment of parent-child interaction. In J.P. Shonkoff and S.J. Meisels (Eds.), *Handbook of early childhood intervention* (pp. 278–302). New York: Cambridge University Press.

Barnes, L.L., Plotnikoff, G.A., Fox, K., and Pendleton, S. (2000). Spirituality, religion, and pediatrics: Intersecting worlds of healing. *Pediatrics, 106*(4), 899.

Barnett, S. (1999). Clinical and cultural issues in caring for deaf people. *Family Medicine, 31*(1), 17–22.

Barnett, W.S. (1995). Long-term effects of early childhood programs on cognitive and school outcomes. *The Future of Children, 5*(3), 25–50.

Baum, C.R., and Shannon, M.W. (1997). The lead concentration of reconstituted infant formula. *Journal of Toxicology—Clinical Toxicology, 35*(4), 371–375.

Baumrind, D. (1971). Current patterns of parental authority. *Development Psychology Monographs, 4*(1, Pt. 2).

Bays J. (1990). Substance abuse and child abuse: Impact of addiction on the child. *Pediatric Clinics of North America, 37*(4), 881–904.

Bearer, C.F., Emerson, R.K., Roitman, E.S., and Shackleton, C. (1997). Maternal tobacco smoke exposure and persistent pulmonary hypertension of the newborn. *Environmental Health Perspectives, 105*, 202–206.

Bearer, C.F., O'Riordan, M.A., and Powers, R. (2000). Lead exposure from blood transfusion in VLBW infants. *Journal of Pediatrics, 137*, 549–554.

Becerra, J.E., Hogue, C.J., Atrash, H.K., and Perez, N. (1991). Infant mortality among Hispanics: A portrait of heterogeneity. *Journal of the American Medical Association, 265*(2), 217–221.

Becker, G.S. (1981). *A treatise on the family.* Cambridge, MA: Harvard University Press.

Beckwith, L., and Rodning, C. (1992). Evaluating effects of intervention with preterm infants. In S.L. Friedmena and M.D. Sigman (Eds.), *The psychological development of low birthweight children* (pp. 389–410). Norwood, NJ: Ablex Publishing Corp.

Behrman, R.E. (1995) Issues in children's health. *Bulletin of the New York Academy of Medicine.* Winter Supplement, 575–585.

Behrman, R.E. (Ed.). (1997). Children and poverty. *Future of Children, 7*(2).

Ben-Shahar, Y., Robichon, A., Sokolowski, M.B., and Robinson, G.E. (2002). Influence of gene action across different time scales on behavior. *Science, 296*(5568), 741–744.

Ben-Shlomo, Y., and Kuh, D. (2002) A life course approach to chronic disease epidemiology: Conceptual models, empirical challenges and interdisciplinary perspectives. *International Journal of Epidemiology, 31*(2), 285–293.

Bensley, L., and Van Eenwyk, J. (2001). Video games and real-life aggression: Review of the literature. *Journal of Adolescent Health, 29*, 244–257.

Bentley, M., Gavin, L., Black, M.M., and Teti, L. (1999). Infant feeding practices of low-income, African-American, adolescent mothers: An ecological, multigenerational perspective. *Social Science and Medicine, 49*, 1085–1100.

Berkman, L.F., and Syme, S.L. (1979). Social networks, host resistance, and mortality: A nine-year follow-up study of Alameda County residents. *American Journal Epidemiology, 109*(2), 186–204.

Bernstein, R.S., Stayner, L.T., Elliot, L.J., Kimbrough, R., Falk, H., and Blade L. (1984). Inhalation exposure to formaldehyde: An overview of its toxicology, epidemiology, monitoring, and control. *American Industrial Hygiene Association, 261*, 1183–1187.

Berry, J.W., and Worthington, E.L., Jr. (2001). Forgivingness, relationship quality, stress while imagining relationship events, and physical and mental health. *Journal of Counseling Psychology, 48*(4), 447–455.

Bertram, C., and Hanson, M.A. (2002). Prenatal programming of postnatal endocrine responses by glucocorticoids. *Reproduction, 124*, 459–467.

Bess, F.H., Dodd-Murphy, J., and Parker, R.A. (1998). Children with minimal sensorineural hearing loss: Prevalence, educational performance and functional status. *Ear and Hearing, 19*, 339–354.

Bethell, C., Klein, J., and Peck, C. (2001a). Assessing health system provision of adolescent preventive services: The Young Adult Health Care Survey. *Medical Care, 39*(5), 478–490.

Bethell, C., Peck, C., and Schor, E. (2001b). Assessing health system provision of well-child care: The promoting healthy development survey. *Pediatrics, 107*(5), 1084–1094.

Bethell, C., Reuland, C.H., Halfon, N., and Schor, E.L. (2004). Measuring the quality of preventive and developmental services for young children: National estimates and patterns of clinicians' performance. *Pediatrics, 113*(6 Suppl), 1973–1983.

Birch, L.L., and Davison, K.K. (2001). Family environmental factors influencing the developing behavioral controls of food intake and childhood overweight. *Pediatric Clinics of North America, 48*, 893–907.

Birch, D.A., and Nybo, V. (1984). Promoting school health education in Maine: The Maine School Health Education Program. *Health Education, 15*(5), 67–68.

Bjorner, J.B., Ware, J.E., Jr., and Kosinski, M. (2003). The potential synergy between cognitive models and modern psychometric models. *Quality of Life Research, 12*, 261–274.

Black, C.P. (2003). Systematic review of the biology and medical management of respiratory syncytial virus infection. *Respiratory Care, 48*(3), 209–233.

Black, D., Morris, J., Smith, C., and Townsend, P. (August 1980). *Inequalities in health: Report of a working group*. London: Department of Health and Social Security.

Black, M.M., and Nitz, K. (1996). Grandmother co-residence, parenting, and child development among low income, urban teen mothers. *Journal of Adolescent Health, 18*(3), 218–226.

Blake, J. (1989). *Family size and achievement, Vol. 3: Studies in demography*, Berkeley: University of California Press.

Blalock, J.E. (1984). The immune system as a sensory organ. *Journal of Immunology, 132*, 1067–1070.

Blot, W.J. (1975). Growth and development following prenatal and childhood exposure to atomic radiation. *Journal of Radiation Research (Tokyo), 16*(Suppl), 82.

Blot, W.J., Xu, Z.Y., Boice, J.D., Jr., Zhao, D.Z., Stone, B.J., Sun, J., Jing, L.B., and Fraumeni, J.F., Jr. (1990). Indoor radon and lung cancer in China. *Journal of the National Cancer Institute, 82*, 1025–1030.

Bogin, B. (2001). *The growth of humanity*. New York: Wiley-Liss.

Bove, F., Shim, Y., and Zeitz, P. (2001). Drinking water contaminants and adverse pregnancy outcomes: A review. *Environmental Health Perspectives, 110*(1, Suppl), 61–74.

Boyce, W., Quas, J., Alkon, A., Smider, N.A., Essex, M.J., Kupfer, D.J., and the MacArthur Assessment Battery Working Group of the MacArthur Foundation Research Network on Psychopathology and Development. (2001). Autonomic reactivity and psychopathology in middle childhood. *British Journal of Psychiatry, 179*, 144–150.

Boyce, W.T., Frank, E., Jensen, P.S., Kessler, R.C., Nelson, C.A., and Steinberg, L. (1998). Social context in developmental psychopathology: Recommendations for future research from the MacArthur Network on Psychopathology and Development. *Development and Psychopathology, 10*(1), 143–164.

Boykin, A.W., and Toms, F.D. (1985). Black child socialization: A conceptual framework. In H.P. McAdoo and J.H. McAdoo (Eds.), *Black children: Social, educational, and parental environments* (pp. 33–51). Newbury Park, CA: Sage.

Bradley, R.H., and Caldwell, B.M. (1980). The relation of home environment, cognitive competence, and IQ among males and females. *Child Development, 51*(4), 1140–1148.

Bradley, R.H., and Caldwell, B.M. (1984). The HOME Inventory and family demographics. *Developmental Psychology, 20*(2), 315–320.

Bradley, R.H., Mundfrom, D.J., Whiteside, L., Caldwell, B.M., Casey, P.H., Kirby, R.S., and Hansen, S. (1994). The demography of parenting: A re-examination of the association between HOME scores and income. *Nursing Research, 43,* 260–266.

Brazelton, T.B. (1995). Working with families: Opportunities for early intervention. *Pediatric Clinics of North America, 42*(1),1–9.

Breiter, H.C., Gollub, R.L., Weisskoff, R.M., Kennedy, D.N., Makris, N., Berke, J.D., Goodman, J.M., Kantor, H.L., Gastfriend, D.R., Riorden, J.P., Mathew, R.T., Rosen, B.R., and Hyman, S.E. (1997). Acute effects of cocaine on human brain activity and emotion. *Neuron, 19*(3), 591–611.

Breslow, L. (1999). From disease prevention to health promotion. *Journal of the American Medical Association, 281,* 1030–1033.

Briss, P.A., Zaza, S., and Pappaioanou, M. (2000). Reviews of evidence regarding interventions to improve vaccination coverage in children, adolescents, and adults. *American Journal of Preventive Medicine, 18*(1S), 97–140.

Britt, J., Silver, I., and Rivara, F.P. (1998). Bicycle helmet promotion among low income preschool children. *Injury Prevention, 4,* 280–283.

Brody, G.H., Flor, D.L., Hollett-Wright, N., and McCoy, J.K. (1998). Children's development of alcohol use norms: Contributions of parent and sibling norms, children's temperaments, and parent-child discussions. *Journal of Family Psychology, 12,* 209–219.

Bronfenbrenner, U. (1979). *The ecology of human development: Experiments by nature and design.* Cambridge, MA: Harvard University Press.

Bronfenbrenner, U., and Ceci, S. (1994). Nature-nurture reconceptualized in developmental perspective: A bioecological model. *Psychological Review, 101*(4), 568–586.

Brooks, D.R., Davis, L.K., and Gallagher, S.S. (1993). Work-related injuries among Massachusetts children: A study based on emergency department data. *American Journal of Industrial Medicine, 24*(3), 313–324.

Brooks-Gunn, J., and Duncan, G.J. (1997). The effects of poverty on children and youth. *Future of Children, 7,* 55–71.

Brooks-Gunn, J., Duncan G., and Aber, J.L. (Eds.). (1997). *Neighborhood poverty: Context and consequences for children.* New York: Russell Sage.

Broste, S.K., Hansen, D.A., Strand, R.L., and Stueland, D.T. (1989). Hearing loss among high school farm students. *American Journal of Public Health, 79*(5), 619–622.

Brown, A.K., and Glass, L. (1979). Environmental hazards in the newborn nursery. *Pediatric Annals, 8,* 698–700.

Brown, B.V. (2001). *Tracking the well-being of children and youth at the state and local levels using the federal statistical system.* Child Trends: Assessing the New Federalism (Tech. Rep. No. 52). Washington, DC: The Urban Institute.

Brown, J.D., Steele, J.R., and Walsh-Childers, K. (Eds.). (2002). *Sexual teens, sexual media.* Mahwah, NJ: Lawrence Erlbaum Associates.

Brown, J.R., Cramond, J.K., and Wilde, R.J. (1974). Displacement effects of television and the child's functional orientation to media. In J. Blumler and E. Katz (Eds.), *The uses of mass communications: Current perspectives on gratifications research* (pp. 93–112). Beverly Hills, CA: Sage.

Brunner, E., and Marmot, M. (1999). Social organization, stress, and health. In M. Marmot and R.G. Wilkinson (Eds.), *Social determinants of health.* New York: Oxford University Press.

Buchowski, M.S., and Sun, M. (1996). Energy expenditure, television viewing and obesity. *International Journal of Obesity, 20,* 236–244.

Buehler, B.A., Delimont, D., van Waes, M., and Finnell, R.H. (1990). Prenatal prediction of risk of the fetal hydantoin syndrome. *New England Journal of Medicine, 322*(22), 1567–1572.

Buka, S.L., Stichick, T.L., Birdthistile, I., and Earls, F.J. (2001) Youth exposure to violence: Prevalence, risks, and consequences. *American Journal of Orthopsychiatry, 71,* 298–310.

Bullock, K. (2000). Child abuse: The physician's role in alleviating a growing problem. *American Family Physician, 61*(10), 2977–2985.

Bunker, J. (2001). *Medicine matters after all: Measuring the benefits of medical care, a healthy lifestyle, and a just social environment.* London: The Nuffield Trust.

Burse, V.W., DeGuzman, M.R., Korver, M.P., Najam, A.R., Williams, C.C., Hannon, W.H., and Therrell, B.L. (1997). Preliminary investigation of the use of dried-blood spots for the assessment of in utero exposure to environmental pollutants. *Biochemical and Molecular Medicine,* 61(2), 236–239.

Bushman, B., and Anderson, C.A. (2001). Media violence and the American public. *American Psychologist, 56,* 477–489.

Bushman, B.J., and Huesmann, L.R. (2001). Effects of televised violence on aggression. In D.G. Singer and J.L. Singer (Eds.), *Handbook of children and the media* (pp. 223–254). Thousand Oaks, CA: Sage.

Buston, K. (2002). Adolescents with mental health problems: What do they say about health services? *Journal of Adolescence, 25*(2), 231–242.

Butler, N., and Golding, J. (Eds.). (1986). *From birth to five: A study of the health and behavior of Britain's 5 year olds.* New York: Pergamon Press.

Caldju, C., Tannenbaum, B., Sharma, S., Francis, D., Plotsky, P.M., and Meaney, M.J. (1998). Maternal care during infancy regulates the development of neural systems mediating the expression of fearfulness in the rat. *Proceedings of the National Academy of Sciences, 95*(9), 5335–5340.

Calvert, S.L., and Tan, S.L. (1994). Impact of virtual reality on young adults' physiological arousal and aggressive thoughts: Interaction versus observation. *Journal of Applied Developmental Psychology, 15,* 125–139.

Campbell, S.F. (Ed.). (1976). *Piaget sampler: An introduction to Jean Piaget through his own words.* New York: John Wiley.

Canadian Government. (1974). *A new perspective on the health of Canadians (Lalonde Report).* Ottawa: Department of National Health and Welfare.

Caprara, G., Scabini, E., Barbaranelli, C., Pastorelli, C., Regalia, C., and Bandura, A. (1998). Impact of adolescents' perceived self-regulatory efficacy on familial communication and antisocial conduct. *European Psychologist, 3*(2), 125–132.

Card, D. (1999). The causal effect of education on earnings. In O.C. Ashenfelter and D. Card (Eds.), *Handbook of labor economics, Volume 3a.* Burlington, MA: Elsevier Science and Technology Books.

Carroll, K.M., Libby, B., Sheehan, J., and Hyland, N. (2001). Motivational interviewing to enhance treatment initiation in substance abusers: An effective study. *American Journal of Addictions, 10*(4), 335–339

Carter, C.M., Urbanowicz, M., Hemsley, R., Mantilla, L., Strobel, S., Graham, P.J., and Taylor, E. (1993). Effects of a few food diet in attention deficit disorder. *Archives of Disease in Childhood, 69*(5), 564–568.

Case, A., Lubotsky, D., and Paxon, C. (2002). Economic status and health in childhood: The origins of the gradient. *American Economic Review, 92*(5).

Caspi, A., McClay, J., Moffitt, T.E., Mill, J., Martin, J., Craig, I.W., Taylor, A., and Poulton, R. (2002). Role of genotype in the cycle of violence in maltreated children. *Science, 297*(5582), 851–854.

Cassady, C., Starfield, B., Hurtado, M., Berk, R., Nanda, J., and Friedenburg, L. (2000). Measuring consumer experiences with primary care. *Pediatrics, 105*(4), 998–1003.

Centers for Disease Control and Prevention. (1985). Epidemiologic notes and reports prevalence of cytomegalovirus excretion from children in five day-care centers—Alabama. *Morbidity and Mortality Weekly Report, 34*(4), 49–51.

Centers for Disease Control and Prevention. (1990a). Arboviral infections of the central nervous system—United States, 1989. *Morbidity and Mortality Weekly Report, 39*(24), 413–417.

Centers for Disease Control and Prevention. (1990b). Mercury exposure from interior latex paint—Michigan. *Morbidity and Mortality Weekly Report, 39*(8), 125–126.

Centers for Disease Control and Prevention. (1993). Teenage pregnancy and birth rates—United States, 1990. *Morbidity and Mortality Weekly Report, 42*(38).

Centers for Disease Control and Prevention. (1996). Work-related injuries and illnesses associated with child labor—United States, 1993. *Morbidity and Mortality Weekly Report, 45*(22), 464–468.

Centers for Disease Control and Prevention. (1998a). Arboviral infections of the central nervous system—United States, 1996–1997. *Morbidity and Mortality Weekly Report, 47*(25), 517–522.

Centers for Disease Control and Prevention. (1998b). Coronary heart disease mortality trends among whites and blacks Appalachia and United States, 1980–1993. *Morbidity and Mortality Weekly Report, 47*(46), 1005–1008, 1015.

Centers for Disease Control and Prevention. (1999a). Pedestrian fatalities—Cobb, DeKalb, Fulton, and Gwinnett counties, Georgia, 1994–1998. *Morbidity and Mortality Weekly Report, 48*(28), 601–605.

Centers for Disease Control and Prevention. (1999b). Playground safety, United States 1998–1999. *Morbidity and Mortality Weekly Report, 48*(16), 329–332.

Centers for Disease Control and Prevention. (1999c). Ten great public health achievements—United States, 1900–1999. *Morbidity and Mortality Weekly Report, 48*(12).

Centers for Disease Control and Prevention. (2000a). Blood lead levels in young children—United States and selected states, 1996–1999. *Morbidity and Mortality Weekly Report, 49*(50).

Centers for Disease Control and Prevention. (2000b). Consequences of delayed diagnosis of Rocky Mountain spotted fever in children—West Virginia, Michigan, Tennessee, and Oklahoma, May–July 2000. *Morbidity and Mortality Weekly Report, 49*(39), 885–888.

Centers for Disease Control and Prevention. (2000c). Motor-vehicle occupant fatalities and restraint use among children aged 4–8 years—United States, 1994–1998. *Morbidity and Mortality Weekly Report, 49*(7), 135–137.

Centers for Disease Control and Prevention. (2001). Recommendations for using fluoride to prevent and control dental caries in the United States. *Morbidity and Mortality Weekly Report, 50*(RR14), 1–42.

Centers for Disease Control and Prevention. (2002a). Cat-scratch disease in children—Texas, September 2000–August 2001. *Morbidity and Mortality Weekly Report, 51*(10), 212–214.

Centers for Disease Control and Prevention. (2002b). Lyme disease—United States, 2000. *Morbidity and Mortality Weekly Report, 51*(2), 29–31.

Centers for Disease Control and Prevention. (2002c). Provisional surveillance summary of the West Nile virus epidemic—United States, January–November 2002. *Morbidity and Mortality Weekly Report, 51*(50), 1129–1133.

Centers for Disease Control and Prevention. (2002d). Racial and ethnic disparities in infant mortality rates—60 largest U.S. cities, 1995–1998. *Morbidity and Mortality Weekly Report, 51*(15), 329–332, 343.

Centers for Disease Control and Prevention. (2003a). Public Health Laboratory Biomonitoring Implementation Program: Notice of availability of funds. *Federal Register, 68*(64), 16287.

Centers for Disease Control and Prevention. (2003b). *Second national report on human exposure to environmental chemicals* (Report No. 02-0716). Atlanta: Author.

Cervero, R. (2002). Built environments and mode choice: Toward a normative framework. *Transportation Research Part D: Transport and Environment, 7*(4), 265–284.

Cervero, R., and Ewing, R. (2001). Travel and the built environment: A synthesis. *Transportation Research Record, 1780,* 87–113.

Chaffee, S.H., and McLeod, J.M. (1972). Adolescent television use in the family context. In G.A. Comstock and E.A. Rubinstein (Eds.), *Television and social behavior* (pp. 149–172). Washington, DC: U.S. Government Printing Office.

Champoux, M., Bennett, A., Shannon, C., Higley, J.D., Lesch, K.P., and Suomi, S.J. (2002). Serotonin transporter gene polymorphism, differential early rearing, and behavior in rhesus monkey neonates. *Molecular Psychiatry, 7*(10), 1058–1063.

Chao, R.K. (1994). Beyond parental control and authoritarian parenting style: Understanding Chinese parenting through the cultural notion of training. *Child Development, 65,* 1111–1119.

Chao, J., and Kikano, G.E. (1993). Lead poisoning in children. *American Family Physician, 47,* 113–120.

Chase-Lansdale, P.L., Brooks-Gunn, J., and Zamsky, E. (1994). Young African-American multigenerational families in poverty: Quality of mothering and grandmothering. *Child Development, 65*(2), 373–393.

Chase-Lansdale P.L, Gordon, R.A., Brooks-Gunn, J., and Klebanov, R.A. (1997). Are neighborhood effects on your children mediated by features of the home environment? In J. Brooks-Gunn, G.J. Duncan, and J.L. Aber (Eds.), *Neighborhood poverty: Context and consequences for children* (pp. 119–145). New York: Russell Sage Foundation.

Chase-Lansdale, P.L., Moffitt, R.A., Lohman, B.J., Cherlin, A.J., Coley, R.L., Pittman, L.D., Roff, J., and Votruba-Drzal, E. (2003). Mothers' transitions from welfare to work and the well-being of preschoolers and adolescents. *Science, 299*(5612), 1548–1552.

Chatterji, S., Ustun, B., Sadana, R., Salomon, J.A., Mathers, C.D., and Murray, C.J.L. (2002). *The conceptual basis for measuring and reporting on health.* (Global Programme on Evidence for Health Policy Discussion Paper No. 45). Geneva: World Health Organization.

Chaturvedi, N. (2001). Ethnicity as an epidemiological determinant—Crudely racist or crucially important? *International Journal of Epidemiology, 30,* 925–927.

Check, J.V.P. (1985). *Effects of violent and nonviolent pornography.* Ottawa: Department of Justice for Canada.

Chen, J., and Kennedy, C. (2001). Television viewing and children's health. *Journal of the Society of Pediatric Nurses, 1,* 35–36.

Chester, J.A., Lumeng, L., Li, T.K., and Grahame, N.J. (2003). High- and low-alcohol-preferring mice show differences in conditioned taste aversion to alcohol. *Alcoholism: Clinical and Experimental Research, 27*(1), 12–18.

Chia, S.E., and Shi, L.M. (2002). Review of recent epidemiological studies on paternal occupations and birth defects. *Occupational and Environmental Medicine, 59,* 149–155.

Child Trends. (2003). *Child Trends Databank.* Available: http://www.childtrendsdatabank.org/. [Accessed February 27, 2003].

Church, J., and Williams, H. (2001). Another sniffer dog for the clinic? *Lancet, 358*(9285), 930.

Clark, R., Tyroler, H.A., and Heiss, G. (1999). Orthostatic blood pressure responses as a function of ethnicity and socioeconomic status: The ARIC Study. *Annals of the New York Academy of Sciences, 896,* 316–317.

Cocking, R.R., and Greenfield, P.M. (1996). Effects of interactive entertainment technologies on children's development. In P.M. Greenfield and R.R. Cocking (Eds.), *Interacting with video* (pp. 3–7). Norwood, NJ: Ablex.

Coie, J.D., Lochman, J.E., Terry, R., and Hyman, C. (1992). Predicting early adolescent disorder from childhood aggression and peer rejection. *Journal of Consulting and Clinical Psychology, 60*(5), 783–792.

Coiro, M.J. (2001). Depressive symptoms among women receiving welfare. *Women and Health, 32*(1), 1–12.

Cole, T. (1999). Ebbing epidemic: Youth homicide rate at a 14-year low. *Journal of American Medical Association, 281,* 25–26.

Colt, J.S., and Blair, A. (1998). Parental occupational exposures and risk of childhood cancer. *Environmental Health Perspectives, 106*(3), 909–925.

Committee on Biological Markers of the National Research Council. (1987). Biological markers in environmental health research. *Environmental Health Perspectives, 74,* 3–9.

Conanan, B., London, K., Martinez, L., Modersbach, D., O'Connell, J., O'Sullivan, M., Raffanti, S., Ridolfo, A., Post, P., Santillan Rabe, M., Song, J., and Treherne, L. (2003) *Adapting your practice: Treatment and recommendations for homeless patients with HIV/AIDS.* Nashville: Health Care for the Homeless Clinicians' Network, National Health Care for the Homeless Council, Inc.

Contrada, R.J., Ashmore, R.D., Gary, M.L., Coups, E., Egeth, J.D., Sewell, A., Ewell, K., and Goyal, T.M. (2001). Measures of ethnicity-related stress: Psychometric properties, ethnic group differences, and associations with well-being. *Applied Social Psychology, 31*(9), 1775–1820.

Cooley, M.R., Turner, S.M., and Beidel, D.C. (1995). Assessing community violence: The children's report of exposure to violence. *Journal of American Academy of Child and Adolescent Psychiatry, 34*(2), 201–208.

Corser, N.C. (1996). Sleep of 1- and 2-year old children in intensive care. *Issues in Comprehensive Pediatric Nursing, 19*(1), 17–31.

Cottrell, L., Li, X., Harris, C., D'Alessandri, D., Atkins, M., Richardson, B., and Stanton, B. (2003). Parent and adolescent perceptions of parental monitoring and adolescent risk involvement. *Parenting: Science and Practice, 3,* 179–195.

Coulton, C. (1996). Effects of neighborhoods in large cities on families and children: Implications for services. In A.J. Kahn and S.B. Kamerman (Eds.), *Children and their families in big cities: Strategies for service reform.* New York: Columbia University.

Cowen, E.L., Pedersen, A., Babigian, H., Izzo, L.D., and Trost, M.A. (1973). Long-term follow-up of early detected vulnerable children. *Journal of Consulting and Clinical Psychology, 41*(3), 438–446.

Cravens, H. (1993). Child saving in modern America 1870s–1990s. In R. Wallons (Ed.), *Children at risk in America: History, concepts, and public policy.* Albany: State University of New York Press.

Cummings, E.M., and Davies, P.T. (1994). Maternal depression and child development. *Journal of Child Psychology and Psychiatry, 35*(1):73–112.

Cureton-Lane, R.A., and Fontaine, D.K. (1997). Sleep in the pediatric ICU: An empirical investigation. *American Journal of Critical Care, 6*(1), 56–63.

Currie, J., and Gruber, J. (1996a). Health insurance eligibility, utilization of medical care, and child Health. *The Quarterly Journal of Economics, 111*(2), 431–466.

Currie, J., and Gruber, J. (1996b). Saving babies: The efficacy and cost of recent changes in the Medicaid eligibility of pregnant women. *Journal of Political Economy, 104*(6), 1263–1296.

Currie, J., and Stabile, M. (2002). *Socioeconomic status and health: Why is the relationship stronger for older children?* (NBER Working Paper No. w9098). Cambridge, MA: National Bureau of Economic Research.

Currie, J., and Thomas, D. (1995). Medical care for children: Public insurance, private insurance, and racial differences in utilization. *Journal of Human Resources, 30*(1), 135–162.

Cutler, D., and Gruber, J. (1997). Medicaid and private insurance: Evidence and implications. *Health Affairs, 16*(1), 194–200.

Dafny, L., and Gruber, J. (In Press). Public insurance and child hospitalizations: Access and efficiency effects. *Journal of Public Economics.*

Daly, M., Duncan, G., McDonough, P., and Williams, D. (2002). Optimal indicators of socioeconomic status for health research. *American Journal of Public Health, 92*(7), 1151–1157.

Davidson E.H. (1986). *Gene activity in early development.* Orlando, FL: Academic Press.

Davidson, E.H. (2001). Genomic regulatory systems for development. *Development Growth and Differentiation, 43*(Suppl 1):S10.

Davis, C.L., Delamater, A.M., Shaw, K.H., La Greca, A.M., Eidson, M.S., Perez-Rodriguez, J.E., and Nemery, R. (2001). Parenting styles, regimen adherence, and glycemic control in 4- to 10-year-old children with diabetes. *Journal of Pediatric Psychology, 26,* 123–129.

Dawson, G., Hessel, D., and Frey, K. (1994). Social influences on early developing biological and behavioral systems related to risk for affective disorder. *Development and Psychopathology, 6,* 759–779.

Dawson, G., Ashman, S.B., and Carver, L.J. (2000). The role of early experience in shaping behavioral and brain development and its implications for social policy. *Development and Psychopathology, 12*(4), 695–712.

Day, N., Cornelius, M., Goldschmidt, L., Richardson, G., Robles, N., and Taylor, P. (1992). The effects of prenatal tobacco and marijuana use on offspring growth from birth through 3 years of age. *Neurotoxicology and Teratology, 14*(6), 407–414.

De Joy, D.M. (1983). Environmental noise and children: Review of recent findings. *Journal of Auditory Research, 23,* 181–194.

Deaton, A., and Paxson, C. (2001). *Mortality, income, and income inequality over time in Britain and the United States.* (NBER Working Paper No. w8534). Cambridge, MA: National Bureau of Economic Research.

DeCasper, A.J., and Fifer, W.P. (1980). Of human bonding: Newborns prefer their mothers' voices. *Science, 6,* 1174–1176.

Delamater, A.M., Jacobson, A.M., Anderson, B., Cox, D., Fisher, L., Lustman, P., Rubin, R., and Wysocki, T. (2001). Psychosocial therapies in diabetes. *Diabetes Care, 24,* 1286–1292.

Dellinger, A.M., and Staunton, C.E. (2002). Barriers to children walking and biking to school—United States, 1999. *Morbidity and Mortality Weekly Report, 51*(32), 701–704.

Demissie, K., Hanley, J.A., Menzies, D., Joseph, L., and Erns, P. (2000). Agreement in measuring socio-economic status: Area-based versus individual measures. *Chronic Diseases in Canada, 21*(1), 1–7.

Derksen, D.J., and Strasburger, V.C. (1994). Children and the influence of the media. *Primary Care, 21,* 747–758.

Derstine, B. (1996). Job-related fatalities involving youths, 1992–1995. *Compensation and Working Conditions* (December), 1–3.

Dick, A.W., Klein, J.D., Shone, L.P., Zwanziger, J., Yu, H., and Szilagyi, P.G. (2003). The evolution of the State Children's Health Insurance Program (SCHIP) in New York: Changing program features and enrollee characteristics. *Pediatrics, 112*(6pt2), e542.

Dickinson, D.K., and DeTemple, J. (1998). Putting parents in the picture: Maternal reports of preschool literacy as a prediction of early reading. *Early Childhood Research Quarterly, 13*(2), 241–261.

Dickstein, S., Seifer, R., Magee, K.D., Mirsky, K.D.E., and Lynch, M.M. (1998). *Timing of maternal depression, family functioning, and infant development: A prospective view.* Paper presented at the biennial meeting of the MARCE Society, Iowa City, IA.

Dietz, W.H. (2001). The obesity epidemic in young children: Reduce television viewing and promote playing. *British Medical Journal, 322,* 313–314.

Dietz, W.H., and Gortmaker, S.L. (1985). Do we fatten our children at the television set? Obesity and television viewing in children and adolescents. *Pediatrics, 75,* 807–812.

Dietz, W.H., Bandini, L.G., Morelli, J.A., Peers, K.F., and Ching, P. (1994). Effect of sedentary activities on resting metabolic rate. *American Journal of Clinical Nutrition, 59,* 556–559.

Diez-Roux, A. (2001). Investigating neighborhood and area effects on health. *American Journal of Public Health, 91,* 1783–1789.

DiMaggio, C., and Durkin, M. (2002). Child pedestrian injury in an urban setting: Descriptive epidemiology. *Academic Emergency Medicine, 9*(1), 54–62.

DiMatteo, M.R. (2000). Practitioner-family-patient communication in pediatric adherence: Implications for research and clinical practice. In D. Drotar (Ed.), *Promoting adherence to medical treatment in chronic childhood illness: Concepts, methods and interventions* (pp. 237–258). Mahwah, NJ: Erlbaum.

DiPrete, T.A., and Forristal, J.D. (1994). Multilevel models: Methods and substance. *Annual Review of Sociology, 20,* 331–357.

Dodge, K.A., Lansford, J.E., Burks, V.S., Bates, J.E., Pettit, G.S., Fontaine, R., and Price, J.M. (2003). Peer rejection and social information-processing factors in the development of aggressive behavior problems in children. *Child Development, 74,* 374–393.

Doll, J., and Ajzen, I. (1992). Accessibility and stability of predictors in the theory of planned behavior. *Journal of Personality and Social Psychology, 63*(5), 754–765.

Dornbusch, S.M., Carlsmith, J.M., Bushwall, S.J., Ritter, P.L., Leiderman, H., Hastorf, A.H., and Gross, R.T. (1985). Single parents, extended households, and the control of adolescents. *Child Development, 56,* 326–341.

Dorr, A., and Kunkel, D. (1990). Children in the media environment: Change and constancy amid change. *Communication Research, 17,* 5–25.

Downey, G., and Coyne, J. (1990). Children of depressed parents: An integrative review. *Psychological Bulletin, 108,* 50–76.

Duncan, G.J. (1988). The volatility of family income over the life course. In P.B. Baltes, D. Featherman, and R.M. Lerner (Eds.), *Life-span development and behavior, volume 9* (pp. 317–358). Hillsdale, NJ: Lawrence Erlbaum Associates.

Duncan, G.J., and Chase-Lansdale, L.P. (2001). *For better and for worse: Welfare reform and the well-being of children and families.* New York: Russell Sage.

Duncan, G.J., and Magnuson, K. (2002). Economics and parenting. *Parenting: Science and Practice, 2*(4), 437–450.

Duncan, G., and Peterson, E. (2001). The long and short of asking questions about income, wealth and labor supply. *Social Science Research, 30*(2), 248–263.

Duncan, G.J., and Raudenbush, S. (1999). *Neighborhoods and adolescent development: How we can determine the links?* Evanston, IL: Northwestern University and University of Chicago, Joint Center for Poverty Research.

Duncan, G.J., and Raudenbush, S. (2001a). Getting context right in studies of child development. In A. Thornton (Ed.), *The well-being of children and families: Research and data needs* (pp. 356–383). Ann Arbor: University of Michigan Press.

Duncan, G.J., and Raudenbush, S. (2001b). Neighborhoods and adolescent development: How can we determine the links? In A. Booth and A.C. Crouter (Eds.), *Does it take a village? Community effects on children, adolescents, and families* (pp. 105–136). State College: Pennsylvania State University Press.

Duncan, T.E., Duncan, S.C., Strycker, L.A., Li, F., and Alpert, A. (1999). *An introduction to latent variable growth curve modeling: Concepts, issues, and applications.* Mahwah, NJ: Lawrence Erlbaum Associates.

Durant, R.H., Baranowski, T., Johnson, M., and Thompson W.O. (1994). The relationship among television watching, physical activity, and body composition of young children. *Pediatrics, 94,* 449–455.

Durbin, D.R. (1999). Preventing motor vehicle injuries. *Current Opinion in Pediatrics, 11*(6), 583–587.

Dyson, J.L. (1990). The effect of family violence on children's academic performance and behavior. *Journal of the National Medical Association, 82*(1), 17–22.

Earls, F., and Buka, S. (1997) *A research report from the Project on Human Development in Chicago Neighborhoods from the National Institute of Justice.* Washington, DC: U.S. Department of Justice.

Ebrahim, S.H., and Gfroerer, J. (2003). Pregnancy-related substance use in the United States during 1996–1998. *Obstetrics and Gynecology, 101*(2), 374–379.

Egbuonu, L., and Starfield, B. (1982). Child health and social status. *Pediatrics, 69,* 550–555.

Eisen, M., Ware, J., Donald C., and Brook, R. (1979). Measuring components of children's health status. *Medical Care, 17,* 902–921.

Eiser, C. (1997). Children's quality of life measures. *Archives of Disease in Childhood, 77*, 350–354.

Eiser, C., and Morse, R.B. (2001). The measurement of quality of life in children: Past and future perspectives. *Journal of Developmental and Behavioral Pediatrics, 22*(4), 248–256.

Ellen, I.G., Mijanovich, T., and Dillman, K.N. (2001). Neighborhood effect on health: Exploring the links and assessing the evidence. *Journal of Urban Affairs, 23*, 391–408.

Elliot, M.R., Drummond, J., and Bernard, K.E. (1996) Subjective appraisal of infant crying. *Clinical Nursing Research, 5*(2), 237–250.

Ellis, J.A., Stebbing, M., and Harrap, S.B. (2001). Significant population variation in adult male height associated with the Y chromosome and the aromatase gene. *Journal of Clinical Endocrinology and Metabolism, 86*(9), 4147–4150.

Eng, T.R. (2001). *The eHealth landscape: A terrain map of emerging information and communication technologies in health and health care.* Princeton, NJ: The Robert Wood Johnson Foundation.

Engle, G. (1977). The need for a new medical model: A challenge for biomedicine. *Science, 197*(4286), 129–196.

Enwisle, D., and Astone, N.M. (1994). Some practical guidelines for measuring youth's race/ethnicity and socioeconomic status. *Child Development, 65*, 1521–1540.

Epstein, F.H. (1996). Cardiovascular disease epidemiology. A journey from the past into the future. *Circulation, 93*, 1755–1764.

Erickson, J.D. (2002). Folic acid and prevention of spina bifida and anencephaly: 10 years after the U.S. Public Health Service recommendation. *Morbidity and Mortality Weekly Report, 51*, 1–3.

Erickson, J.D., Mulinare, J., Yang, Q., Johnson, C.L., Pfeiffer, C., Gunter, E.W., Giles, W.H., and Bowman, B.A. (2002). Folate status in women of childbearing age, by race/ethnicity—United States 1999–2000. *Morbidity and Mortality Weekly Report, 51*(36), 808–810.

Erkut, S., Alarcón, O., and García Coll, C. (1999a). *Normative study of Puerto Rican adolescents: Final report.* (Report No. CRW 23). Wellesly, MA: Wellesley Centers for Women.

Erkut, S., Alarcón, O., García Coll, C., Tropp, L.R., and Vazquez García, H.A. (1999b). The dual focus approach to creating bilingual measures. *Journal of Cross-Cultural Psychology, 30*(2), 206–218.

Erkut, S., Szalacha, L.A., García Coll, C., and Alarcón, O. (2000). Puerto Rican early adolescents' self-esteem patterns. *Journal of Research on Adolescence, 10*(3), 343–368.

Esterick, P.V. (2002). *Risks, rights, and regulations communicating about risks and infant feeding.* Penang, Malaysia: World Alliance for Breastfeeding Action.

Etzel, R., and Balk, S. (Eds.). (1999). *Handbook of pediatric environmental health.* Elk Grove Village, IL: American Academy of Pediatrics.

Evans, G.W., Lercher, P., Meis, M., Ising, H., and Kofler, W.W. (2001). Community noise exposure and stress in children. *The Journal of the Acoustical Society of America, 109*(3), 1023–1027.

Evans, R.G., and Stoddart, G.L. (1990). Producing health, consuming health care. *Social science and medicine, 31*(12), 1347–1363.

Evans, R.G., and Stoddart, G.L. (2003). Consuming research, producing policy? *American Journal of Public Health, 93*(3), 371–379.

Faith, M.S., Berman, N., Heo, M., Pietrobelli, A., Gallagher, D., Epstein, H.L., Eiden, M.T., and Allison, D.B. (2001). Effects of contingent television on physical activity and television viewing in obese children, *Pediatrics, 107*, 1043–1048.

Falk, S.A., and Woods, N.F. (1973). Hospital noise—Levels and potential health hazards. *New England Journal of Medicine, 289*, 774–781.

Falkner, B. (2002). Birth weight as a predictor of future hypertension. *American Journal of Hypertension, 15*, 43S–45S.

Farmer, C.M., Retting, R.A., and Lund, A.K. (1999). Changes in motor vehicle occupant fatalities after repeal of the national maximum speed limit. *Accident Analysis and Prevention 31*, 537–543.

Farran, D. (2000). Another decade of intervention for children who are low income or disabled: What do we know now? In J. Shonkoff and S. Meisels (Eds.), *Handbook of early childhood intervention* (2nd ed., pp. 510–548). New York: Cambridge University Press.

Fawcett, S.B., Paine, A.L., Francisco, V.T., and Vliet, M. (1993). Promoting health through community development. In D.S. Glenwick and L.A. Jason (Eds.), *Promoting health and mental health in children, youth, and families*, (pp. 233–255). New York: Springer.

Feachem, R.G.A. (2000). Poverty and inequity: A proper focus for the new century. *Bulletin of the World Health Organization, 78*(1), 1–2. Available: http://www.who.int/bulletin/pdf/2000/issue1/Editorial.pdf.

Federal Interagency Forum on Child and Family Statistics. (July 2003). *America's children: Key national indicators of well-being*. Health Resources and Services Administration Information Center. Washington, DC: U.S. Government Printing Office.

Fenske, R.A., Black, K.G., Elkner K.P., Lee, C.L., Methner, M.M., and Soto, R. (1990). Potential exposure and health risks of infants following indoor residential pesticide applications. *American Journal of Public Health, 80*, 689–693.

Ferrante, R.J., Andreassen, O.A., Dedeoglu, A., Ferrante, K.L., Jenkins, B.G., Hersch, S.M., and Beal, M.F. (2002). Therapeutic effects of coenzyme Q10 and remacemide in transgenic mouse models of Huntington's disease. *Journal of Neuroscience, 22*(5), 1592–1599.

Feychting, M., Plato, N., Nise, G., and Ahlbom, A. (2001). Paternal occupational exposures and childhood cancer. *Environmental Health Perspectives, 109*, 193–196.

Field, T. (1995). Psychologically depressed parents. In M.H. Bornstein (Ed.), *Handbook of parenting, Vol. 4: Applied and practical parenting* (pp. 85–99). Hillsdale, NJ: Erlbaum.

Field, T. (2002). Preterm infant massage therapy studies: An American approach. *Seminars in Neonatology, 7*, 487–494.

Fielding, J.E., Sutherland, C.E., and Halfon, N. (1999). Community health report cards. Results of a national survey. *American Journal of Preventive Medicine, 17*(1), 79–86.

Finnell, R.H., Waes, J.G., Eudy, J.D., and Rosenquist, T.H. (2002). Molecular basis of environmentally induced birth defects. *Annual Review of Pharmacology and Toxicology, 42*, 181–208.

Fireman, B., Black, S.B., Shinefield, H.R., Lee, J., Lewis, E., and Ray, P. (2003). Impact of the pneumococcal conjugate vaccine on otitis media. *Pediatric Infectious Disease Journal, 22*(1), 10–16.

Fletcher, R.H., and Fairfield, K.M. (2002). Vitamins for chronic disease prevention in adults: Clinical applications. *Journal of American Medical Association, 287*(23), 3127–3129.

Forrest, C., Glade, G., Baker, A., Bocian, A., Kang, M., and Starfield, B. (1999). The pediatric primary-specialty care interface: How pediatricians refer children and adolescents to specialty care. *Archives of Pediatric and Adolescent Medicine, 153*(7), 705–714.

Forrest, C., Glade, G., Baker, A., von Schrader, S., and Starfield, B. (2000). Coordination of specialty referrals and physician satisfaction with referral care. *Archives of Pediatric and Adolescent Medicine, 154*, 499–506.

Forrest, C., Rebok, G., Riley, A., Starfield, B., Green, B., Robertson, J., and Tambor, E. (2001). Elementary school-aged children's reports of their health: A cognitive interviewing study. *Quality of Life Research, 10*(1), 59–70.

Forrest, C., Majeed, A., Weiner, J., Carroll, K., and Bindman, A. (2002a). Comparison of specialty referral rates in the United Kingdom and the United States: Retrospective cohort analysis. *British Medical Journal, 325*(7360), 370–371.

Forrest, C., Nutting, P., Starfield, B., and von Schrader, S. (2002b). Family physicians' referral decisions: Results from the ASPN referral study. *Journal of Family Practitioner, 51*, 515–522.

Francis, D., Diorio, J., Liu, D., and Meaney, M.J. (1999). Nongenomic transmission across generations of maternal behavior and stress responses in the rat. *Science, 286*(5442), 1155–1158.

Francis, D.D., Young, L.J., Meaney, M.J., and Insel, T.R. (2002). Naturally occurring differences in maternal care are associated with the expression of oxytocin and vasopressin (V1a) receptors: Gender differences. *Journal of Neuroendocrinology, 14*(5), 349–353.

Francis, M.M., Mellem, J.E., and Maricq, A.V. (2003). Bridging the gap between genes and behavior: Recent advances in the electrophysiological analysis of neural function in *Caenorhabditis elegans*. *Trends in Neuroscience, 26*(2), 90–99.

Frankel, K.A., and Harmon, R.J. (1996). Depressed mothers: They don't always look as bad as they feel. *Journal of the American Academy of Child and Adolescent Psychiatry, 35*(3), 289–298.

Frankenhaeuser, M., and Lundberg, U. (1974). Immediate and delayed effects of noise on performance and arousal. *Biological Psychology, 2*(2), 127–133.

Fridman, M.S., Powell, K.E., Hutwagner, L., Graham, L.M., and Teague, W.G. (2001). Impact of changes in transportation and commuting behaviors during the 1996 summer olympic games in Atlanta on air quality and childhood asthma. *Journal of American Medical Association, 285*, 897–905.

Freedman, S.A., Pierce, P.M., and Reiss, J.G. (1987). Model program REACH: A family-centered community-based case management model for children with special health care needs. *Child Health Care, 16*(2), 114–117.

Friedrich-Cofer, L., and Huston, A.C. (1986). Television violence and aggression: The debate continues. *Psychological Bulletin, 100*, 364–371.

Frumkin, H. (2002). Urban Sprawl and Public Health. *Public Health Reports, 117*, 201–217.

Frumkin, H. (2003). Child Health and the Built Environment. Paper prepared for the Committee on Evaluation of Children's Health. Commissioned jointly by the National Research Council and the Institute of Medicine.

Fuchs, V. (1983). *How We Live.* Cambridge, MA: Harvard University Press.

Fuligni, A.J. (1997). The academic achievement of adolescents from immigrant families: The roles of family background, attitudes, and behavior. *Child Development, 68*, 261–273.

Furstenberg, F.F., Jr., Cook, T.D., Eccles, J., Elder, G.H., Jr., and Sameroff, A.J. (1999). *Managing to make it: Urban families and adolescent success.* Chicago: University of Chicago Press.

Gallimore, R., Weisner, T.S., Bernheimer, L.P., Guthrie, D., and Nihira, K. (1993). Family responses to young children with developmental delays: Accommodation activity in ecological and cultural context. *American Journal of Mental Retardation, 98*(2), 185–206.

Galster, G., Hanson, R., Wolman, H., Coleman, S., and Freihage, J. (2000). Wrestling sprawl to the ground: Defining and measuring an elusive concept. *Housing Facts and Findings, 2*(4).

García, J.A., and Weisz, J.R. (2002).When youth mental health care stops: Therapeutic relationship problems and other reasons for ending youth outpatient treatment. *Journal of Consulting and Clinical Psychology, 70*(2), 439–443.

García Coll, C.T., and Magnuson, K. (2000). Culture, ethnicity, and minority status as sources of developmental risks and resources. In J. Shonkoff and S. Miesels (Eds.), *Handbook of early childhood intervention, Vol. II* (pp. 94–114). Cambridge: Cambridge University Press.

García Coll, C., and Pachter, L. (2002). Ethnic and minority parenting. In M.H. Borstein (Ed.), *Handbook of parenting.* 2nd Edition. Mahwah, NJ: Lawrence Erlbaum Publishers.

García Coll, C.T., Lamberty, G., Jenkins, R., McAdoo, H.P., Crnic, K., Wasick, B.H., and Vazquez Garcia, H. (1996). An integrative model for the study of developmental competencies in minority children. *Child Development, 67*(5), 1891–1914.

Gazmararian, J.A., James, S.A., and Lepowski, J.M. (1995). Depression and black and white women: The role of marriage and socioeconomic status. *Annals of Epidemiology, 5*, 455–463.

Gelernter, J., Page, G.P., Bonvicini, K., Woods, S.W., Pauls, D.L., and Kruger, S.A. (2003) Chromosome 14 risk locus for simple phobia: Results from a genomewide linkage scan. *Molecular Psychiatry, 8*(1), 71–82.

Gennetian, L., Duncan, G., Knox, V.W., Vargas, W., Clark-Kaufman, E., and London, A.S. (2002). *How welfare and work policies for parents affect adolescents.* New York: Manpower Demonstration Research Corporation.

Geronimus, A.T., Bound, J., and Neidert, L.J. (1996). On the validity of using census geocode characteristics to proxy individual socioeconomic characteristics. *Journal of the American Statistical Association, 91*, 529–537.

Gilbert, S.F. (2000). *Developmental biology.* 6th Edition. Sunderland, MA: Sinauer Associates.

Gill, A.G., Vega, W.A., and Dimas, J.M. (1994). Acculturative stress and personal adjustment among Hispanic adolescent boys. *Journal of Community Psychology, 22*, 45–53.

Gold, R., Kennedy, B., Connell, F., and Kawachi, I. (2002). Teen births, income inequality and social capital: Developing a understanding of the causal pathway. *Health Place, 8*, 77–83.

Golding, J. (1997). Sudden infant death syndrome and parental smoking—A literature review. *Pediatric and Perinatal Epidemiology, 11*(1), 67–77.

Goldman, L.R., and Koduru, S. (2000). Chemicals in the environment and developmental toxicity to children: A public health and policy perspective. *Environmental Health Perspectives, 108*(Suppl 3), 443–448.

Gomaa, A., Hu, H., Bellinger, D., Schwartz, J., Tsaih, S.W., Gonzalez-Cossio, T., Schnaas, L., Peterson, K., Aro, A., and Hernandez-Avila, M. (2002). Maternal bone lead as an independent risk factor for fetal neurotoxicity: A prospective study. *Pediatrics, 110*(1), 110–118.

Gonzalez, C.A., Sala, N., and Capella, G. (2002). Genetic susceptibility and gastric cancer risk. *International Journal of Cancer, 100*(3), 249–260.

Goodman, E., Slap, G., and Huang, B. (2003). The public health impact of socioeconomic status on adolescent depression and obesity. *American Journal of Public Health, 93*, 1844–1850.

Gorn, G.J., and Goldberg, M.E. (1982). Behavioral evidence for the effects of televised food messages to children. *Journal of Consumer Research, 9*, 200–205.

Graber, J.A., and Brooks-Gunn, J. (1996). Transition and turning points: Navigating the passage from childhood to adolescents. *Developmental Psychology, 32*(4), 768–776.

Green, M., and Palfrey, J.S. (2002). *Bright futures: Guidelines for health supervision of infants, children and adolescents.* Arlington, VA: National Center for Education in Maternal and Child Health.

Greenfield, P.M. (1994). Video games as cultural artifacts. *Journal of Applied Developmental Psychology, 15*, 3–11.

Greydanus, D.E., Farrell, E.G., Sladkin, K., and Rypma, C.B. (1990). The gang phenomenon and the American teenager. *Adolescent Medicine, 1*(1), 55–70.

Groce, N.E., and Zola, I.K. (1993). Multiculturalism, chronic illness, and disability. *Pediatrics, 91*(5), 1048–1055.

Grossman, D.C. (2000). The history of injury control and epidemiology of child and adolescent injuries. *The Future of Children, 10*(1), 23–52.

Groves, B.M., Zuckerman, B., Marans, S., and Cohen, D.J. (1993). Silent victims: Children who witness violence. *Journal of the American Medical Association, 269*(2), 262–264.

Gunter, B. (2001). *Media sex: What are the issues?* Mahwah, NJ: Lawrence Earlbaum Associates.

Guo, G., and VanWey, L.K. (1999). Sibship size and intellectual development: Is the relationship causal? *American Sociological Review, 64*(2), 169–187.

Guthrie, R. (2001). Compensation: Problems with the concept of disability and the use of American Medical Association guides. *Journal of Law Medicine, 9*(2), 185–199.

Gutierrez, J., Sameroff, A., and Karrer, B. (1988). Acculturation and SES effects on Mexican-American parents' concepts of development. *Child Development, 59*, 250–255.

Hack, M., Flannery, D.J., Schluchter, M., Cartar, L., Borawski, E., and Klein, N. (2002). Outcomes in young adulthood for very-low-birth-weight infants. *New England Journal of Medicine, 346*, 149–157.

Haines, M.M., Standfeld, S.A., Brentnall, S., Head, J., Berry, B., Jiggins, M., and Hygge, S. (2001). The West London Schools Study: The effects of chronic aircraft noise exposure on child health. *Psychological Medicine, 31*(8), 1385–1396.

Halfon, N., and Hochstein M. (2002). Life course health development: An integrated framework for developing health policy and research. *The Milbank Quarterly, 80*(3), 433–479.

Halfon, N., and Klee, L. (1987). Health services for California's foster children: Current practices and policy recommendations. *Pediatrics, 80*(2), 183–191.

Halfon, N., and Lawrence, W. (2003). Health Services Working Group Report to the National Advisory Committee, National Children Study.

Halfon, N., Berkowitz, G., and Klee, L. (1992). Mental health service utilization by children in foster care in California. *Pediatrics, 89,* 1238–1244.

Halfon, N., Inkelas, M., and Wood, D. (1995). Nonfinancial barriers to care for children and youth. *Annual Reviews of Public Health, 16,* 447–472.

Halfon, N., Inkelas, M., Wood, D., and Schuster, M. (1996). Health care reform for children and families: Refinancing and restructuring the U.S. child health system. In R.M. Rice et al. (Eds.), *Changing the U.S. health care system: Key issues in health services, policy, and management* (pp. 227–254). San Francisco: Jossey-Bass.

Halfon, N., Wood, D.L., Valdez, R., Pereyra, M., and Duan, N. (1997). Medicaid enrollment and health services access by Latino children in inner-city Los Angeles. *Journal of American Medical Association, 277*(8), 636–641.

Halfon, N., Newacheck, P., Hughes, D., and Brindis, C. (1998). Community health monitoring: Taking the pulse of America's children. *Maternal and Child Health Journal, 2*(2), 95–109.

Halfon, N., Inkelas, M., Wood, D.L., and Schuster, M.A. (2001). Health reform for children and families. In R. Andersen, T. Rice, and G. Kominsky (Eds.), *Changing the U.S. health care system: Key issues in health services policy and management.* San Francisco: Jossey-Bass.

Halfon, N., Olson, L., Inkelas, M., Mistry, R., Sareen, H., Lange, L., and Wright, J. (2002). Summary statistics from the National Survey of Early Childhood Health, 2000. National Center for Health Statistics. *Vital Health Statistics, 15*(3).

Halfon, N., Uyeda, K., Inkelas, M., and Rice, T. (2004). Building bridges: A comprehensive system for healthy development and school readiness. In N. Halfon, T. Rice, and M. Inkelas (Eds.), *Building state early childhood comprehensive systems series.* Los Angeles, CA: National Center for Infant and Early Childhood Health Policy.

Hall, L.A., Gurley, D.N., Sachs, B., and Kryscio, R.J. (1991). Psychosocial predictors of maternal depressive symptoms, parental attitudes, and child behavior in single-parent families. *Nursing Research, 40*(4), 214–220.

Hansen, K.K. (1998). Folk remedies and child abuse: A review with emphasis on caída de mollera and its relationship to shaken baby syndrome. *Child Abuse and Neglect, 22*(2), 117–127.

Harada, M. (1978). Methyl mercury poisoning due to environmental contamination ("Minamata disease"). In F.W. Oehme (Ed.), *Toxicity of heavy metals in the environment* (pp. 261–302). New York: Marcel Dekker.

Hardy, R., Kuh, D., Langenberg, C., and Wadsworth, M. (2003). Birth weight, childhood social class, and change in adult blood pressure in the 1946 British birth cohort. *Lancet, 362,* 1179–1183.

Harpin, V.A., and Rutter, N. (1983). Barrier properties of the newborn infant's skin. *Journal of Pediatrics, 102*(3), 419–425.

Harrell, J., Hall, S., and Taliferro, J. (2003). Physiological responses to racism and discrimination: An assessment of the evidence. *American Journal of Public Health, 93,* 243–248.

Harris, E.S., Canning, R.D., and Kelleher, K.J. (1996). A comparison of measures of adjustment, symptoms, and impairment among children with chronic medical conditions. *Journal of the American Academy of Child and Adolescent Psychiatry, 35*(8), 1025–1028.

Hart, B., and Risley, T.R. (1995). *Meaningful experiences in the everyday experiences of young American children.* Baltimore: Brookes.

Hart, K., Bishop, J., and Truby, H. (2003). Changing children's diets: Developing methods and messages. *Journal of Human Nutrition and Dietetics, 16,* 365–366.

Harter, S. (1982). The perceived competence scale for children. *Child Development, 53,* 87–97.

Hartup, W.W., and Laursen, B. (1993). Conflict and context in peer relations. In C. Hart (Ed.), *Children on playgrounds: Research perspectives and applications* (pp. 44–84). Albany: State University of New York Press.

Harwood, R. (1992). The influence of culturally deprived values on Anglo and Puerto Rican mothers' perceptions of attachment behavior. *Child Development, 63*(4), 822–839.

Harwood, R.L., Schoelmerich, A., Schulze, P.A., and Gonzalez, Z. (1999). Cultural differences in maternal beliefs and behaviors: A study of middle-class Anglo and Puerto Rican mother-infant pairs in four everyday situations. *Child Development, 70*(4), 1005–1016.

Haugland, S.W., and Wright, J.L. (1997). *Young children and technology: A world of discovery.* Boston: Allyn and Bacon.

Hauser, R., and Warren, J. (1997). Socioeconomic indexes for occupations: A review, update and critique. In A. Raftery and J. Wilt (Eds.), *Sociological methodology* (pp. 177–298). Cambridge, MA: Blackwell Publishing.

Hauser, S.T., Jacobson, A.M., Lavori, P., Wolfsdorf, J.I., Herskowitz, R.D., Milley, J.E., Bliss, R., Wertlieb D., and Stein, J. (1990). Adherence among children and adolescents with insulin-dependent diabetes mellitus over a four-year longitudinal follow-up: II. Immediate and long-term linkages with the family milieu. *Journal of Pediatric Psychology, 15,* 527–542.

Haverman, R., and Wolfe, B. (1994). *Succeeding generations: On the effect of investments in children.* New York: Russell Sage Foundation.

Hawkins, J.D., Catalano, R.F., Morrison, D., O'Donnell, J., Abbott, R., and Day, E. (1992). The Seattle Social Development Project: Effects of the First Four Years on Protective Factors and Problem Behaviors. In J. McCord and R.E. Tremblay (Eds.), *Preventing Antisocial Behavior: Interventions from Birth through Adolescence* (pp. 139–161). New York: Guilford Press.

Hay, D.F., and Ross, H. (1982). The social nature of early conflict. *Child Development, 53*(1), 105–113.

Hayes-Bautista, D. (2003). Research on culturally competent health care systems: Less sensitivity, more statistics. *American Journal of Preventive Medicine, 24*(3S), 8–9.

Hayes-Bautista, D.E., Hsu, P., Hayes-Bautista, M., Iniguez, D., Chamberlin, C.L., Rico, C., and Solorio, R. (2002). An anomaly within the Latino epidemiological paradox: The Latino adolescent male mortality peak. *Archives of Pediatrics and Adolescent Medicine, 156*(5), 480–484.

Hays, R.D., Morales, L.S., and Reise, S.P. (2000). Item response theory and health outcomes measurement in the 21st century. *Medical Care, 38*(2), 28–42.

Hazuda, H.P., Stern, M.P., and Haffnen, S.M. (1988). Acculturation and assimilation among Mexican Americans: Scales and population-based data. *Social Sciences, 69,* 687–706.

Health Resources and Service Administration. (2002). *Child Health USA 2002.* Maternal and Child Health Bureau. Washington, DC: U.S. Department of Health and Human Services.

Healy, J. (1990). *Endangered minds: Why our children don't think.* New York: Simon and Schuster.

Heckman, J. (1999). *Policies to foster human capital.* (NBER Working Paper No. w7288). Cambridge, MA: National Bureau of Economic Research.

Hegarty, C.M., Jonassen, J.A., and Bittman, E.L. (1990). Influences of photoperiod and testosterone on pituitary hormone gene expression in golden hamsters. *Journal of Neuroendocrinology, 5,* 567–573.

Hendricks, T.J., Fyodorov, D.V., Wegman, L.J., Lelutiu, N.B., Pehek, E.A., Yamamoto, B., Silver, J., Weeber, E.J., Sweatt, J.D., and Deneris, E.S. (2003). Pet-1 ETS gene plays a critical role in 5-HT neuron development and is required for normal anxiety-like and aggressive behavior. *Neuron, 3*(2), 233–247.

Henkin, R.I., and Knigge, K.M. (1963). Effect of sound on hypothalamic pituitary-adrenal axis. *American Journal of Physiology, 204,* 701–704.

Herbert, T., and Cohen, S. (1993). Stress and immunity in humans: A meta-analytic review. *Psychosomatic Medicine, 55,* 364–379.

Hertzman, C. (1999). The biological embedding of early experience and its effects on health in adulthood. *Annals of the New York Academy of Sciences, 896,* 85–95.

Hertzman, C. (2000). The case for an early childhood developmental strategy. *Isuma, 1*(2), 11–18.

Hertzman, C., McLean, S.A., Kohen, D.E., Dunn, J., and Evans, T. (2002). *Early learning in Vancouver: Report of the Community Asset Mapping Project (CAMP).* Vancouver, BC: Human Early Learning Partnership (HELP), University of British Columbia.

High, P., Hopman, M., LaGasse, L., Sege, R., Moran, J., Gutierrez, C., and Becker, S. (1999) Child centered literacy orientation: A form of social capital? *Pediatrics, 103*(4), 55e.

High, P.C., LaGasse, L., Becker, S., Ahlgren, I., and Gardner, A. (2000). Literacy promotion in primary care pediatrics: Can we make a difference? *Pediatrics, 105,* 927–934.

Hilton, B.A. (1976). Quantity and quality of patients' sleep and sleep-disturbing factors in a respiratory intensive care unit. *Journal of Advanced Nursing, 1,* 453–468.

Hochbaum, G.M. (1956). Why people seek diagnostic x-rays. *Public Health Reports, 71*(4), 377–380.

Hoff-Ginsberg, E., and Tardif, T. (1995). *Socioeconomic status and parenting.* In M.H. Bornstein (Ed.), *Handbook of parenting, volume 4* (pp. 161–187). Mahwah, NJ: Lawrence Erlbaum.

Hogan, D.P., Rogers, M.L., and Msall, M.E. (2000). Functional limitations and key indicators of well-being in children with disability. *Archives of Pediatrics and Adolescent Medicine, 154*(10), 1042–1048.

Holliday, R. (1990). Genomic imprinting and allelic exclusion. *Development,* (Suppl), 125–129.

Holmberg, M. (1980). The development of social interchange patterns from 12 to 42 months. *Child Development, 51,* 448–456.

Holtzclaw, J., Clear, R., Dittmar, H., Goldstein, D., and Haas, P. (2002). Location efficiency: Neighborhood and socio-economic characteristics determine auto ownership and use-studies in Chicago, Los Angeles and San Francisco. *Transportation Planning and Technology, 25*(1), 29–48.

Holtzman, N. (2002). Genetics and social class. *Journal of Epidemiology and Community Health, 56,* 529–535.

Holtzman, N.A. (2001). Putting the search for genes in perspective. *International Journal of Health Services, 31*(2), 445–461.

Horwitz, S.M., Simms, M.D., and Farrington, R. (1994). Impact of developmental problems on young children's exits from foster care. *Journal of Developmental and Behavioral Pediatrics, 15,* 105–110.

Howes, C., and Unger, O.A. (1989). Play with peers in child care settings. In M. Bloch and A. Pelligrini (Eds.), *The ecological contexts of children's play* (pp. 104–119). Norwood, NJ: Ablex.

Huesmann, L.R., and Eron, L.D. (1986). The development of aggression in American children as a consequence of television violence viewing. In L.R. Huesmann and L.D. Eron (Eds.), *Television and the aggressive child: A cross-national comparison* (pp. 45–80). Hillsdale, NJ: Lawrence Erlbaum.

Huston, A.C., and Wright, J.C. (1997). Mass media and children's development. In W. Damon (Series Ed.), I. Siegel, and A. Remminger (Volume Eds.), *Handbook of child psychology, Vol. 4: Child psychology in practice* (pp. 999–1058). 5th Edition. New York: Wiley.

Huston, A.C., Duncan, G.J., Granger, R., Bos, J., McLoyd, V., Mistry, R., Crosby, D., Gibson, C., Magnuson, K., Romich, J., and Ventura, A. (2001). Work-based antipoverty programs for parents can enhance the school performance and social behavior of children. *Child Development, 72*(1), 318–336.

Hutchins, V.L. (1997). A history of child health and pediatrics in the United States. In R. Stein (Ed.), *Health care for children: What's right, what's wrong, what's next.* New York: United Hospital Fund.

Huttenlocher, J., Haight, W., Bryk, A., Seltzer, M., and Lyons, T. (1991). Early vocabulary growth: Relation to language input and gender. *Developmental Psychology, 27,* 236–248.

Huxley, R., Neil, A., and Collins, R. (2002). Unraveling the fetal origins hypothesis: Is there really an inverse association between birthweight and subsequent blood pressure? *Lancet, 360*(9334), 659–665.

Ingelfinger, J.R. (2003). Is microanatomy destiny? *New England Journal of Medicine, 348*(2), 99–100.

Ingelfinger, J.R., and Woods, L.L. (2002). Prenatal programming, renal development, and adult renal function. *American Journal of Hypertension, 15,* 46S–49S.

Institute of Medicine. (1988). *The future of public health.* Committee for the Study of the Future of Public Health, Division of Health Care Services. Washington, DC: National Academy Press.

Institute of Medicine. (1996). *Fetal alcohol syndrome: Diagnosis, epidemiology, prevention, and treatment.* Washington, DC: National Academy Press.

Institute of Medicine. (1997). *Improving health in the community: A role for performance monitoring.* J.S. Durch, L.A. Bailey, M.A. Stoto (Eds.), Committee on Using Performance Monitoring to Improve Community Health. Washington, DC: National Academy Press.

Institute of Medicine. (1999). *Leading health indicators for Healthy People 2010: Final report.* C.A. Chrvala and R.J. Bulger (Eds.), Committee on Leading Health Indicators for Healthy People 2010, Division of Health Promotion and Disease Prevention. Washington, DC: National Academy Press.

Institute of Medicine. (2000). *Promoting health: Intervention strategies from social and behavioral research.* Committee on Capitalizing on Social Science and Behavioral Research to Improve the Public's Health, Division of Health Promotion and Disease Prevention. Washington, DC: National Academy Press.

Institute of Medicine. (2001a). *Crossing the quality chasm: A new health system for the 21st century.* Committee on Quality of Health Care in America. Washington, DC: National Academy Press.

Institute of Medicine. (2001b). *Health and behavior: The interplay of biological, behavioral, and societal influences.* Washington, DC: National Academy Press.

Institute of Medicine. (2002a). *Fostering rapid advances in health care: Learning from system demonstrations.* J.M. Corrigan, A. Greiner, and S.M. Erickson (Eds.), Committee on Rapid Advance Demonstration Projects: Health Care Finance and Delivery Systems, Board on Health Care Services. Washington, DC: The National Academies Press.

Institute of Medicine. (2002b). *Guidance for the National Healthcare Disparities Report.* E.K. Swift, (Ed.), Committee on Guidance for Designing a National Healthcare Disparities Report, Board on Health Care Services. Washington, DC: The National Academies Press.

Institute of Medicine. (2003). *Unequal treatment: Confronting racial and ethnic disparities in health care.* B. Smedley, A. Stith, and A. Nelson (Eds.), Committee on Understanding and Eliminating Racial and Ethnic Disparities in Health Care, Board on Health Science Policy. Washington, DC: The National Academies Press.

Institute of Medicine and National Research Council. (1998). *America's children: Health insurance and access to care.* Committee on Children, Health, and Access to Care, Division of Health Care Services and Board on Children, Youth, and Families. Washington, DC: National Academy Press.

Ireys, H.T., and Perry, J.J. (1999). Development and evaluation of a satisfaction scale for parents of children with special health care needs. *Pediatrics, 104*(5), 1182–1191.

Ireys, H., Wehr, E., and Cooke, R. (1999). *Defining medical necessity: Strategies for promoting access to quality care for persons with developmental disabilities, mental retardation, and other special health care needs.* Arlington, VA: National Center for Education in Maternal and Child Health.

Ireys, H.T., Chernoff, R., DeVet, K.A., and Kim, Y. (2001). Maternal outcomes of a randomized controlled trial of a community-based support program for families of children with chronic illnesses. *Archives of Pediatrics and Adolescent Medicine, 155*(7), 771–777.

Isabella, R.A. (1995). The origins of infant-mother attachment: Maternal behavior and infant development. In R.Vasta (Ed.), *Annals of child development* (pp. 57–81). Bristol, PA: Jessica Kingsley.

Jacobson, J.L., and Jacobson, S.W. (2002). Breast-feeding and gender as moderators of teratogenic effects on cognitive development. *Neurotoxicology and Teratology, 24*(3), 349–358.

Jameson, E.J., and Wehr, E. (1994) Drafting national health care reform legislation to protect the health interests of children. *Stanford Law and Policy Review, 5*, 152–176.

Janus, M., and Offord, D. (2000). Readiness to learn at school. *Isuma, 1*(2), 71–75.

Jarrett, R.L. (1997). Bringing families back in: Neighborhood effects on child development. In J. Brooks-Gunn, G. Duncan, and J.L. Aber (Eds.), *Neighborhood poverty: Context and consequences for children* (pp. 104–138). New York: Russell Sage.

Jemmott, J.B., and Jemmott, L.S. (1994). Interventions for adolescents in community settings. In R.J. DiClemente and J.L. Peterson (Eds.), *Preventing AIDS: Theories and methods of behavioral interventions* (pp. 141–174). New York: Plenum Press.

Jensen, P., Roper, M., Fisher, P., Piacentini, J., Canino, G., Richters, J., Rubio-Stipec, M., Dulcan, M., Goodman, S., Davies, M., Rae, D., Shaffer, D., Bird, H., Lahey, B., and Schwab-Stone, M. (1995). Test-retest reliability of the Diagnostic Interview Schedule for Children (DISC-2.1), parent, child, and combined algorithms. *Archives of General Psychiatry, 52*, 61–71.

Jensen, P., Rubio-Stipec, M., Canino, G., Bird, H., Dulcan, M., Schwab-Stone, M., and Lahey, B. (1999). Parent and child contributions to child psychiatric diagnosis: Are both informants always needed? *Journal of the American Academy of Child and Adolescent Psychiatry, 38*, 1569–1579.

Jessor, R., and Jessor, S.L. (1977). *Problem behavior and psychosocial development: A longitudinal study of youth.* New York: Academic Press.

Jester, J.M., Jacobson, S.W., Sokol, R.J., Tuttle, B.S., and Jacobson, J.L. (2000). The influence of maternal drinking and drug use on the quality of the home environment of school-aged children. *Alcoholism Clinical and Experimental Research, 24*(8), 1187–1197.

Johnson, M.O. (2001). Mother-infant interaction and maternal substance use/abuse: An integrative review of research literature in the 1990s. *Online Journal of Knowledge Synthesis for Nursing, 8*(2).

Johnston, C., Rivara, F.P., and Soderberg, R. (1994). Children in car crashes: Analysis of data for injury and use of restraints. *Pediatrics, 93*(6 Pt 1), 960–965.

Kagan, J., Reznick, J.S., and Snidman, S. (1987). The physiology and psychology of behavioral inhibition in children. *Child Development, 58*(6), 1459–1473.

Kagan, J., Snidman, N., and Arcus, D. (1998). Childhood derivatives of high and low reactivity in infancy. *Child Development, 69*, 1483–1493.

Kahleova, R., Palyzova, D., Zvara, K., Zvarova, J., Hrach, K., Novakova, I., Hyanek, J., Bendlova, B., and Kozich, V. (2002). Essential hypertension in adolescents: Association with insulin resistance and with metabolism of homocysteine and vitamins. *American Journal of Hypertension, 15*(10 Pt 1), 857–864.

Kahn, R.S., Khoury, J., Nichols, W.C., and Lanphear, B.P. (2003). Role of dopamine transporter genotype and maternal prenatal smoking in childhood hyperactive-impulsive, inattentive, oppositional behaviors. *Journal of Pediatrics, 143*, 104–110.

Kajino, H., Chen, Y.Q., Seidner, S.R., Waleh, N., Mauray, F., Roman, C., Chemtob, S., Koch, C.J., and Clyman, R.I. (2001). Factors that increase the contractile tone of the ductus arteriosus also regulate its anatomic remodeling. *American Journal of Physiology. Regulatory: Integrative and Comparative Physiology, 281*(1), R291–R301.

Kam, P.C., Kam, A.C., and Thompson, J.F. (1994). Noise pollution in the anesthetic and intensive care environment. *Anesthesia, 49*, 982–986.

Karlson, T., and Noren, J. (1979). Farm tractor fatalities: The failure of voluntary safety standards. *American Journal of Public Health, 69*, 146–149.

Karoly, L.A., Greenwood, P.W., Everingham, S.S., Houbé, J., Kilburn, M.R., Rydell, C.P., Sanders, M., and Chiesa, J. (1998). *Investing in our children: What we know and don't know about the costs and benefits of early childhood interventions.* Santa Monica, CA: RAND Corporation.

Katz, L., Kling, J., and Liebman, J. (1999). *Moving to Opportunity in Boston: Early impacts of a housing mobility program.* Paper presented at the conference Neighborhood Effects on Low Income Families. Joint Center for Poverty Research, Northwestern University, University of Chicago.

Katz, L.F., Kling, J.R., and Liebman, J.B. (2001). Moving to opportunity in Boston: Early results of a randomized mobility experiment. *Quarterly Journal of Economics*, 607–654.

Katz, M.B. (1997). *In the shadow of the poorhouse: A social history of welfare in America.* New York: Basic Books.

Kauffman, K.S., Seidler, F.J., and Slotkin, T.A. (1994). Prenatal dexamethasone exposure causes loss of neonatal hypoxia tolerance: Cellular mechanisms. *Pediatric Research, 35*(5), 515–522.

Kaufman, R.H., Adam, E., Hatch, E.E., Noller, K., Herbst, A.L., Palmer, J.R., and Hoover, R.N. (2000). Continued follow-up of pregnancy outcomes in diethylstilbestrol-exposed offspring. *Obstetrics and Gynecology, 96*(4), 483–489.

Kawachi, I., Kennedy, B.P., Lochner, K., and Prothrow-Stith, D. (1997). Social capital, income inequality, and mortablity. *American Journal of Public Health, 87*(9), 1491–1498.

Keating, D., and Hertzman, C. (Eds.). (1999). *Developmental health and the wealth of nations.* New York: Guilford Press.

Keipert, J.A. (1985). The harmful effects of noise in a children's ward. *Australian Pediatric Journal, 21*(2), 101–103.

Kellem, S.G., Ensminger, M.E., and Turner, R.J. (1977). Family structure and the mental health of children: Concurrent and longitudinal community-wide studies. *Archives of General Psychiatry, 34,* 1012–1022.

Keller, G., Zimmer, G., Mall, G., Ritz, E., and Amann, K. (2003). Nephron number in patients with primary hypertension. *New England Journal of Medicine, 348*(2), 101–108.

Kendall-Tackett, K. (2002). The health effects of childhood abuse: Four pathways by which abuse can influence health. *Child Abuse and Neglect, 26*(6–7), 715–729.

Kenrick, D.T., Gutierres, S.E., and Goldberg, L.L. (1989). Influence of popular erotica on judgments of strangers and mates. *Journal of Experimental Social Psychology, 25,* 159–167.

Kessler, R., and Cleary, P.D. (1980). Social class and psychological distress. *American Sociological Review, 45,* 463–478.

Kessler, R.A. (1982). A disaggregation of the relationship between socioeconomic status and psychological distress. *American Sociological Review, 47,* 752–764.

Kiecolt-Glaser, J.K. (1999). Stress, personal relationships, and immune function: Health implications. *Brain, Behavior, and Immunity, 13,* 61–72.

Kitman, J.L. (2000, March 2). The secret history of lead. *The Nation.*

Klaus, M.H., Jerauld, R., Kreger, N.C., McAlpine, W., Steffa, M., and Kennel, J.H. (1972). Maternal attachment: Importance of the first post-partum days. *New England Journal of Medicine, 286,* 460–463.

Klebanov, P.K., Brooks-Gunn, J., and Duncan, G.J. (1994). Does neighborhood and family poverty affect mothers' parenting, mental health, and social support? *Journal of Marriage and the Family, 56*(2), 441–455.

Klepeis, N.E., Nelson, W.C., Ott, W.R., Robinson, J.P., Tsang, A.M., Switzer, P., Behar, J.V., Hern, S.C., and Engelmann, W.H. (2001). The National Human Activity Pattern Survey (NHAPS): A resource for assessing exposure to environmental pollutants. *Journal of Exposure Analysis and Environmental Epidemiology, 11*(3), 231–252.

Klesges, R.C., Shelton, M.L., and Klesges, L.M. (1993). Effects of television on metabolic rate: Potential implications for childhood obesity. *Pediatrics, 91,* 281–286.

Kline, J., Stein, Z., and Hutzler, M. (1987). Cigarettes, alcohol and marijuana: Varying associations with birthweight. *International Journal of Epidemiology, 16,* 41–51.

Klip, H., Verloop, J., van Gool, J.D., Koster, M.E., Burger, C.W., and van Leeuwen, F.E. (2002). Hypospadias in sons of women exposed to diethylstilbestrol in utero: A cohort study. *Lancet, 359,* 1102–1107.

Klopman, G., and Chakravarti, S.K. (2003). Screening of high production volume chemicals for estrogen receptor binding activity (II) by the MultiCASE expert system. *Chemosphere, 51*(6), 461–468.

Kosnett, M. (Ed.). (1990). *Case studies in environmental medicine: Arsenic toxicity.* Atlanta: U.S. Department of Health and Human Services.

Kozel, P.J., Davis, R.R., Krieg, E.F., Shull, G.E., and Erway, L.C. (2002). Deficiency in plasma membrane calcium ATPase isoform 2 increases susceptibility to noise-induced hearing loss in mice. *Hearing Research, 164*(1–2), 231–239.

Kraus, J.F., Hooten, E.G., Brown, K.A., Peed-Asa, C., Heye, C., and McArthur, D.L. (1996). Child pedestrian and bicyclist injuries: Results of community surveillance and a case-control study. *Injury Prevention, 2*(3), 212–218.

Krieger, N. (2000). Discrimination and health. In L. Berkman and I. Kawachi (Eds.), *Social epidemiology* (pp. 36–75). New York: Oxford University Press.

Krieger, N. (2003). Does racism harm health? Did child abuse exist before 1962? On explicit questions, critical science, and current controversies: An ecosocial perspective. *American Journal of Public Health, 93*(2), 194–199.

Krieger, N., Williams, D., and Moss, N. (1997). Measuring social class in U.S. public health research: Concepts, methodologies, and guidelines. *Annual Review Public Health, 18*, 341–378.

Kuhlthau, K., Walker, D.K., Perrin, J.M., Bauman, L., Gortmaker, S.L., Newacheck, P.W., and Stein, R.E.K. (1998). Assessment of managed care for children with chronic conditions. *Health Affairs, 17*, 42–52.

Kunitz, S.J. (2002). Holism and the idea of general susceptibility to disease. *International Journal of Epidemiology, 31*(4), 722–729.

Kuo, M., Mohler, B., Raudenbush, S.L., and Earls, F.J. (2000). Assessing exposure to violence using multiple informants: Application of hierarchical linear model. *Journal of Child Psychology and Psychiatry, 41*(8), 1049–1056.

Kupersmidt, J., and Coie, J.D. (1990). Preadolescent peer status, aggression, and school adjustment as predictors of externalizing problems in adolescence. *Child Development, 61*(5), 1350–1362.

Kuttner, M.J., Delamater, A.M., and Santiago, J.V. (1990). Learned helplessness in diabetic youths. *Journal of Pediatric Psychology, 15*, 581–594.

Kyngas, HA. (1999). Compliance of adolescents with asthma. *Nursing and Health Sciences, 1*(3), 195–202.

Kyngas, H.A., Kroll, T., and Duffy, M.E. (2000). Compliance in adolescents with chronic diseases: A review. *Journal of Adolescent Health, 26*(6), 379–388.

Kyngas, H. (2001). Predictors of good compliance in adolescents with epilepsy. *Seizure, 10*(8), 548–553.

La Greca, A.M., and Bearman, K.J. (2002). The diabetes social support questionnaire—Family version: Evaluating adolescents' diabetes-specific support from family members. *Journal of Pediatric Psychology, 27*(8), 665–676.

La Greca, A.M., Bearman, K.J., and Moore, H. (2002). Peer relations of youth with pediatric conditions and health risks: Promoting social support and healthy lifestyles. *Journal of Developmental and Behavioral Pediatrics, 23*(4), 271–280.

Laframboise, H.L. (1973). Health policy: Breaking the problem down into more manageable segments. *Canadian Medical Association Journal, 108*, 388–393.

LaFramboise, T., Coleman, H.L.K., and Gerton, J. (1993). Psychological impact of biculturalism: Evidence and theory. *Psychological Bulletin, 114*, 395–412.

LaFreniere, P.J., and Sroufe, L.A. (1985). Profiles of peer competence in the preschool: Interrelations between measures, influence of social ecology, and relations to attachment history. *Developmental Psychology, 21*, 56–69.

Lagasse, L.L., Seifer, R., and Lester, B.M. (1999). Interpreting research on prenatal substance exposure in the context of multiple confounding factors. *Clinics in Perinatology, 26*(1), 39–54.

Lai, T.J., Liu, X., Guo, Y.L., Guo, N.W., Yu, M.L., Hsu, C.C., and Rogan W.J. (2002). A cohort study of behavioral problems and intelligence in children with high prenatal polychlorinated biphenyl exposure. *Archives of General Psychiatry, 59*(11), 1061–1066.

Lamberts, H., Wood, M., and Hofmans-Okkes, I.M. (1993). *The international classification of primary care in the European community: With a multi-language layer.* Oxford: Oxford University Press.

Lane, H., and Bahan, B. (1998). Ethics of cochlear implantation in young children: A review and reply from a deaf-world perspective. *Otolaryngology and Head and Neck Surgery, 119*(4), 297–313.

Lanphear, B.P., Dietrich, K.N., and Berger, O. (2003). Prevention of lead toxicity in U.S. children. *Ambulatory Pediatrics, 3*(1), 27–36.

Lantz, P.M., House, J.S., Lepkowski, J.M., Williams, D.R., Mero, R.P., and Chen, J. (1998). Socioeconomic factors, health behaviors, and mortality: Results from a nationally representative prospective study of U.S. adults. *Journal of the American Medical Association, 279*(21), 1703–1780.

Laosa, L. (1980). Maternal teaching strategies in Chicano and Anglo-American families: The influence of culture and education on maternal behavior. *Child Development, 51,* 759–765.

Lapidge, K.L., Oldroyd, B.P., and Spivak, M. (2002). Seven suggestive quantitative trait loci influence hygienic behavior of honey bees. *Naturwissenschaften, 89*(12), 565–568.

Larson, L.E. (1974). An examination of the salience hierarchy during adolescence: The influence of the family. *Adolescence, 35,* 317–332.

Lawler, K.A., Younger, J., Piferi, R.A., Jones, W.H. (2000). *A physiological profile of forgiveness.* Paper presented at the annual meeting of the Society for Behavioral Medicine, Nashville, TN.

Layde, P.M., Maas, L.A, Teret, S.P., Brasel, K.J., Kuhn, E.M., Mercy, J.A., Hargarten, S.W., and Maas, L.A. (2002). Patient safety efforts should focus on medical injuries. *Journal of American Medical Association, 287*(15), 1993–1997.

Leaderer, B.P. (1990). Assessing exposures to environmental tobacco smoke. *Risk Analysis, 10,* 19–26.

Lesko, S.M., Corwin, M.J., Vezina, R.M., Hunt, C.E., Mandell, F., McClain, M., Heeren, T., and Mitchell, A.A. (1998). Changes in sleep position during infancy: A prospective longitudinal assessment. *Journal of American Medical Association, 280*(4), 336–340.

Levine, M., and Levine, A. (1992). *Helping children: A social history.* Oxford: Oxford University Press.

LeVine, R.A. (1977). Child rearing as cultural adaptation. In P.H. Leiderman, S. Tulkin, and A. Rosenfeld (Eds.), *Culture and infancy: Variations in the human experience* (pp. 15–27). New York: Academic Press.

Leyden, K.M. (2003). Social capital and the built environment: The importance of walkable neighborhoods. *American Journal of Public Health, 93*(9).

Li, X., Stanton, B., and Feigelman, S. (2000). Impact of perceived parental monitoring on adolescent risk behavior over 4 years. *Journal of Adolescent Health, 27,* 49–56.

Liabo, K., Lucas, P., and Roberts, H. (2003). Can traffic calming measures achieve the Children's Fund objective of reducing inequalities in child health? *Archives of Disease in Childhood, 88,* 235–236.

Lightstone, A.S., Dhillon, P.K., Peek-Asa, C., and Kraus, J.F. (2001). A geographic analysis of motor vehicle collisions with child pedestrians in Long Beach, California: Comparing intersection and midblock incident locations. *Injury Prevention, 7*(2), 155–160.

Liss, D.S., Waller, D.A., Kennard, B.D., McIntire, D., Capra, P., and Stephens, J. (1998). Psychiatric illness and family support in children and adolescents with diabetic ketoacidosis: A controlled study. *Journal of American Academy of Child and Adolescent Psychiatry, 37*(5), 536–544.

Lohr, K.N., Aaronson, N., Alonso, J., Burnam, A., Patrick, D., Perrin, E., and Stein, R. (2002). Assessing health status and quality-of-life instruments: Attributes and review criteria. *Quality of Life Research, 11,* 193–205.

Long, N., Starfield, B., and Kelleher, K. (1994). Childhood co-morbidity of psychiatric disorders in pediatric primary care. In J. Miranda, A. Hohmann, C. Attkisson, and D. Larson (Eds.), *Mental disorders in primary care.* San Francisco, CA: Jossey-Bass.

LoSasso, A.T., and Buchmueller, C. (2002). *The effect of the State Children's Health Insurance Program on health insurance coverage.* (NBER Working Paper No. 9405). Cambridge, MA: National Bureau of Economic Research.

Lowe, J.B., McDermott, L.J., Stanton, W.R., Clavarino, A., Balanda, K.P., and McWhirter, B. (2002). Behavior of caregivers to protect their infants from exposure to the sun in Queensland, Australia. *Health Education Research, 17*(4), 405–414.

Lowry, R., Wechsler, H., Kann, L., and Collins, J.L. (2001). Recent trends in participation in physical education among US high school students. *Journal of School Health, 71*(4), 145–152.

Lozoff, B. (1989). Nutrition and behavior. *American Psychologist, 44*(2), 231–236.

Lu, M.C., and Halfon, N. (2003). Racial and ethnic disparities in birth outcomes: A life course perspective. *Maternal and Child Health Journal, 7*(1), 13–30.

Lucas, A., Fewtrell, M.S., and Cole, T.J. (1999). Fetal origins of adult disease: The hypothesis revisited. *British Medical Journal, 319*(7204), 245–249.

Lukens, J.N. (1987). The legacy of well-water methemoglobinemia. *Journal of the American Medical Association, 257*, 2793–2795.

Lunt, T.F., Denning, D.E., Schell, R.R., Heckman, M., and Shockley, W.R. (1990). The SeaView Security Model. *IEEE Transactions on Software Engineering, 16*(6), 593–607.

Luttenbacher, M. (2002). Relationships between psychosocial factors and abusive parental attitudes in low-income single mothers. *Nursing Research, 51*(3), 158–167.

Macciardi, F., Morenghi, E., and Morabito, A. (1999). Alcoholism as a complex trait: Comparison of genetic models and role of epidemiological risk factors. *Genetic Epidemiology, 17*(1), S247–S252.

MacDorman, M.F., Minino, A.M., Strobino, D.M., and Guyer, B. (2002). Annual summary of vital statistics. *Pediatrics, 110*(6), 1037–1052.

Mack, K.J., and Mack, P.A. (1992). Induction of transcription factors in somatosensory cortex after tactile stimulation. *Molecular Brain Research, 12*, 141–147.

Magnuson, K., and McGroder, S. (2002). *The effect of increasing welfare mothers' education on their young children's academic problems and school readiness.* (JCPR Working Paper 280). Evanston, IL: Insitute for Policy Research.

Malamuth, N.M., and Impett, E.A. (2001). Research on sex in the media: What do we know about effects on children and adolescents? In D.G. Singer and J.L. Singer (Eds.), *Handbook of children and the media* (pp. 269–287). Thousand Oaks, CA: Sage.

Mallett, R., Leff, J., Bhugra, D., Pang, D., and Zhao, J.H. (2002). Social environment, ethnicity and schizophrenia: A case-control study. *Society for Psychiatry and Psychiatric Epidemiology, 37*(7), 329–335.

Malmstron, M., Sundquist, J., and Johansson, S.E. (1999). Neighborhood environment and self-reported health status: A multilevel analysis. *American Journal of Public Health, 89*(8), 1181–1186.

Manitoba Centre for Health Policy. (2002). Improving children's health: How population-based research can inform policy. *Canadian Journal of Public Health, 93*(2).

Manne, S.L. (1998). Treatment adherence and compliance. In R.T. Ammerman and J.V. Campo (Eds.), *Handbook of pediatric psychology and psychiatry* (pp. 103–132). Boston: Allyn and Bacon.

Manski, C. (1993). Identification of endogenous social effects: The reflection problem. *Review of Economic Studies, 60*, 531–542.

Manuel, J. (1999). A healthy home environment? *Environmental Health Perspectives, 107*(7), A352–A357.

Markides, K.S., and Coreil, J. (1986). The health of Hispanics in the southwestern United States: An epidemiologic paradox. *Public Health Reports, 101*(3), 253–265.

Marmot, M. (1999). Epidemiology of socioeconomic status and health: Are determinants within countries the same as between countries? In N. Adler, M. Marmot, B. McEwen, and J. Stewart (Eds.), *Socioeconomic status and health in industrial nations: Social, psychological, and biological pathways.* New York: New York Academy of Sciences.

Marmot, M.G., and Syme, S.L. (1976). Acculturation and coronary heart disease in Japanese-Americans. *American Journal Epidemiology, 104*(3), 225–247.

Marmot, M.G., Shipley, M.J., and Rose, O. (1984). Inequalities in death: Specific explanations of a general pattern. *Lancet, 1*, 1003–1006.

Marmot, M.G., Ryff, C., Bumpass, L., Sipley, M.J., and Marks, N.F. (1997). Social inequalities in health: Next questions and converging evidence. *Social Science and Medicine, 44*, 901–910.

Martin, J.A., Hamilton, B.E., Ventura, S.J., Menacker, F., and Park, M.M. (2002). Births: Final data for 2000. *National Vital Statistics Reports, 50*(5).

Martinez, G.M., and Day, J.C. (1999). *Current population reports: School-enrollment—social and economic characteristics of students, October 1997.* Washington, DC: U.S. Census Bureau.

Martinez, P., and Richters, J.E. (1993). The NIMH community violence project II: Children's distress symptoms associated with violence exposure. *Psychiatry, 56*(1), 22–35.

Matalon, S., and O'Brodovich, H. (1999). Sodium channels in alveolar epithelial cells: Molecular characterization, biophysical properties, and physiological significance. *Annual Review of Physiology, 61*, 627–661.

Matheson, M.P., Stansfeld, S.A., and Haines, M.M. (2003). The effects of chronic aircraft noise exposure on children's cognition and health: 3 field studies. *Noise and Health, 5*(19), 31–40.

McAdoo, H.P. (1981). Upward mobility and parenting in middle-income black families. *Journal of Black Psychology, 8*(1), 1–22.

McEwen, B.S. (1998). Stress, adaptation, and disease: Allostasis and allostatic load. *Annals of the New York Academy of Sciences, 840*, 33–44.

McGauhey, P.J., and Starfield, B. (1993). Child health and the social environment of white and black children. *Social Science Medicine, 36*(7), 867–874.

McGauhey, P.J., Starfield, B., Alexander, C., and Ensminger, M.E. (1991). Social environment and vulnerability of low birth weight children: A social-epidemiological perspective. *Pediatrics, 88*(5), 943–953.

McGinnis, J.M., and Foege, W.H. (1999). Mortality and morbidity attributable to use of addictive substances in the United States. *Proceedings of the Association of American Physicians, 111*(2), 109–118.

McGinnis, J.M., Williams-Russo, P., and Knickman, J.R. (2002). The case for more active policy attention to health promotion. *Health Affairs, 21*(2), 78–93.

McGinnis, M., and Foege, W. (1993). Actual causes of death in the United States. *Journal of the American Medical Association, 270*, 2207–2212.

McGue, M., Iacono, W.G., Legrand, L.N., and Elkins, I. (2001). Origins and consequences of age at first drink. II: Familial risk and heritability. *Alcoholism Clinical and Experimental Research, 25*(8), 1166–1173.

McKenzie, K. (2003). Racism and health. *British Medical Journal, 326*, 65–66.

McKenzie, T.L., Marshall, S.J., Sallis, J.F., and Conway, T.L. (2000). Student activity levels, lesson context, and teacher behavior during middle school physical education. *Research Quarterly for Exercise and Sport, 71*(3), 249–259.

McKenzie-Mohr, D., and Zanna, M. (1990). Treating women as sexual objects: Look to the (gender schematic) male who has viewed pornography. *Personality and Social Psychology Bulletin, 16*, 296–308.

McLanahan, S., and Sandefur, G. (1994). *Growing up with a single parent: What hurts, what helps.* Cambridge, MA: Harvard University Press.

Mcleod J.D., and Kessler, R. (1990). Socioeconomic status differences in vulnerability to undesirable life events. *Journal of Health and Social Behavior, 31*, 162–172.

McMurray, R.G., Harrel, J.S., Deng, S., Bradley, C.B., Cox, L.M., and Bangdiwala, S.I. (2000). The influence of physical activity, socioeconomic status, and ethnicity on the weight status of adolescents. *Obesity Research, 8*, 130–139.

McQuaid, E.L., Kopel, S.J., Klein, R.B., and Fritz, G.K. (2003). Medication adherence in pediatric asthma: Reasoning, responsibility, and behavior. *Journal of Pediatric Psychology, 28*, 323–333.

Mehler, J., Bertoncini, J., and Barriere, M. (1978). Infant recognition of mother's voice. *Perception, 7*, 491–497.

Mendoza, F.S., Takata, G.S., and Martorell, R. (1994). Health status and health care access for mainland Puerto Rican children: Results from the Hispanic Health and Nutrition Examination Survey. In G. Lamberty and C. Garcia Coll (Eds.), *Puerto Rican women and children: Issues in health, growth, and development* (pp. 211–227). New York: Plenum Press.

Miller, H. (1997). Prenatal cocaine exposure and mother-infant interaction: Implications for occupational therapy intervention. *American Journal of Occupational Therapy, 51*(2), 119–131.

Milunsky, A. (1992). Maternal heat exposure and neural tube defects. *Journal of American Medical Association, 68*, 882.

Milyo, J., and Millar, J. (2002). Income inequality and health status in the United States: Evidence from the Current Population Survey. *Journal of Human Resources, 37*(3), 510–539.

Mohamed, E.I., Linder, R., Perriello, G., Di Daniele, N., Poppl, S.J., and De Lorenzo, A. (2002). Predicting type 2 diabetes using an electronic nose-based artificial neural network analysis. *Diabetes, Nutrition and Metabolism, 15*(4), 215–221.

Moll, L.C., Amanti, C., Neff, D., and Gonzalez, N. (1992). Funds of knowledge for teaching: Using a qualitative approach to connect homes and classrooms. *Theory into Practice. 31*(2), 132–141.

Moore, K.T., Halle, T., Vandivere, S., and Mariner, C. (2002). Scaling back survey scales: How short is too short? *Sociological Methods and Research, 30*(4), 530–567.

Morales, L.S., Lara, M., Kington, R.S., Valdez, R.O., and Escarce, J.J. (2002). Socioeconomic, cultural, and behavioral factors affecting Hispanic health outcomes. *Journal of Health Care for the Poor and Underserved, 13*(4), 477–503.

Morland, K., Wing, S., Diex Roux, A., and Poole, C. (2002). Neighborhood characteristics associated with the location of food stores and food service places. *American Journal of Preventive Medicine, 22*, 23–29.

Morris, P.A., Huston, A.C., Duncan, G.J., Crosby, D.A., and Bos, J.M. (2001). *How welfare and work policies affect children: A synthesis of research.* New York: Manpower Demonstration Research Corporation.

Morrison, F.J., Griffith, E.M., and Alberts, D.M. (1997). Nature-nurture in the classroom: Entrance age, school readiness, and learning in children. *Developmental Psychology, 33*, 254–262.

Morrongiello, B.A., Midgett, C., and Shields, R. (2001). Don't run with scissors: Young children's knowledge of home safety rules. *Journal of Pediatric Psychology, 26*(2), 105–115.

Moy, J.A. (2003). Cultural aspects in the treatment of patients with skin disease. *Dermatologic Clinics, 21*(4), 733–742.

Msall, M.E., DiGaudio, K., Rogers, B.T., LaForest, S, Catanzaro, N.L., Cambell, J., Wilczenski, F., and Duffy, L.C. (1994). Functional Independence Measure for Children (Wee-FIM). Conceptual basis and pilot use in children with developmental disabilities. *Clinical Pediatrics, 33*(7), 421–430.

Mueller, E., and Silverman, N. (1989). Peer relations in maltreated children. In D. Cicchetti and V. Carlson (Eds.), *Child maltreatment: Theory and research on the causes and consequences of child abuse and neglect* (pp. 529–578). New York: Cambridge University Press.

Muronzomi, M., Chow, T.J., and Patterson, C. (1969). Chemical concentrations of pollutant lead aerosols, terrestrial dusts and sea salts in Greenland and Antartic snow strata. *Geochimica et Cosmochimica Acta, 33*, 1247.

Murphy, D.A., Wilson, C.M., Durako, S.J., Muenz, L.R., Belzer, M. (2001). Adolescent Medicine HIV/AIDS Research Network. Antiretroviral medication adherence among the REACH HIV-infected adolescent cohort in the USA. *AIDS Care, 13*(1), 27–40.

Murphy, J.M. (1998). Child passenger safety. *Journal of Pediatric Health Care, 12*(3), 130–138.

Murray, C.J., and Lopez, A.D. (1996). Evidence-based health policy—Lessons from the Global Burden of Disease Study. *Science, 274*(5288), 740–743.

Nathanielsz, P.W. (1999). *Life in the womb: The origin of health and disease.* Ithaca, NY: Promethean Press.

National Center for Health Statistics. (2002a). *National Survey of Early Childhood Health 2000.* Hyattsville, MD: Centers for Disease Control and Prevention. Available: http://www.cdc.gov/nchs/about/major/slaits/nsech.htm. [Accessed January 1, 2004].

National Center for Health Statistics. (2002b). *Prevalence of overweight among children and adolescents: United States, 1999–2000.* Available: http://www.cdc.gov/nchs/products/pubs/pubd/hestats/overwght99.htm.

National Center for Health Statistics. (2004). Deaths: Injuries, 2001. R.N. Anderson, A.M. Minino, L.A. Fingerhut, M. Warner, and M.A. Heinen. *National Vital Statistics Reports, 52*(21). Available: http://www.cdc.gov/nchs/data/nvsr/nvsr52/nvsr52_21acc.pdf.

National Education Goals Panel. (1997). *Getting a good start in school.* Washington, DC: Author.

National Highway Traffic Safety Administration. (2001). *Traffic safety facts 2000: A compilation of motor vehicle crash data from the fatality analysis reporting system and the general estimates system.* Washington, DC: U.S. Department of Transportation.

National Institute of Justice. (1989). *Drug use forecasting (DUF) fourth quarter: 1988* (pp. 6–7). Washington, DC: U.S. Department of Justice.

National Research Council. (1984). Ecocultural niches of middle childhood: A cross-cultural perspective. T.S. Weisner. In W.A. Collins (Ed.), *Development during middle childhood: The years from six to twelve.* Committee on Child Development Research and Public Policy. Washington, DC: National Academy Press.

National Research Council. (1989). *Biological Markers in Reproductive Toxicology.* Subcommittee on Reproductive and Neurodevelopmental Toxicology, Committee on Biologic Markers, Board on Environmental Studies and Toxicology. Washington, DC: National Academy Press.

National Research Council. (1990). The social consequences of growing up in a poor neighborhood. C. Jencks and S.E. Mayer. In L.E. Lynn and M.G.H. McGeary (Eds.), *Inner-City Poverty in the United States* (pp. 111–186). Committee on National Urban Policy. Washington, DC: National Academy Press.

National Research Council. (1993). *Pesticides in the diets of infants and children.* Committee on Pesticides in the Diets of Infants and Children, Board on Agriculture and Board on Environmental Studies and Toxicology, Commission on Life Sciences. Washington, DC: National Academy Press.

National Research Council. (2000). *Toxicological effects of methylmercury.* Committee on the Toxicological Effects of Methylmercury, Board on Environmental Studies and Toxicology, Commission on Life Sciences. Washington, DC: National Academy Press.

National Research Council. (2001). *New horizons in health: An integrative approach.* Committee on Future Directions for Behavioral and Social Sciences Research at the National Institutes of Health, B.H. Singer and C.D. Ryff (Eds.). Washington, DC: National Academy Press.

National Research Council. (2004). *Measuring Racial Discrimination.* Panel on Methods for Assessing Discrimination. R.M. Blank, M. Dabady, and C.F. Citro (Eds.). Washington, DC: The National Academies Press.

National Research Council Committee on Biological Markers. (1987). Biological markers in environmental health research. *Environmental Health Perspectives, 74,* 3–9.

National Research Council and Institute of Medicine. (1995a). *Integrating federal statistics on children: Report of a workshop.* Committee on National Statistics and Board on Children and Families, Commission on Behavioral and Social Sciences and Education. Washington, DC: National Academy Press.

National Research Council and Institute of Medicine. (1995b). Child development in the context of family and community resources: An agenda for national data collections. J. Brooks-Gunn, B. Brown, G.J. Duncan, and K.A. Moore. In *Integrating federal statistics on children: Report of a workshop.* Committee on National Statistics and Board on Children and Families, Commission on Behavioral and Social Sciences and Education. Washington, DC: National Academy Press.

National Research Council and Institute of Medicine. (2000). *From neurons to neighborhoods. The science of early childhood development.* Committee on Integrating the Science of Early Childhood Development, J.P. Shonkoff and D.A. Phillips (Eds.). Washington, DC: National Academy Press.

National Research Council and Institute of Medicine. (2001). Vulnerability, risk, and protection. R.W. Blum, C. McNeely, and J. Nonnemaker. In B. Fischhoff, E.O. Nightingale, and J.G. Iannotta (Eds.), *Adolescent risk and vulnerability: Concepts and measures.* Board on Children, Youth, and Families. Washington, DC: National Academy Press.

National Research Council and Institute of Medicine. (2003). *Working families and growing kids: Caring for children and adolescents.* Committee on Family and Work Policies. E. Smolinsky and J. Gootman (Eds.). Board on Children, Youth, and Families, Division of Behavioral and Social Sciences and Education. Washington, DC: The National Academies Press.

National Research Council and Social Science Research Council. (1993). *Private lives and public policies: Confidentiality and accessibility of government statistics.* Panel on Confidentiality and Data Access, G.T. Duncan, T.B. Jabine, and V.A. de Wolf (Eds.). Washington, DC: National Academy Press.

Nazroo, J. (2003). The structuring of ethnic inequalities in health: Economic position, racial discrimination, and racism. *American Journal of Public Health, 93,* 277–284.

Needleman, H.L., McFarland, C., Ness, R.B., Fienberg, S.E., and Tobin, M.J. (2002). Bone lead levels in adjudicated delinquents. A case control study. *Neurotoxicology Teratology, 24*(6), 711–717.

Newacheck, P., and Halfon, N. (1998). Prevalence and impact of disabling childhood chronic conditions. *American Journal of Public Health, 88*(4), 610–617.

Newacheck, P., Stein, R., Bauman, L., and Hung, Y. (2003). Disparities in the prevalence of disability between black and white children. *Archives of Pediatrics and Adolescent Medicine, 157*(3), 244–248.

Newacheck, P.W., Stein, R.E.K., Walker, D.K., Gortmaker, S.L., Kuhlthau, K., and Perrin, J.M. (1996). Monitoring and evaluating managed care for children with chronic illnesses and disabilities. *Pediatrics, 98*(5), 952–958.

Newacheck, P.W., Hung, Y.Y., and Wright, K.K. (2002). Racial and ethnic disparities in access to care for children with special health care needs. *Ambulatory Pediatrics, 2*(4), 247–254.

Newbrun, E. (1989). Effectiveness of water fluoridation. *Journal of Public Health Dentistry, 49,* 279–289.

Nicholl, J.P. (1989). Epidemiology of babies dying at different ages from the sudden infant death syndrome. *Journal of Epidemiology and Community Health, 43,* 133.

Nichols, T.R., Graber, J.A., Brooks-Gunn, J., and Botvin, G.J. (2004). Maternal influences on smoking initiation among urban adolescent girls. *Journal of Research on Adolescence, 14*(1), 73–97.

Niskar, A.S., Kieszak, S.M., Holmes, A.E., Esteban, E., Rubin, C., and Brody, D.J. (2001). Estimated prevalence of noise-induced hearing threshold shifts among children 6 to 19 years of age: The Third National Health and Nutrition Examination Survey, 1988–1994, United States. *Pediatrics, 108*(1), 40–43.

Nordio, S. (1978). Needs in child and maternal care: Rational utilization and social-medical resources. *Rivista Italiana di Pediatria, 4,* 3–20.

Nuñez, A.E., and Taft, M.L. (1985). A chemical burn simulating child abuse. *American Journal of Forensic Medicine and Pathology, 6,* 181–183.

O'Connor, M.J., Kogan, N., and Findlay, R. (2002). Prenatal alcohol exposure and attachment behavior in children. *Alcoholism: Clinical and Experimental Research, 26*(10):1592–1602.

Odegaard, G., Lindbladh, E., and Hovelius, B. (2003). Children who suffer from headaches—A narrative of insecurity in school and family. *The British Journal of General Practice, 53*(488), 210–213.

Ogbu, J.U. (2003). *Black American students in an affluent suburb: A study of academic disengagement.* Mahwah, NJ: Lawrence Erlbaum Associates.

Olds, D.L., and Kitzman, H. (1993). Review of research on home visiting for pregnant women and parents of young children. *Future of Children, 3*(3), 53–92.

Olds, D.L., Eckenrode, J.J., Henderson, C.R., Jr., Kitzman, H., Powers, J., Cole, R., Sidora, K., Morris, P., Pettitt, L.M., and Luckey, D. (1997). Long-term effects of home visitation on maternal life course and child abuse and neglect: Fifteen-year followup of a randomized trial. *Journal of the American Medical Association, 278*(8), 637–643.

Olds, D.L., Henderson, C.R., Jr., Kitzman, H., Eckenrode, J.J., Cole, R., Tatelbaum, R., Robinson, J., Pettitt, L.M., O'Brien, R., and Hill, P. (1998). Prenatal and infancy home visitation by nurses: A program of research. In C. Rovee-Collier, L.P. Lipsitt, and H. Hayne (Eds.), *Advances in infancy research, volume 12* (pp. 79–130). Stamford, CT: Ablex.

Olds, D.L., Henderson, C.R., Jr., Kitzman, H., Eckenrode, J.J., Cole, R.E., and Tatelbaum, R. (1999). Prenatal and infancy home visitation by nurses: Recent findings. *Future of Children: Home Visiting: Recent Program Evaluations, 9*(1), 44–65.

Omar, H., Fowler, A., and D'Angelo, S. (2002). Improved continuation rate of depot-medroxyprogesterone acetate in adolescent mothers. *International Journal of Adolescent Medicine and Health, 14*(2), 149–152.

Ong, C.N., Phoon, W.O., Law, H.Y., Tye, C.Y., and Lim, H.H. (1985). Concentrations of lead in maternal blood, cord blood, and breast milk. *Archives of Diseases in Childhood, 60,* 756–759.

ORC Macro. (2000). *Evaluation of state-based integrated health information systems.* Report sponsored by the Centers for Disease Control and Prevention, Epidemiology Program Office. Atlanta: Author.

Organisation for Economic Cooperation and Development. (2002). *Table 2: Infant mortality, deaths per 1000 live births: Health data 2002.* Available: http://www.oecd.org/xls/M00031000/M00031359.xls.

Orr, L., Feins, J., Jacob, R., Beecroft, E., Sanbonmatsu, L., Katz, L.F., Liebman, J.B., and Kling, J.R. (2003). *Moving to opportunity: Interim impacts evaluation.* Washington, DC: U.S. Department of Housing and Urban Development.

Osofsky, J.D., Wewers, S., Hann, D.M., and Fick, A.C. (1993). Chronic community violence: What is happening to our children? *Psychiatry, 56*(1), 36–45.

Ott, J., Greening, L., Palardy, N., Holderby, A., and DeBell, W.K. (2000). Self-efficacy as a mediator variable for adolescents' adherence to treatment for insulin-dependent diabetes mellitus. *Children's Health Care, 29*(1), 47–63.

Ottawa Charter for Health Promotion. (1986). *First International Conference on Health Promotion.* Presented on November 21, 1986. Available: http://www.who.int/hpr/NPH/docs/ottawa_charter_hp.pdf. [Accessed December 30, 2003].

Ownby, D.R., Johnson, C.C., and Peterson, E.L. (2002). Exposure to dogs and cats in the first year of life and risk of allergic sensitization at 6 to 7 years of age. *Journal of the American Medical Association, 288*(8), 963–972.

Paik, H., and Comstock, G. (1994). The effects of television violence on antisocial behavior: A meta-analysis. *Communication Research, 24,* 516–546.

Pastor, D.L. (1981). The quality of mother-infant attachment and its relationship to toddlers: Initial sociability with peers. *Developmental Psychology, 17,* 326–335.

Patterson, C., Ericson, J., Manea-Krichten, M., and Shirahata, H. (1991). Natural skeletal levels of lead in homo sapiens: Sapiens uncontaminated by technological lead. *Science of the Total Environment, 107.*

Patterson, G.R. (1982). *Coercive family process: A social learning approach.* (Vol. 3). Eugene, OR: Castalia.

Patterson, G.R. (1995). Coercion as a basis for early age of onset for arrest. In J. McCord (Ed.), *Coercion and punishment in long-term perspectives* (pp. 81–105). New York: Cambridge University Press.

Patterson, G.R., and Fisher, P.A. (2002). Recent developments in our understanding of parenting: Bidirectional effects, causal models, and the search for parsimony. In M. Bornstein (Ed.), *Handbook of parenting: Practical issues in parenting*. Second Edition, Volume 5. Mahwah, NJ: Lawrence Erlbaum.

Patterson, G.R., and Stouthamer-Loeber, M. (1984). The correlation of family management practices and delinquency. *Child Development, 55*, 1299–1307.

Patterson, G.R., Capaldi, D.M., and Bank, L. (1991). An early starter model for predicting delinquency. In D.J. Pepler and K.H. Rubin (Eds.), *The development and treatment of childhood aggression* (pp. 139–168). Hillsdale, NJ: Erlbaum.

Patterson, G.R., Reid, J., and Dishion, T. (1992). *Antisocial boys*. Eugene, OR: Castalia.

Pearlin, L.I., and Schooler C. (1978). The structure of coping. *Journal of Health and Social Behavior, 19*, 2–21.

Perdue, W.C., Stone, L.A., and Gostin, L.O. (2003). The built environment and its relationship to the public's health: The legal framework. *American Journal of Public Health, 93*(9), 1390–1394.

Perera, F.P., Mooney, L.A., and Stampfer, M. et al. (2002). Associations between carcinogen-DNA damage, glutathione S-transferase genotypes, and risk of lung cancer in the prospective Physicians' Health Cohort Study. *Carcinogenesis, 23*(10), 1641–1646.

Perrin, J.M., Kuhlthau, K., Walker, D.K., Stein, R.E.K., Newacheck, P.W., and Gortmaker, S.L. (1997). Monitoring health care for children with chronic conditions in a managed care environment. *Maternal and Child Health Journal, 1*, 15–23.

Perry, C.L., and Silvis, G.L. (1987). Smoking prevention: Behavioral prescriptions for the pediatrician. *Pediatrics, 79*, 790–799.

Pettit, G.S. (1997). The developmental course of violence and aggression. *Psychiatric Clinics of North America, 20*(2), 283–299.

Philadelphia Safe and Sound. (2001). *Report Card 2001: The well-being of children and youth in Philadelphia*. Philadelphia: Philadelphia Coalition for Kids.

Pillow, B., Hill, V., Boyce, A., and Stein, C. (2000) Understanding inference as a source of knowledge: Children's ability to evaluate the certainty of deduction, perception, and guessing. *Developmental Psychology, 36*(2), 169–179.

Pitt, R., Guyer, B., Hsieh, C.C., and Malek, M. (1990). The severity of pedestrian injuries in children: An analysis of the Pedestrian Injury Causation Study. *Accident Analysis and Prevention, 22*(6), 549–559.

Pluim, H.J., Koppe, J.G., Olie, K., van-der-Slikke, J.W., Slot, P.C., and van-Boxtel, C.J. (1994). Clinical laboratory manifestations of exposure to background levels of dioxins in the perinatal period. *Acta Paediatrica, 83*, 583–587.

Politzer, R.M., Yoon, J., Shi, L., Hughes, R.G., Regan, J., and Gaston, M.H. (2001). Inequality in America: The contribution of health centers in reducing and eliminating disparities in access to care. *Medical Care Research and Review, 58*(2), 234–248.

Pollack, H.A., and Frohna, J.G. (2002). Infant sleep placement after the back to sleep campaign. *Pediatrics, 109*(4), 608–614.

Pollack, S.H., Landrigan, P.H., and Mallino, D.L. (1990). Child labor in 1990: Prevalence and health hazards. *Annual Reviews in Public Health, 11*, 359–375.

Portes, A., and Rumbaut, R. (2001). *Legacies: The story of the immigrant second generation*. Berkley: University of California Press.

Posner, J.C., Liao, E., Winston, F.K., Cnaan, A., Shaw, K.N., and Durbin, D.R. (2002). Exposure to traffic among urban children injured as pedestrians. *Injury Prevention, 8*(3), 231–235.

Public Health Policy Advisory Board. (May 1999). *Health and the American child: Part 1: A focus on mortality among children: Risks, trends, and priorities for the twenty-first century*. Washington, DC: Author.

Purugganan, O.H., Stein, R.E.K., Silver, E.J., and Benenson, B.S. (2000). Exposure to violence among urban school-aged children: Is it only on television? *Pediatrics, 106*(4), 949–953.

Pynoos, R.S., Frederick, C., Nader, K., Arroyo, W., Steinberg, A., Eth, S., Nunez, F., and Fairbanks, L. (1987). Life threat and posttraumatic stress in school-age children. *Archives of General Psychiatry, 44*(12), 1057–1063.

Radziszewka, B., Richardson, J.L., Dent, C.W., and Flay, B.R. (1993). Parenting style and adolescent depressive symptoms, smoking and academic achievement: Ethnic, gender and class differences. *Journal of Behavioral Medicine, 19,* 289–305.

Ramey, C.T., Bryant, D.M, Wasik, B.H., Sparling, J.J., Fendt, K.H., and LaVange, L.M. (1992). Infant Health and Development Program for low birth weight, premature infants: Program elements, family participation, and child intelligence. *Pediatrics, 89*(3), 454–465.

Rao, R., and Georgieff, M.K. (2001). Neonatal iron nutrition. *Seminars in Neonatology, 6*(5), 425–435.

Rao, R., Hawkins, M., and Guyer, B. (1997). Children's exposure to traffic and risk of pedestrian injury in an urban setting. *Bulletin of the New York Academy of Medicine, 74*(1), 65–80.

Raudenbush, S.W., and Bryk, A.S. (2002). *Hierarchical linear models: Applications and data analysis methods.* Newbury Park, CA: Sage Publications.

Raudenbush, S.W., and Sampson, R.J. (1999). Ecometrics: Toward a science of assessing ecological settings, with application to the systematic social observation of neighborhoods. *Sociological Methodology, 29,* 1–41.

Regalado, M., Sareen, H., Inkelas, M., Wissow, L., and Halfon, N. (2004). Parents' discipline of young children: Results from the National Survey of Early Childhood Health. Pediatrics, 113(6), 1952–1958.

Regecova, V., and Kellerova, E. (1995). Effects of urban noise pollution on blood pressure and heart rate in preschool children. *Journal of Hypertension, 13*(4), 405–412.

Reichenbach, E.M., Clark, N., Lopez, P., and Loschen, D.J. (1996). C.A.T.C.H.: Community Access to Coordinated Healthcare. *Journal of Nebraska Medicine, 81*(12), 400–405.

Reiss, A.J., Jr. (1971). Systematic observations of natural social phenomena. In H. Costner (Ed.), *Sociological Methodology,* Volume 3 (pp. 3–33). San Francisco: Jossey-Bass.

Repetti, R.L., Taylor, S.E., and Seeman, T.E. (2002). Risky families: Family social environments and the mental and physical health of offspring. *Psychological Bulletin, 128*(2), 330–366.

Resnick, M., Bearmen, P., Blum, R., Bauman, K., Harris, K.M., Jones, J., Tabor, J., Beuhring, T., Sieving, R.E., Shew, M., Ireland, M., Bearinger, L.H., and Udry, J.R. (1997). Protecting adolescents from harm: Findings from the National Longitudinal Study on Adolescent Health. *Journal of the American Medical Assocation, 278*(10), 823–837.

Reszka, E., and Wasowicz, W. (2002). Genetic polymorphism of N-acetyltransferase and glutathione S-transferase related to neoplasm of genitourinary system. Minireview. *Neoplasma, 49*(4), 209–216.

Rice, M.L., Huston, A.C., Truglio, R., and Wright, J. (1990). Words from "Sesame Street": Learning vocabulary while viewing. *Developmental Psychology, 26,* 421–428.

Rietveld, S., and Prins, P.J. (1998). The relationship between negative emotions and acute subjective and objective symptoms of childhood asthma. *Psychological Medicne, 28,* 407–415.

Rigby, M., and Kohler, L. (2002). *Child Health Indicators of Life Development (CHILD): Report to the European Commission.* Luxembourg: European Union Community Health Monitoring Programme.

Riley, A.W., Forrest, C.B., Starfield, B., Green, B., Kang, M., and Ensminger, M. (1998a). Reliability and validity of the adolescent health profile-types. *Medical Care, 36*(8), 1237–1248.

Riley, A.W., Green, B.F., Forrest, C.B., Starfield, B., Kang, M., and Ensminger, M.E. (1998b). A taxonomy of adolescent health: Development of the adolescent health profile-types. *Medical Care, 36*(8), 1228–1236.

Riley, A.W., Starfield, B., Forrest, C.B., Robertson, J. (Submitted). *The value of a global assessment of child by parents and children.*

Riley, J.C., Lennon, M.A., and Ellwood, R.P. (1999). The effect of water fluoridation and social inequalities on dental caries in 5-year-old children. *International Journal of Epidemiology, 28*(2), 300–305.

Risser, A.L., and Mazur, L.J. (1995). Use of folk remedies in a Hispanic population. *Archives of Pediatric and Adolescent Medicine, 149*, 978–981.

Rivara, F.P. (1999). Pediatric injury control in 1999: Where do we go from here? *Pediatrics, 103*(4 pt. 2), 883–888.

Rivara, F.P., and Aitken, M. (1998). Prevention of injuries to children and adolescents. *Advances in Pediatrics, 45*, 37–72.

Rivara, F.P., and Barber, M. (1985). Demographic analysis of childhood pedestrian injuries. *Pediatrics, 76*(3), 375–381.

Roberts, D.F., Foehr, U.G., Rideout, V.J., and Brodie, M. (1999). *Kids and media at the new millennium.* Menlo Park, CA: Kaiser Family Foundation.

Roberts, I., Ashton, T., Dunn, R., and Lee-Joe, T. (1994). Preventing child pedestrian injury: Pedestrian education or traffic calming? *Australian Journal of Public Health, 18*(2), 209–212.

Roberts, I., Norton, R., Jackson, R., Dunn, R., and Hassall, I. (1995). Effect of environmental factors on risk of injury of child pedestrians by motor vehicles: A case-control study. *British Medical Journal, 310*(6972), 91–94.

Robinson, T.N. (2001). Television viewing and childhood obesity. *Pediatric Clinics of North America, 48*(4), 1017–1025.

Robinson, T.N., and Killen, J.D. (1995). Ethnic and gender differences in the relationships between television viewing and obesity, physical activity, and dietary fat intake. *Journal of Health Education, 26*, S91–S98.

Robinson, T.N., Hammer, L.D., Killen, J.D., Kramer, H.C., Wilson, D.M., Hayward, C., and Taylor, C.B. (1993). Does television viewing increase obesity and reduce physical activity? Cross-sectional and longitudinal analyses among adolescent girls. *Pediatrics, 91*, 273–280.

Roche, A.F., Chumleawe, R.M., and Siervogel, R.M. (1982). *Longitudinal study of human hearing, its relationship to noise and other factors. III. Results from the first 5 years.* Washington, DC: U.S. Environmental Protection Agency.

Rodman, D.M., and Zamudio, S. (1991). The cystic fibrosis heterozygote—Advantage in surviving cholera? *Medical Hypotheses, 36*(3), 253–258.

Rodriguez, C.M., and Green, A.J. (1997). Parenting stress and anger expression as predictors of child abuse potential. *Child Abuse and Neglect, 21*(4), 367–377.

Rodriguez, E., Allen, J.A., Frongillo, E.A., Jr., and Chandra, P. (1999). Unemployment, depression, and health: A look at the African-American community. *Journal of Epidemiology and Community Health, 53*, 335–342.

Rogan, W.J., and Ware, J.H. (2003). Exposure to lead in children: How low is low enough? *New England Journal of Medicine, 348*(16), 1515–1516.

Rogan, W.J., Gladen, B.C., McKinney, J.D., Carreras, N., Hardy, P., Thullen, J., Tingelstad, J., and Tully, M. (1986). Polychlorinated biphenyls (PCBs) and dichlorodiphenyl dichloroethene (DDE) in human milk: Effects on growth, morbidity, and duration of lactation. *American Journal of Public Health, 76*, 172–177.

Rogers, R.W. (1983). Cognitive and psychological processes in fear appeals and attitude change: A revised theory of protection motivation. In J. Cacioppi and R. Petty (Eds.), *Social psychophysiology: A sourcebook* (pp. 153–176). New York: Guilford Press.

Rogoff, B. (1990). *Apprenticeship in thinking: Cognitive development in social context.* Oxford: Oxford University Press.

Romer, D. (1994). Using mass media to reduce adolescent drug involvement in drug trafficking. *Pediatrics, 93*, 1073–1077.

Romer, D., Black, M., Ricardo, I., Feigelman, S., Kaljee, L., Galbraith, J., Nesbit, R., Hornik, R.C., and Stanton, B. (1994). Social influences on the sexual behavior of youth at risk for HIV exposure. *American Journal of Public Health, 84,* 977–985.

Roseboom, T.J., van der Meulen, J.H.P., van Montfrans, G.A., Ravelli, A.C.J., Osmond, C., Barker, D.J.P., and Bleker, O.P. (2001). Maternal nutrition during gestation and blood pressure in later life. *Journal of Hypertension, 19*(1), 29–34.

Rosenberg, J. (1991). Jets over Labrador and Quebec: Noise effects on human health. *Canadian Medical Association Journal, 144,* 869–875.

Rosenberg, M., and Pearlin, L.I. (1978). Social class and self-esteem among children and adults. *American Journal of Sociology, 84,* 53–77.

Rosenberg, M.L., and Mercy, J.A. (1986). Homicide: Epidemiologic analysis at the national level. *Bulletin of the New York Academy of Medicine, 62*(5), 376–399.

Rosenthal, R., and Rubin, D. (1982). Comparing effect sizes of independent studies. *Psychology Bulletin, 92,* 500–504.

Ross, N.A., Wolfson, M.C., Dunn, J.R., Berthelot, J.M., Kaplan, G.A., and Lynch, J.W. (2000). Relation between income inequality and mortality in Canada and in the United States: Cross sectional assessment using census data and vital statistics. *British Medical Journal, 320*(7239), 898–902.

Ross, R.P., Campbell, T., Huston-Stein, A., and Wright, J.C. (1981). Nutritional misinformation of children: A developmental and experimental analysis of the effects of televised food commercials. *Journal of Applied Developmental Psychology, 1,* 329–347.

Rubin, D.M., Alessandrini, E.A., Feudtner, C., Mandell, D.S., Localio, A.R., and Hadley, T. (2004). Placement stability and mental health costs for children in foster care. *Pediatrics, 112,* 1336–1341.

Ruby, N.F., Brennan, T.J., Xie, X., Cao, V., Franken, P., Heller, H.C., and O'Hara, B.F. (2002). Role of melanopsin in circadian responses to light. *Science, 298*(5601), 2211–2213.

Rutter, M. (1990). Psychosocial resilience and protective mechanisms. In J. Rolf, A.S. Masten, D. Cicchetti, K. Neuchterlein, and S. Weintraub (Eds.), *Risk and protective factors in the development of psychopathology* (pp. 181–215). Cambridge, UK: Cambridge University Press.

Rutter, M. (1994). Epidemiologic/longitudinal strategies and causal research in child psychiatry. In J.E. Mezzich, M.J. Jorge, and I.M. Salloum (Eds.), *Psychiatric epidemiology: Assessment concepts and methods. The Johns Hopkins series in psychiatry and neuroscience* (pp. 139–166). Baltimore: Johns Hopkins University Press.

Rutter, M. (1998). Developmental catch-up, and deficit, following adoption after severe global early privation. *Journal of Child Psychology and Psychiatry, 39*(4), 465–476.

Rutter, M., Dunn, J., Plomin, R., Simonoff, E., Pickles, A., Maughan, B., Ormel, J., Meyer, J., and Eaves, L. (1997). Integrating nature and nurture: Implications of person-environment correlations and interactions for developmental psychopathology. *Development and Psychopathology, 9*(2), 335–364.

Sachs, B., Hall, L.A., Lutenbacher, M., and Rayens, M.K. (1999). Potential for abusive parenting by rural mothers with low-birth weight children. *Image: Journal of Nursing Scholarship, 31*(1), 21–25.

Saluja, G., Scott-Little, C., and Clifford, R.M. (2000). Readiness for school: A survey of state policies and definitions. *Early Childhood Research and Practice, 2*(2), internet journal. Available: http://ecrp.uiuc.edu/v2n2/Saluja.html.

Sameroff, A., and Fiese, B. (2000). Transactional regulation: The developmental ecology of early interventions. In J.P. Shonkoff and S.J. Meisels (Eds.), *Handbook of early childhood intervention* (pp. 135–159). Cambridge, UK: Cambridge University Press.

Sameroff, A.J., and Fiese, B.H. (Eds.). (1989). *Relationships disturbances in early childhood: A developmental approach.* New York: Basic Books.

Sampson, R.J. (1992). Family management and child development: Insights from social disorganization theory. In J. McCord (Ed.), *Facts, frameworks, and forecasts: Advances in criminological theory, volume 3* (pp. 63–93). New Brunswick, NJ: Transaction Publishers.

Sampson, R.J. (2001). How do communities under gird or undermine human development? Relevant contexts and social mechanisms. In A. Booth and A.C. Crouter (Eds.), *Does it take a village?: Community effects on children, adolescents, and families* (pp. 3–30). Mahwah, NJ: Lawrence Erlbaum.

Sampson, R.J., and Groves, W.B. (1989). Community structure and crime: Testing social disorganization theory. *American Journal of Sociology, 94,* 774–802.

Sampson, R.J., and Raudenbush, S.W. (1999). Systematic social observation of public spaces: A new look at disorder in urban neighborhoods. *American Journal of Sociology, 105*(3), 603–651.

Sampson, R.J., Raudenbush, S.W., and Earls, F. (1997). Neighborhoods and violent crime: A multilevel study of collective efficacy. *Science, 277,* 918–924.

Sampson, R.J., Morenoff, J.D., and Gannon-Rowley, T. (2002). Assessing neighborhood effects: Social processes and new directions in research. *Annual Review of Sociology, 28,* 443–478.

Santos, J., Yang, P.-C., Soderholm, J.D., Benjamin, M., Perdue, M.H. (2001). Role of mast cells in chronic stress induced colonic epithelial barrier dysfunction in the rat. *Gut, 48,* 630–636.

Saraiya, M., Glanz, K., Briss, P., Nichols, P., White, C., and Das, D. (2003). Preventing skin cancer: Findings of the Task Force on Community Preventive Services on reducing exposure to ultraviolet light. *Morbidity and Mortality Weekly Report: Recommendations and Reports, 52*(RR-15), 1–12.

Satcher, D. (2001). Sharing an agenda for children: Progress and challenges related to the 1990 World Summit for Children goals. *Journal of American Medical Association, 286*(11), 1305.

Schardein, J.L. (2000). *Chemically induced birth defects.* New York: Marcel Deckker.

Schechter, M. (2003). Non-genetic influences on cystic fibrosis lung disease: The role of sociodemographic characteristics, environmental exposures, and healthcare interventions. *Seminars in Respiratory and Critical Care Medicine: Cystic Fibrosis and Bronchiectasis, 24*(6), 639–652.

Schieber, R.A., and Thompson, N.J. (1996). Developmental risk factors for childhood pedestrian injuries. *Injury Prevention, 2*(3), 228–236.

Schlesinger, M.J., and Eisenberg, L. (1990). Little people in a big policy world: Lasting questions and new directions in health policy for children. In M.J. Schlesinger and L. Eisenberg (Eds.), *Children in a changing health system.* Baltimore: Johns Hopkins University Press.

Schultz, D., Izard, C.E., and Ackerman, B.P. (2000). Children's anger attribution bias: Relations to family environment and social adjustment. *Social Development, 9,* 284–301.

Schuster M., McGlynn, E., and Brook, R. (1998). How good is the quality of health care in the United States? *The Milbank Quarterly, 76,* 517–563.

Searle, A., Vedhara, K., Norman, P., Frost, A., and Harrad, R. (2000). Compliance with eye patching in children and its psychosocial effects: A qualitative application of protection motivation theory. *Psychology Health and Medicine, 5*(1), 43–54.

Seckl, J.R. (1998). Physiologic programming of the fetus. *Emerging Concepts in Perinatal Endocrinology, 25*(4), 939–962.

Seeman, T.E., Singer, B., Rowe, J.W., Horowitz, R., and McEwen, B.S. (1997). The price of adaptation—Allostatic load and its health consequences: MacArthur studies of successful aging. *Archives of Internal Medicine, 15,* 2259–2268.

Seifer, R., Sameroff, A.J., Dickstein, S., Keitner, G., Miller, I., Rasmussen, S., and Hayden, L.C., (1996). Parental psychopathology, multiple contextual risks, and one-year outcomes in children. *Journal of Clinical Child Psychology, 25,* 423–435.

Selevan, S.G., Kimmel, C.A., and Mendola, P. (2000). Identifying critical windows of exposure for children's health. *Environmental Health Perspectives, 108,* 451–455.

Selevan, S.G., Rice, D.C., Hogan, K.A., Euling, S.Y., Pfahles-Hutchens, A., and Bethel, J. (2003). Blood lead concentration and delayed puberty in girls. *New England Journal of Medicine, 348*(16), 1527–1536.

Selner-O'Hagan, M.B., Kindlon, D.J., Buka, S.L., Raudenbush, S.W., and Earls, F.J. (1998). Assessing exposure to violence in urban youth. *Journal of Child Psychology and Psychiatry, 39*(2), 215–224.

Senechal, M., and LeFevre, J.A. (2002). Parental involvement in the development of children's reading: A five year longitudinal study. *Child Development, 73,* 445–460.

Shaffer, D., and Craft, L. (1999). Methods of adolescent suicide prevention. *Journal of Clinical Psychiatry, 60*(2), 70–74.

Shaffer, D., Fisher, P., Dulcan, M.K., Davies, M., Piacentini, J., Schwab-Stone, M.E., Lahey, B.B., Bourdon, K., Jensen, P.S., Bird, H.R., Canino, G., and Regier, D.A. (1996). The NIMH Diagnostic Interview Schedule for Children Version 2.3 (DISC-2.3): Description, acceptability, prevalence rates, and performance in the MECA Study. Methods for the Epidemiology of Child and Adolescent Mental Disorders Study. *Journal of American Academy of Child and Adolescent Psychiatry, 35*(7), 865–877.

Shah, C.P., Kaham, M., and Krauser, J. (1987). The health of children of low-income families. *Canadian Medical Association Journal, 137,* 485–490.

Shannon, M.W., and Graef, J.W. (1992). Lead intoxication in infancy. *Pediatrics, 89,* 87–90.

Shaw, R.J. (2001). Treatment adherence in adolescents: Development and psychopathology. *Clinical Child Psychology and Psychiatry, 6*(1), 137–150.

Shedler, J., and Block, J. (1990). Adolescent drug use and psychological health. A longitudinal inquiry. *American Psychologist, 45,* 612–630.

Sherry, J.L. (2001). The effects of violent video games on aggression: A meta-analysis. *Human Communication Research, 27,* 409–431.

Shi, L., and Starfield, B. (2000). Primary care, income equality, and self-rated health in the United States: A mixed-level analysis. *International Journal of Health Services, 30*(3), 541–555.

Shi, L., and Starfield, B. (2002). Primary care, self-rated heatlh, and reductions in social disparities in health. *Health Services Research, 37*(3), 529–550.

Shi, L., Starfield, B., and Xu, J. (2003). Primary care quality: Community health center and health maintenance organizations. *Southern Medical Journal, 96*(8), 787–795.

Shi, L., Regan, L., Politzer, R., and Luo, J. (2001). Community health centers and racial/ethnic disparities in healthy life. *International Journal of Health Services, 31,* 567–582.

Sibbald, B. (2002). Arsenic and pressure-treated wood: The argument moves to the playground. *Canadian Medical Association Journal, 166*(1), 79.

Siegel, M.J., Bauman, L.J., and Stein, R.E.K. (2004, May). *Racial/Ethnic Disparities in Child Health: Another Failed Explanation.* Poster Presentation at the Annual Meeting of Pediatric Academic Societies, San Francisco, CA.

Silver, E.J., Stein, R.E.K., and Dadds, M.R. (1996). Moderating effects of family structure on the relationship between physical and mental health in urban children with chronic illness. *Journal of Pediatric Psychology, 21,* 43–56.

Simeonsson, R.J., Leonardi, M., Bjorck-Akesson, E., Hollenweger, J., Lollar, D.J., and Matinuzzi, A. (2003). Measurement of disability in children and youth: Implications of the ICF. *Disability and Rehabilitation, 25*(11–12), 602–610.

Simms, M.D., Dubowitz, H., and Szilagyi, M.A. (2000). Health care needs of children in the foster care system. *Pediatrics, 106*(4 Suppl), 909–918.

Singer, B., and Ryff, C.D. (1999). Hierarchies of life histories and associate health risks. *Annals of the New York Academy of Sciences, 896,* 96–115.

Singer, L.T., Arendt, R., Minnes, S., Farkas, K., and Salvator, A. (2000). Neurobehavioral outcomes of cocaine-exposed infants. *Neurotoxicology and Teratology, 22*(5), 653–666.

Singer, L.T., Arendt, R., Minnes, S., Salvator, A., Siegel, A.C., and Lewis, B.A. (2001). Developing language skills of cocaine-exposed infants. *Pediatrics, 107*(5), 1057–1064.

Singer, L.T., Arendt, R., Minnes, S., Farkas, K., Salvator, A., Kirchner, H.L., and Kliegman, R. (2002a). Cognitive and motor outcomes of cocaine-exposed infants. *Journal of the American Medical Association, 287*(15), 1990–1991.

Singer, L.T., Salvator, A., Arendt, R., Minnes, S., Farkas, K., and Kliegman, R. (2002b). Efffects of cocaine/polydrug exposure and maternal psychological distress on infant birth outcomes. *Neurotoxicology and Teratology, 24*(2), 127–135.

Skuse, D.H., Albanese, A., Stanhope, R., Gilmour J., and Voss, L. (1996). A new stress-related syndrome of growth failure and hyperphagia in children associated with reversibility of growth-hormone insufficiency. *Lancet, 348*(9024), 353–358.

Sleet, D.A., Schieber, R.A., and Gilchrist, J. (2003). Health promotion policy and politics: Lessons from childhood injury prevention. *Health Promotion Practice, 4*(2), 103–108.

Small, S., and Supple, A. (2001). Communities as systems: Is a community more than the sum of its parts. In A. Booth and A.C. Crouter (Eds.), *Does it take a village? Community effects on children, adolescents, and families,* (pp. 61–70). State College: Pennsylvania State University Press.

Smith, D.W., Hopper, A.Q., Shahin, S.M., Cohen, R.S., Ostrander, C.R., Ariagno, R.L., and Stevenson, D.K. (1984). Neonatal bilirubin production estimated from "end-tidal" carbon monoxide concentration. *Journal of Pediatric Gastroenterology & Nutrition, 3*(1), 77–80.

Smith, M., and Martin, F. (1995). Domestic violence: Recognition, intervention, and prevention. *Medical Surgery Nurse, 4*(1), 21–25.

Sokol, R.J., Delaney-Black, V., and Nordstrom, B. (2003). Fetal alcohol spectrum disorder. *Journal of the American Medical Association, 290*(22), 2996–2999.

Solis, J.M., Marks, G., Garcia, M., and Shelton, D. (1990). Acculturation, access to care, and use of preventive services by Hispanics: Findings from HHANES 1982–84. *American Journal of Public Health, 80,* 11–19.

St. Lawrence, J.S., Brasfield, T.L., Jefferson, K.W., Alleyne, E., O'Bannon, R.E., 3rd, and Shirley, A. (1995). Cognitive–behavioral intervention to reduce African-American adolescents' risk for HIV infection. *Journal of Consulting and Clinical Psychology, 63*(2), 221–237.

Stanken, B.A. (2000). Promoting helmet use among children. *Journal of Community Health Nursing, 17,* 85–92.

Stansbury, K., and Zimmermann, L.K. (1999). Relations among child language skills, maternal socialization of emotion regulation, and child behavior problems. *Child Psychiatry and Human Development, 30*(2), 121–142.

Stansfeld, S., Haines, M., and Brown, B. (2000). Noise and health in the urban environment. *Reviews on Environmental Health, 15*(1–2), 43–82.

Stanton, B., Black, R., Engle, P., and Pelto, G. (1992). Theory-driven behavioral intervention research for the control of diarrheal diseases. *Social Science and Medicine, 35,* 1405–1420.

Stanton, B., Li, X., Black, M., Ricardo, I., Galbraith, J., Kaljee, L., and Feigelman, S. (1994). Sexual practices and intentions among preadolescent and early adolescent low-income urban African-Americans. *Pediatrics, 93,* 966–973.

Stanton, B.F., Li X., Black, M.M., Ricardo, I., Galbraith, J., Feigelman, S., and Kaljee, L. (1996). Longitudinal stability and predictability of sexual perceptions, intentions, and behaviors among early adolescent African-Americans. *Journal of Adolescent Health, 18*(1), 10–19.

Stanton, B.F., Li, X., Galbraith, J., Cornick, G., Fiegelman, S., Kaljee, L., and Zhou, Y. (2000). Parental underestimates of adolescent risk behavior: A randomized, controlled trial of a parental monitoring intervention. *Journal of Adolescent Health, 26*(1), 18–26.

Starfield, B. (1974). Measurement of outcome: A proposed scheme. *The Milbank Quarterly, 52,* 39–50.

Starfield, B. (1985a). *The effectiveness of medical care: Validating clinical wisdom.* Baltimore: Johns Hopkins University Press.

Starfield, B. (1985b). Motherhood and apple pie: The effectiveness of medical care for children. *Milbank Memorial Fund Quarterly, 63*(3), 523–546.

Starfield, B. (1988). *Primary care: Balancing health needs, services, and technology.* New York: Oxford University Press.

Starfield, B. (1991). Childhood morbidity: Comparisons, clusters, and trends. *Pediatrics, 88*(3), 519–526.

Starfield, B. (1992). Child and adolescent health status measures. *Future of Children, 2*(2), 25–39.

Starfield, B. (2000a). Evaluating the State Children's Health Insurance Program: Critical considerations. *Annual Review of Public Health, 21*, 569–585.

Starfield, B. (2000b). Is U.S. health really the best in the world? *Journal of American Medical Association, 284*(4), 483–485.

Starfield, B. (2001). New paradigms for quality in primary care. *British Journal of General Practice, 51*(465), 303–309.

Starfield, B., and Shi, L. (1999). Determinants of health: Testing of a conceptual model. *Annals of the New York Academy of Sciences, 896*, 344–346.

Starfield, B., Bergner, M., Ensminger, M., Riley, A., Ryan, S., Green, B., McGauhey, P., Skinner, A., and Kim, S. (1993). Adolescent health status measurement: Development of the Child Health and Illness Profile. *Pediatrics, 91*(2), 430–435.

Starfield, B., Cassady, C., Nanda, J., Forrest, C., and Berk, R. (1998). Consumer experiences and provider perceptions of the quality of primary care: Implications for managed care. *Journal of Family Practice, 46*(3), 216–226.

Starfield, B., Riley, A.W., Witt, W.P., and Robertson, J. (2002a). Social class gradients in health during adolescence. *Journal of Epidemiology and Community Health, 6*(5), 354–361.

Starfield, B., Robertson, J., and Riley, A.W. (2002b). Social class gradients and health in childhood. *Ambulatory Pediatrics, 2*(4), 238–246.

Stattin, H., and Kerr, M. (2000). Parental monitoring: A reinterpretation. *Child Development, 71*(4), 1072–1085.

Steele, C.M. (1997). A threat in the air: How stereotypes shape the intellectual identities and performance of women and African-Americans. *American Psychologist, 52*, 613–629.

Steele, C.M., and Aronson, J. (1995). Stereotype threat and intellectual performance of African Americans. *Journal of Personality and Social Psychology, 69*, 797–811.

Stein, M.B., Jang, K.L., Taylor, S., Vernon, P.A., and Livesley, W.J. (2002). Genetic and environmental influences on trauma exposure and posttraumatic stress disorder symptoms: A twin study. *American Journal of Psychiatry, 159*(10), 1675–1681.

Stein, R.E., and Jessop, D.J. (1990). Functional status II(R): A measure of child health status. *Medical Care, 28*(11), 1041–1055.

Stein, R.E.K. (Ed.). (1997). *Health care for children: What's right what's wrong what's next.* New York: United Hospital Fund Publishers.

Stein, R.E.K., and Jessop, D.J. (1984). Relationship between health status and psychological adjustment among children with chronic conditions. *Pediatrics, 73*, 169–174.

Stein, R.E.K., and Silver, E.J. (2002). Comparing different definitions of children with chronic conditions in a national data set. *Ambulatory Pediatrics, 2*, 63–70.

Stein, R.E.K., Gortmaker, S., Perrin, E., Perrin, J., Pless, I.B., Walker, D.K., and Weitzman, M. (1987). Severity of illness: Concepts and measurements. *Lancet, 2*(8574), 1506–1509.

Steinberg, L. (1999). *Adolescence (5th edition).* New York: McGraw-Hill.

Steinberg, L., Mounts, N.S., Lamborn, S.D., and Dornbusch, S.M. (1989). Authoritative parenting, psychosocial maturity, and academic success among adolescents. *Child Development, 60*(6), 1424–1436.

Steinberg, L., Mounts, N.S., and Lamborn, S. (1991). Authoritative parenting and adolescent adjustment across varied ecological niches. *Journal of Research on Adolescence, 1*, 19–36.

Steinberg, L., Dornbusch, S.M., and Brown, B.B. (1992). Ethnic differences in adolescent achievement: An ecological perspective. *American Psychologist, 47*, 723–729.

Stevenson, M.R., Rimajova, M., Edgecombe, D., and Vickery, K. (2003). Childhood drowning: Barriers surrounding private swimming pools. *Pediatrics, 111*(2), E115–E119.

Stevens-Simon, C., Kelly, L., and Kulick, R. (2001). A village would be nice but... it takes a long-acting contraceptive to prevent repeat adolescent pregnancies. *American Journal of Preventive Medicine, 21*(1), 60–65.

Story, M., and Faulkner, P. (1990). The prime time diet: A content analysis of eating behavior and food messages in television program content and commercials. *American Journal of Public Health, 80,* 736–740.

Stronks, K., van de Mheen, H.D., and Mackenbach, J.P. (1998). A higher prevalence of health problems in low income groups: Does it reflect relative deprivation? *Journal of Epidemiology and Community Health, 52,* 548–57.

Svensson, A., and Hansson, L. (1985). Blood pressure and response to "stress" in 11–16 year old children. *Acta Medica Scandinavia Supplement, 693,* 51–55.

Szalacha, L.A., Erkut, S., Garcia Coll, C., Alarcon, O., Fields, J.P., and Ceder, I. (2003). Discrimination and Puerto Rican children's and adolescents' mental health. *Cultural Diversity and Ethnic Minority Psychology, 9*(2), 141–55.

Szapocznik, J., Kurtines, W.M., and Fernandez, T. (1981). Bicultural involvement and adjustment in Hispanic-American youth. *International Journal of Intercultural Relations, 4,* 353–375.

Tafalla, R.J., and Evans, G.W. (1997). Noise, physiology, and human performance: The potential role of effort. *Journal of Occupational Health Psychology, 2*(2), 148–55.

Takayama, J.I., Bergman, A.B., and Connell, F.A. (1994). Children in foster care in the state of Washington: Health care utilization and expenditures. *Journal of the American Medical Association, 271,* 1905–1950.

Taras, H.L., Sallis, J.F., Patterson, T.L., Nader, P.R., and Nelson, J.A. (1989). Television's influence on children's diet and physical inactivity. *Journal of Development and Behavioral Pediatrics, 10,* 176–180.

Tatum, B. (1987). *Assimilation blues.* Westport, CT: Greenwood.

Tauber, E., Roe, H., Costa, R., Hennessy, J.M., and Kyriacou, C.P. (2003). Temporal mating isolation driven by a behavioral gene in drosophila. *Current Biology, 13*(2), 140–145.

Taylor, L., Zuckerman, B., Harik, V., and Groves, B.M. (1994) Witnessing violence by young children and their mothers. *Developmental and Behavioral Pediatrics, 15,* 120–123.

Taylor, P.R., Lawrence, C.E., Hwang, H.L., and Paulson, A.S. (1984). Polychlorinated biphenyls: Influence on birthweight and gestation. *American Journal of Public Health, 74,* 1153–1154.

Terrell, F., and Terrell, S. (1984). Race of counselor, client sex, cultural mistrust level, and premature termination from counseling among black clients. *Journal of Counseling Psychology, 31,* 371–375.

Thomas, A.M., Peterson, L., and Goldstein, D. (1997). Problem solving and diabetes regimen adherence by children and adolescents with IDDM in social pressure situations: A reflection of normal development. *Journal of Pediatric Psychology, 22,* 541–561.

Thompson, C.E., Worthington, R., and Atkinson, D.R. (1994). Counselor content orientation, counselor race, and black women's cultural mistrust and self-disclosures. *Journal of Counseling Psychology, 41,* 155–161.

Thompson, G.N. (1985). Lead mobilization during pregnancy (letter). *Medical Journal of Australia, 143,* 131.

Tilson, H.A., Jacobson, J.L., and Rogan, W.J. (1990). Polychlorinated biphenyls and the developing nervous system: Cross-species comparisons. *Neurotoxicology and Teratology, 12,* 239–248.

Tinsley, B. (2003). *How children learn to be healthy.* Cambridge: Cambridge University Press.

Towner, E., and Ward, H. (1998). Prevention of injuries to children and young people: The way ahead for the U.K. *Injury Prevention, 4*(4), 17–25.

Tronick, E.Z., and Beeghly, M. (1999). Prenatal cocaine exposure, child development, and the compromising effects of cumulative risk. *Clinics in Perinatology, 26*(1), 151–171.

United Nations Children's Fund. (2001). *A league table of child deaths by injury in rich nations.* (Innocenti Report Care No. 2). Florence: UNICEF Innocenti Research Center.

Urbano, R.C. (2001). *Linking data to overcome barriers: The Tennessee approach to coordination of services for children.* Washington, DC: The Association of State and Territorial Health Officials.

U.S. Census Bureau. (2002). Table 3: Poverty status of people, by age, race, and hispanic origin: 1959 to 2001: Historical poverty tables. Available: http://www.census.gov/hhes/poverty/histpov/hst pov3.html.

U.S. Department of Health and Human Services. (1981). *Better health for our children: A national strategy* (Volume III). Select Panel for the Promotion of Child Health. A Statistical Profile. Washington, DC: Author.

U.S. Department of Health and Human Services. (1999). *Mental health: A report of the surgeon general.* Substance Abuse and Mental Health Services Administration, Center for Mental Health Services, National Institutes of Health, National Institute of Mental Health. Rockville, MD: Author.

U.S. Department of Health and Human Services. (2000, November). *Healthy People 2010: Understanding and improving health.* 2nd edition. Washington, DC: U.S. Government Printing Office.

U.S. Department of Health and Human Services. (2001a). *A strategy for building the national health information infrastructure.* National Committee on Vial and Health Statistics. Washington, DC: Author.

U.S. Department of Health and Human Services. (2001b). *Trends in the well-being of America's children and youth.* Office of the Assistant Secretary for Planning and Evaluation. Washington, DC: U.S. Government Printing Office.

U.S. Department of Health and Human Services. (2003). *Summary of the HIPAA Privacy Rule.* Office for Civil Rights. Washington, DC: Author.

U.S. Environmental Protection Agency, Office of Research and Development. (1992). *Respiratory health effects of passive smoking: Lung cancer and other disorders.* Washington, DC: Author.

U.S. Environmental Protection Agency. (1987). Asbestos-Containing Materials in Schools. Final Rule and Notice (40 CFR Part 763). *Federal Register, 23,* 637–638.

U.S. Environmental Protection Agency. (1998). *Chemical hazard data availability study: What do we really know about the safety of high production volume chemicals?* Office of Prevention Pesticides and Toxic Substances. Washington, DC: Author.

U.S. Environmental Protection Agency. (2000a). *America's children and the environment: A first view of available measures.* Washington, DC: Author.

U.S. Environmental Protection Agency. (2000b). *Child-specific exposure factors handbook.* (Report No. USEPA NCEA-W-0853). Office of Research and Development, National Center for Environmental Assessment. Washington, DC: Author.

U.S. Environmental Protection Agency. (2000c). *Mercury research strategy.* (Report No. EPA/600/R-00/073). Office of Research and Development. Washington, DC: Author.

U.S. Environmental Protection Agency. (2001). *Our built and natural environments: A technical review of the interactions between land use, transportation, and environmental quality.* (Pub. No. EPA 231-R-01-002). Washington, DC: Author.

U.S. Environmental Protection Agency. (2003). *America's children and the environment: Measures of contaminants, body burdens, and illnesses.* (Report No. 240-R-03-001). Washington, DC: Author.

U.S. General Accounting Office. (1995). *School facilities: Condition of America's schools.* Washington, DC: Author.

U.S. Public Health Service. (2000). *Report of the Surgeon General's Conference on Children's Mental Health: A national action agenda.* Washington, DC: U.S. Department of Health and Human Services.

Ustun, B., Rehm, J., and Chatterji, S. (2002). Are disability weights universal? Ranking of the disabling effects of different health conditions in 14 countries by different informants. In C.J.L. Murray, J.A. Salomon, C.D. Mathers, and A.D. Lopez (Eds.), *Summary measures of population health.* Geneva: World Health Organization.

van den Akker, M., Buntinx, F., Metsemakers, J.F., Roos, S., and Knottnerus, J.A. (1998). Multi-morbidity in general practice: Prevalence, incidence, and determinants of co-occurring chronic and recurrent diseases. *Journal of Clinical Epidemiology, 51*(5), 367–375.

van Dyck, P.C., McPherson, M., Strickland, B.B., Nesseler, K., Blumberg, S.J., Cynamon, M.L., Newacheck, P.W. (2002). The national survey of children with special health care needs. *Ambulatory Pediatrics, 2*(1), 29–37.

van Ryn, M., and Fu, S. (2003). Paved with good intentions: Do public health and human service providers contribute to racial/ethnic disparities in health? *American Journal of Public Health, 93*, 248–255.

Ventura, S.J., Abma, J.C., Mosher, W.D., Henshaw, S. (2003). Revised pregnancy rates, 1990–97, and new rates for 1998–99: United States. *National Vital Statistics Reports, 52*(7), 1–16.

Volovitz, B., Duenas-Meza, E., Chmielewska-Szewczyk, D.A., Kosa, L., Astafieva, N.G., Villaran, C., Pinacho-Daza, C., Laurenzi, M., Jasan, J., Menten, J., and Leff, J.A. (2000). Comparison of oral montelukast and inhaled cromolyn with respect to preference, satisfaction, and adherence: A multicenter, randomized, open-label, crossover study in children with mild to moderate persistent asthma. *Current Therapeutic Research, Clinical and Experimental, 61*, 490–506.

Wade, T.J., Pai, N., Eisenberg, J.N., and Colford, J.M., Jr. (2003). Do U.S. Environmental Protection Agency water quality guidelines for recreational waters prevent gastrointestinal illness? A systematic review and meta-analysis. *Environmental Health Perspectives, 111*(8), 1102–1109.

Wadsworth, M.E.J. (1999). Early life. In M. Marmot and R.G. Wilkinson (Eds.), *Social determinants of health.* New York: Oxford University Press.

Wagstaff, A., and van Doorslaer, E. (2000). Income inequality and health: What does the literature tell us? *Annual Review of Public Health, 21*, 543–567.

Wald, D.S., Law, M., Morris, J.K. (2002). Homocysteine and cardiovascular disease: Evidence on causality from a meta-analysis. *British Medical Journal, 325*(7374), 1202.

Wald, N.J., Morris, J.K., and Wald, D.S. (2001). Quantifying the effect of folic acid. *Lancet, 358*, 2069–2073.

Waldron, I., Weiss, C.C., and Hughes, M.E. (1998). Interacting effects of multiple roles on women's health. *Journal of Health and Social Behavior, 39*(3), 216–236.

Wall, T.L., Carr, L.G., and Ehlers, C.L. (2003). Protective association of genetic variation in alcohol dehydrogenase with alcohol dependence in Native American mission Indians. *American Journal of Psychiatry, 160*(1), 41–46.

Wallace, J.M., and Forman, T.A. (1998). Religion's role in promoting health and reducing risk among American youth. *Health Education and Behavior, 25*(6), 721–741.

Wallace, J.M., Brown, T.N., Bachman, J.G., and LaViest, T.A. (2003). *Religion, race, and abstinence from drug use among American adolescents.* Monitoring the future occasional paper 58. Ann Arbor: Institute for Social Research, University of Michigan.

Ware, J. (2003). Conceptualization and measurement of health-related quality of life: Comments on an evolving field. *Archives of Physical Medicine and Rehabilitation, 84*(4pt2), S43–S51.

Wartella, E.A., Heintz, K.E., Aidman, A.J., and Mazzarella, S.R. (1990). Television and beyond: Children's video media in one community. *Communication Research, 17*, 45–64.

Watkins, C.E., Jr., and Terrell, F. (1988). Mistrust level and its effects on counseling expectations in Black client-White counselor relationships: An analogue study. *Journal of Counseling Psychology, 35*, 194–197.

Watkins, C.E, Jr., Terrell, F., Miller, F.S., and Terrell, S.L. (1989). Cultural mistrust and its effects on expectational variables in black client-white counselor relationships. *Journal of Counseling Psychology, 36*, 447–450.

Wazana, A., Rynard, V.L., Raina, P., Krueger, P., and Chambers, L.W. (2000). Are child pedestrians at increased risk of injury on one-way compared to two-way streets? *Canadian Journal of Public Health, 91*(3), 201–206.

Weatherall, R., Joshi, H., and Macran, S. (1994). Double burden or double blessing? Employment, motherhood, mortality in the Longitudinal Study of England and Wales. *Social Science and Medicine, 38*(2), 285–297.

Weaver, J.B., Masland, J.L., and Zillman, D. (1984). Effects of erotica on young men's aesthetic perception of their female sexual partners. *Perceptual and Motor Skills, 58,* 929–930.

Weich, S., Burton, E., Blanchard, M., Prince, M., Sproston, K., and Erens, B. (2001). Measuring the built environment: Validity of a site survey instrument for use in urban settings. *Health and Place, 7,* 283–292.

Weiler, R.M., Pigg, R.M., Jr., McDermott, R.J. (2003). Evaluation of the Florida coordinated school health program pilot schools project. *Journal of School Health, 73*(1), 3–8.

Weisner, T.S. (1997). The ecocultural project of human development: Why ethnography and its findings matter. *Ethos, 25*(2), 177–190.

Weisner, T.S. (2002). Ecocultural understandings of children's development pathways. *Human Development, 45,* 275–281.

Weiss, B.D. (1986). Prevention of bicycle-related head injuries. *American Journal of Preventative Medicine, 2,* 330–333.

Weller, S.C., and Romney, A.K. (1988). *Systematic data collection.* Beverly Hills, CA: Sage Publications.

Werner, E.E. (1993). Risk, resilience, and recovery: Perspectives from the Kauai Longitudinal Study. *Development and Psychopathology, 5,* 503–515.

Wijnen, H., Boothroyd, C., Young, M.W., and Claridge-Chang, A. (2002). Molecular genetics of timing in intrinsic circadian rhythm sleep disorders. *Annals of Medicine, 34*(5), 386–393.

Wilkinson, R.G. (1992). Income distribution and life expectancy. *British Medical Journal, 304*(6820), 165–168.

Williams, D., Neighbors, H., and Jackson, J. (2003). Racial/ethnic discrimination and health: Findings from community studies. *American Journal of Public Health, 93,* 200–208.

Williams, T.M. (Ed.). (1986). *The impact of television: A natural experiment in three communities.* Orlando, FL: Academic Press.

Wilson, W.J. (1987). *The truly disadvantaged: The inner city, the underclass and the public policy.* Chicago: University of Chicago Press.

Wind, T.W., and Silvern, L. (1994). Parenting and family stress as mediators of the long-term effect on child abuse. *Child Abuse and Neglect, 118*(5), 439–453.

Winn, M. (1985). *The plug-in drug.* New York: Viking.

Wise, B.K., Cuffe, S.P., and Fischer, T. (2001). Dual diagnosis and successful participation of adolescents in substance abuse treatment. *Journal of Substance Abuse Treatment, 21*(3), 161–165.

Wise, P.H. (2003). The anatomy of a disparity in infant mortality. *Annual Review of Public Health, 24,* 341–362.

Woodard, E.H., and Gridina, N. (2000). *Media in the home 2000: The fifth annual survey of parents and children.* Philadelphia: University of Pennsylvania, Annenberg Public Policy Center.

World Health Organization. (1986). *Environmental Health Criteria 59: Principles for evaluating health risks from chemicals during infancy and early childhood: The need for a special approach.* Geneva: Author.

World Health Organization. (2000). *Health systems: Improving performance.* The World Health Report. Geneva: Author.

Wright, A.L., Holbert, C.J., Martinez, F.D., Morgan, W.J., and Taussig, L.M. (1989). Breast feeding and lower respiratory tract illness in the first year of life. Group Health Medical Associates. *British Medical Journal, 299*(6705), 946–949.

Wright, J.C., Huston, A.C., Scantlin, R., and Kotler, J. (2000). The Early Window Project: Sesame Street prepares children for school. In S.M. Fisch and R.T. Truglio (Eds.), *"G" is for growing: Thirty years of research on children and Sesame Street.* Mahwah, NJ: Lawrence Erlbaum.

Wu, Y., Stanton, B., Galbraith, J., Kaljee, L., Cottrell, L., Li, X., Harris, C.V., D'Alessandri, D., and Burns, J.M. (2003). Sustaining and broadening intervention impact: A longitudinal randomized trial of 3 adolescent risk reduction approaches. *Pediatrics, 111*(1), 32–38.

Wysocki T., Harris, M.A., Greco, P., Bubb, J., Danda, C.E., Harve, L.M., McDonnell, K., Taylor, A., and White, N.H. (2000). Randomized, controlled trial of behavior therapy for families of adolescents with insulin-dependent diabetes mellitus. *Journal of Pediatric Psychology, 25*(1), 23–33.

Yazdanbakhsh, M., Kremsner, P.G., and van Ree, R. (2002). Allergy, parasites, and the hygiene hypothesis. *Science, 296*(5567), 490–494.

Yen, I.H., and Syme, S.L. (1999). The social environment and health: A discussion of the epidemiologic literature. *Annual Review of Public Health, 20*, 287–308.

Yoshimoto, Y. (1988). Risk of cancer among children exposed in utero to A-bomb radiations, 1954–1980. *Lancet, 2*, 665.

Young, K. (1998). Population health: Concepts and methods. In *Chapter 2: Measuring health and disease in populations I, section on demographic and health transition* (pp. 41–44). Oxford: Oxford University Press.

Yu, M.L, Chen-Chin, H., Gladen, B.C., and Rogan, W.J. (1991). In utero PCB/PCDF exposure: Relation of developmental delay to dysmorphology and dose. *Neurotoxicology and Teratology, 13*(2), 195–202.

Zeise, L., Painter, P., Berteau, P.E., Fan, A.M., Jackson, R.J. (1991). Alar in fruit: Limited regulatory action in the face of uncertain risks. In B.J. Garrick and W.C. Gekler (Eds.), *The analysis, communication, and perception of risk* (pp. 275–284). New York: Plenum Press.

Zelier, V. (1994). *Pricing the priceless child.* Princeton, NJ: Princeton University Press.

Zill, N. (1996). Parental schooling and children's health. *Public Health Reports, 111*, 34–43.

Zill, N. (2000). Does Sesame Street enhance school readiness?: Evidence from a national survey of children. In S.M. Fisch and R.T. Truglio (Eds.), *"G" is for growing: Thirty years of research on children and Sesame Street.* Mahwah, NJ: Lawrence Erlbaum.

Zuckerman, B., Augustyn, M., Groves, B.M., and Parker, S. (1995). Silent victims revisited: The special case of domestic violence. *Pediatrics, 96*(3), 511–513.

Appendix A

Datasets for Measuring Children's Health and Influences on Children's Health

1. *National Health Interview Survey* (Centers for Disease Control and Prevention)—A survey that assess family demographics, income, and health care accessibility. http://www.cdc.gov/nchs/nhis.htm
2. *National Health and Nutrition Examination Survey* (Centers for Disease Control and Prevention)—A survey conducted by the National Center for Health Statistics that collects information regarding the health and diet of people in the United States through the use of interviews and a health test. http://www.cdc.gov/nchs/nhanes.htm
3. *National Mortality Data* (Centers for Disease Control and Prevention)—Data collected through death certificates related to cause of death and basic demographics. http://www.cdc.gov/nchs/about/major/dvs/desc.htm
4. *National Child Abuse and Neglect Data System* (U.S. Department of Health and Human Services)—Data collected annually on child maltreatment from state child protective services agencies. http://nccanch.acf.hhs.gov/pubs/fact sheets/canstats.cfm
5. *Current Population Survey* (Bureau of Labor Statistics and the Census Bureau—A monthly survey of about 55,000 households, the CPS is the primary source of information on the labor force characteristics of the noninstitutionalized U.S. population. Periodic supplements provide information on school enrollment, income, health, employee benefits, and work schedules. http://www.bls.census.gov/cps/overmain.htm
6. *Survey of Children with Special Health Care Need* (Centers for Disease Control and Prevention)—A one-time survey designed to produce estimates of the number of children with special health care needs in each state, to de-

scribe the types of services that they need and use, to assess shortcomings in the system of care, and to provide estimates of health care coverage for all children. It is unclear whether it will be repeated. http://www.cdc.gov/nis/faq_chscn.htm

7. *Disease Surveillance Systems* (Centers for Disease Control and Prevention)— Disease surveillance systems provide for the ongoing collection, analysis, and dissemination of data to prevent and control disease. Disease surveillance data are used by public health professionals, medical professionals, private industry, and interested members of the public. http://www.cdc.gov/ncidod/osr/

8. *National Health Care Survey* (Centers for Disease Control and Prevention)— The survey collects data on the health care field and monitors health care use, the impact of medical technology, and the quality of care provided to a changing U.S. population. http://www.cdc.gov/nchs/nhcs.htm

9. *National Survey of America's Families* (Urban Institute)—The National Survey of American Families periodically gathers data on the well-being of children and adults for both a national sample and for large state samples 13 states. The survey provides quantitative measures of child, adult, and family well-being in America, with an emphasis on persons in low-income families. The survey incorporates ways of measuring changes in child well-being designed by Child Trends. http://www.urban.org/Content/Research/NewFederalism/AboutANF/AboutANF.htm

10. *Decennial Census* (U.S. Census Bureau)—The decennial census collects population and housing data from the entire U.S. population and selective demographic data (e.g., ancestry, disability, income) from a 1-in-6 sample population subsample. http://factfinder.census.gov/servlet/BasicFactsServlet?_lang=en

11. *National Household Survey on Drug Use and Health* (formerly National Household Survey of Drug Abuse; Substance Abuse and Mental Health Services Administration)—A survey on the prevalence, patterns, and consequences of drug and alcohol use and abuse in the United States. http://www.samhsa.gov/oas/nhsda.htm

12. *Global Youth Tobacco Survey* (Centers for Disease Control and Prevention)— World Health Organization and CDC developed the Global Youth Tobacco Survey (GYTS) to track tobacco use among youth across countries using a common methodology and core questionnaire. The surveillance system is intended to enhance the capacity of countries to design, implement, and evaluate tobacco control and prevention programs. http://www.cdc.gov/tobacco/global/gyts/GYTS_intro.htm

13. *Youth Risk Behavior Survey* (Centers for Disease Control and Prevention)—A nationally coordinated survey of each state that identifies high-risk youth behaviors through the use of school and classroom samples. Data from this survey are available for participating states every 2 years, enabling the moni-

toring of trends in risky youth behavior. http://www.cdc.gov/nccdphp/dash/yrbs/yrbsaag.htm

14. *Monitoring the Future* (Survey Research Center, University of Michigan)—Monitoring the Future is an ongoing study of the behaviors, attitudes, and values of U.S. secondary school students, college students, and young adults. Each year, a total of about 50,000 8th, 10th, and 12th grade students are surveyed (12th graders since 1975, and 8th and 10th graders since 1991). In addition, annual follow-up questionnaires are mailed to a sample of each graduating class for a number of years after their initial participation. http://monitoringthefuture.org/

15. *National Survey of Family Growth* (Centers for Disease Control and Prevention)—The purpose of this survey is to provide information on marriage, divorce, contraception, infertility, and the health of women and infants in the United States. http://www.cdc.gov/nchs/about/major/nsfg/nsfgback.htm

16. *National Mortality Follow-Back Survey* (Centers for Disease Control and Prevention)—Uses a sample of U.S. residents who die in a given year to supplement the death certificate data with information from the next of kin or another person familiar with the decedent's life history. http://www.cdc.gov/nchs/about/major/nmfs/desc.htm

17. *Pregnancy Risk Assessment Monitoring System* (Centers for Disease Control and Prevention, Washington State Department of Health)—An ongoing survey that collects data before, during, and shortly after pregnancy. It provides information on intendedness of pregnancy, use of alcohol and tobacco, baby's sleeping position, percentage of women breastfeeding, social support, and battering during pregnancy. http://www.doh.wa.gov/cfh/prams/default.htm#What

18. *National Immunization Survey* (Centers for Disease Control and Prevention)—A list-assisted random-digit-dialing telephone survey that began data collection in April 1994 to monitor childhood immunization. The target population is children between the ages of 19 and 35 months living in the United States at the time of the interview. http://www.cdc.gov/nis/

19. *National Survey of Early Childhood Health* (Maternal and Child Health Bureau and American Academy of Pediatrics)—A national random telephone survey with parents of over 2,000 children ages 4 to 35 months. The goal is to improve the understanding of household experiences in conjunction with preventive pediatric care in addition to the various methods used by families to promote children's health in the household. http://www.cdc.gov/nchs/about/major/slaits/nsech.htm

20. *National Household Education Surveys Program* (U.S. Department of Education)—A data collection system of the National Center for Education Statistics designed to address a wide range of education-related issues. The specific surveys included in this program include Adult Education; Before and After School Programs and Activities; Civic Involvement; Early Childhood Pro-

gram Participation; Household Library Use; Parent and Family Involvement in Education; School Readiness and School Safety and Discipline. http://nces.ed.gov/nhes/

21. *National Survey of Children's Health* (Maternal and Child Health Bureau and National Center for Health Statistics)—A partnership that is currently collecting information on 2,000 children per state through a random-digit-dialing telephone survey intended to identify information on demographics, health and function status, health insurance coverage, health care access and utilization, family and neighboring functioning, and age-specific issues. http://www.cdc.gov/nchs/about/major/slaits/nsch.htm

22. *National Survey of Families and Households* (Center for Demography, University of Wisconsin)—The National Survey of Families and Households consists of three waves. The first wave was 1987–1988, the second was the 5-year follow-up (1992–1994), and the third was from 2001 to 2002. This survey collects information on life history, including the respondent's family living arrangements in childhood, departures and returns to the parental home, and histories of marriage, cohabitation, education, fertility, and employment. http://www.ssc.wisc.edu/nsfh/home.htm

23. *Medical Expenditure Panel Survey* (U.S. Department of Health and Human Services)—The Medical Expenditure Panel Survey (MEPS) has four components: (1) Household (2) Nursing Home (3) Medical Provider and (4) Insurance. MEPS collects data on the specific health services used, frequency of use, the cost of these services, how they are paid for, as well as data on the cost, scope, and breadth of private health insurance held by and available to the U.S. population. http://www.meps.ahrq.gov/WhatIsMEPS/Overview.HTM#Background

24. *Early Childhood Longitudinal Survey—Kindergarten Cohort* (U.S. Department of Education)—An ongoing effort by the U.S. Department of Education, National Center for Education Statistics that follows a nationally representative sample of approximately 22,000 children from kindergarten through 5th grade. Information on children's cognitive, social, emotional, and physical development; children's home environment; home educational practices; school environment; classroom environment; classroom curriculum; and teacher qualifications are provided by the school, teachers, and families. http://nces.ed.gov/ecls/kindergarten/studybrief.asp

25. *National Longitudinal Survey of Adolescent Health* (also known as Add Health; Carolina Population Center)—A school-based longitudinal study of the health-related behaviors of adolescents in grades 7 to 12 designed to explore the causes of these behaviors, with an emphasis on the influence of social context, such as families, friends, schools, and communities. http://www.cpc.unc.edu/projects/addhealth/design

26. *National Longitudinal Survey of Youth 1997* (U.S. Department of Labor)—A longitudinal survey that collects information on adolescents ages 12 to 16

who are transitioning from the school to work environments. http://www.bls.gov/nls/home.htm

Note: The National Longitudinal Survey of Youth 1979 also provides longitudinal data on an adolescent cohort and the children born to them. http://www.bls.gov/nls/nlsy79.htm

27. *National Linked Birth/Death Data* (Centers for Disease Control and Prevention)—Established in 1983, a research dataset comprised of linked birth and death certificates for infants born in the United States who died before reaching 1 year of age. The purpose of this linkage is to use the many additional variables available from the birth certificate in infant mortality analysis in order to provide insight into the major factors influencing infant mortality in the United States. http://www.cdc.gov/nchs/products/elec_prods/subject/linkedbd.htm#description1

28. *Early Childhood Longitudinal Survey—Birth Cohort* (U.S. Department of Education)—A study that provides detailed information on children's development, health, early care, and education that follows a nationally representative sample of approximately 13,500 children born in 2001 from 9 months of age through the 1st grade. http://nces.ed.gov/ecls/Birth/studybrief.asp

29. *Survey of Income and Program Participation* (U.S. Census Bureau)—A primary purpose of this survey is to measure the receipt of benefits from federal, state, and local programs and provide more accurate estimates on the distribution and dynamics of income in the country. http://www.sipp.census.gov/sipp/sippov98.htm

30. *National Vital Statistics Data* (Centers for Disease Control and Prevention, Vital Statistics of the United States)—Statistics collected at birth, marriage, divorce, and death and published on an annual basis. http://www.cdc.gov/nchs/products/pubs/pubd/vsus/vsus.htm

TABLE A-1 Data Sets for Measuring Children's Health and Influences on Children's Health

Data Source	One Time	Periodic	Continuous	Longitudinal
CROSS-SECTIONAL				
National Health Interview Survey		x		
National Health and Nutrition Examination Survey		x		
National Mortality Data		x		
National Child Abuse and Neglect Data System (NCANDS)		x		
Current Population Survey		x		
Survey of Children with Special Health Care Needs	x			
Disease Surveillance Systems		x		
National Health Care Survey		x		
National Survey of America's Families		x		
National Birth Certificate Data		x		
Health Behavior of School-Aged Children				
Decennial Census		x		
National Household Survey of Drug Abuse		x		
Global Youth Tobacco Survey		x		
Youth Risk Behavior Survey		x		
Monitoring the Future		x		
National Survey of Family Growth		x		
National Mortality Follow-Back Survey		x		
Pregnancy Risk Assessment Monitoring System		x		
National Immunization Survey		x		
National Survey of Early Childhood Health	x			
National Household Education Survey		x		
National Child Health Survey	x			
National Survey of Early Childhood Health, Child Well-Being and Welfare		x		
LONGITUDINAL				
National Survey of Families and Households		x		x
Medical Expenditure Panel Survey		x		x
Early Childhood Longitudinal Survey Kindergarten Cohort				
National Longitudinal Survey of Adolescent Health (Add Health)	x			x
National Longitudinal Survey of Youth—1997 Cohort*				x
National Linked Birth/Death Data		x		x
Early Childhood Longitudinal Survey, Birth Cohort				x
Survey of Income and Program Participation		x		

Age			Geographic Level			
0-5	6-11	12-17	National	State	Local	International
x	x	x	x			
x	x	x	x			
x	x	x	x	x	x	
x	x	x	x	x		
x	x	x	x	x		
x	x	x	x	x		
x	x	x	x	x	x	
x	x	x	x			
x	x	x	x			
x		x	x	x	x	
	x	x	x			x
	x	x	x	x	x	
		x	x	x		
		x	x	x		x
		x	x	x	x	
		x	x			
		x	x			
		x	x			
x				x		
x			x	x	x	
x			x			
x			x			
			x			
x						
x	x	x	x			
x	x	x	x			
x	x		x			
		x	x			
		x	x			
x			x	x	x	
x			x			
		x	x			

continued

TABLE A-1 Continued

	Periodicity			
Data Source	One Time	Periodic	Continuous	Longitudinal
ADMINISTRATIVE				
Title V State Block Grant Performance Measurement System, Maternal and Child Health Programs			x	
National Vital Statistics System			x	
OTHER				
Aid to Families with Dependent Children (AFDC)		x		
Birth Defects Surveillance Systems		x		
Women and Infants (WIC)		x		
Immunization Registries		x		

*There is also a NLSY 1979 Cohort

Age				Geographic Level			
0-5	6-11	12-17		National	State	Local	International
x	x	x			x		
x				x			
x	x	x		x	x		
x							
x					x		
x					x		

Appendix B

Gaps Analysis of Measures
of Children's Health and Influences
on Children's Health in Select National Surveys

INTRODUCTION AND PURPOSE

This appendix examines selected national surveys to assess the current status of children's health measurement and monitoring at the national level. This review is intended to inform an assessment of the current national approaches to measuring children's health using survey methods. We examined 12 national surveys that collect information on children's health and both its social and medical influences. Specifically, we gathered data on the design and reach of the surveys (Table B-1) and on the following aspects of child health:

- Health conditions (Table B-2)
- Children's health status, functioning, and health potential (Table B-3)
- Influences on children's health (Table B-4)

The surveys that we reviewed encompass the vast majority of large, nationally representative, and publicly available efforts to collect information about children's health and the individual, social, economic, and medical care influences of health as defined broadly. The review incorporates both public and private initiatives; one-time and ongoing surveys (only the most current version); longitudinal and cross-sectional designs; and surveys focusing on different child age groups. While many other nationally representative studies have been conducted by individual researchers and organizations, most of these are not publicly available and are limited to very narrow topics, making them less useful for monitoring national child health issues over the long term. While these surveys or data collection systems are important sources of child health information, they are not comprehensive enough to allow for detailed examination of patterns, trends, and disparities in health.

The surveys are ordered from left to right according to the design and frequency of the survey. Organized from left to right are ongoing cross-sectional national surveys of children's health, followed by shorter duration or paneled longitudinal design surveys, and then small one-time specialty surveys. For each survey, we summarize key aspects of the design, including the frequency, origin date, sponsor, research design, sample size, age-group focus, and respondent (Table B-1). We then review, in Tables B-2 through B-4, the child health measures and influences on child health. Each child health topic is coded with a somewhat arbitrary system that indicates whether the topic is measured "comprehensively" (defined as three or more questions), "adequately" (defined as one or two questions), through a biological or physical mechanism (e.g., blood test), using data from a birth certificate, or not at all. The variables examined in the tables are organized and correspond with the structure of the report. Note: Some questions included in the tables (e.g., MEPS) are asked only of specific age groups (e.g., ages 5-17).

SUMMARY RESULTS OF THE REVIEW

The review identifies patterns of health topics that are commonly covered in national health surveys as well as gaps in which topics have rarely or never been addressed. We discuss the results with respect to whether the survey was a one-time endeavor or an ongoing initiative in order to analyze the consistency of data on specific topics. We also briefly discuss the measurement of race and ethnicity across surveys because of the national focus on eliminating racial and ethnic disparities in health.

Measurement of Children's Health Conditions

Many of the national surveys ask parents to report on specific health conditions that are common among children and adolescents. The most common conditions are asthma, mental disorders (measured broadly), infectious diseases, pregnancy among teens, and child injuries. These conditions, however, were measured in no more than half of all the surveys. While the National Health Interview Survey (NHIS) and the National Health and Nutrition Examination Survey (NHANES) assess the greatest breadth of conditions, NHANES collects the most comprehensive and detailed information on specific conditions. Because NHANES collects biological samples from children (usually a blood test) to assess the presence of certain conditions, it also has the potential to collect things such as biomarkers.

Despite the comprehensiveness of NHIS and NHANES, there remain some gaps in the measurement of children's health conditions across surveys. Among the newer morbidities are mental health conditions such as Attention Deficit Disorder and Attention Deficit Hyperactivity Disorder (ADD/ADHD) and depression, and these conditions (though commonly diagnosed) are usually not included in national surveys of child health. Difficulty in identifying and measuring these conditions (beyond parent report of diagnosis) is likely to be a barrier to more frequent inclusion in large national surveys. Screening for the presence of a condition, such as depression or ADHD, often involves the use of 10 or more questions, which can take up a relatively large amount of scarce interview time. There are other nonsurvey data sources, however, that exist for monitoring child health conditions, including the annual National Ambulatory Medical Care Survey that collects data from medical offices about patient symptoms, diagnoses, and ambulatory care provided.

Measures of Child Health Status, Functioning, and Health Potential

Nearly every national survey assesses some aspect of a child's physical health. The majority of the measures currently in national surveys relate to aspects of physical functioning and impairments or deficits in mobility, ability to do usual activities, or more specific deficits in hearing, vision, or speech. Some more recent surveys have tended to adopt broader perspectives on children's health, evaluating aspects of cognitive, emotional, and even social functioning. The broader perspective of what constitutes health is not routinely included in ongoing surveys but is rather the focus of more detailed and topic-specific one-time surveys.

The largest apparent gaps in the assessment of children's health are in the evaluation of health potential (or rather more positive aspects of development and functioning). While many surveys asked about impairments in functioning, only a handful of one-time studies actually incorporated questions about positive developmental and functional trajectories, such as positive personal affect or self-sufficiency. Refined understandings of health and well-being recognize that health is more than merely the absence of illness, although this is yet to be reflected in ongoing national surveys of children's health.

Measures of Family and Community Influences on Health

National surveys of child health have made tremendous steps in recognizing the importance of family determinants on child development. Nearly every survey measures race and ethnicity and some aspect of socioeconomic status (most commonly income and education) of the family. Many of the one-time special surveys have also recognized the contribution of family composition to children's health and the threats to development that are potentially associated with family disruptions (such as divorce), parent health status, and aspects of parenting (such as discipline and providing rich learning environments). Of particular interest is the recent attention given to the role of child care (both formal and informal) in national surveys. For example, the Early Childhood Longitudinal Study—Birth Cohort (ECLS-B) not only asks a series of questions to parents about their child care needs and beliefs, but also interviews the care providers and directors of the child care centers themselves. Interestingly, the ECLS-B also incorporates direct observation of child care practices to assess the quality of care that is provided.

While substantial progress has been made with the evaluation of family influences on health, few national surveys incorporate questions about community factors that may influence children's health and development. Add Health is one of the few surveys to ask questions about community socioeconomic level, community unemployment rates, physical safety in the community (e.g., school and housing safety), and aspects of the social organization of the neighborhood (e.g., social cohesion, diversity, and social networks). Uniquely, Add Health further incorporates the use of direct observation of neighborhoods to note the safety of the neighborhood, housing adequacy, and other factors. While these community factors are increasingly known to influence children's health, they are rarely included in ongoing national surveys.

Measurement of Health System Influences on Health

National surveys of child health also frequently assess the influences of health systems on children's health and development, most often incorporating measures of access to care and health service use. Ongoing surveys also seem to focus on childhood immunizations in order to support national efforts to monitor children's immunization status. Health insurance is covered in all but three of the surveys.

Measures of quality of health care, particularly those examining more qualitative aspects of care (e.g., patient-provider interpersonal factors), are underrepresented in the ongoing national surveys. Coordination of care is nearly nonexistent in the surveys, with the exception of the National Survey of Children with Special Health Care Needs, which examines experiences of children with special health care needs. Relatively little information is provided on the content of care, particularly the receipt of childhood preventive services other than immunizations. The National Survey of Early Childhood Health (NSECH) comprehensively asks parents about preventive services they have received, and uniquely ascertains whether the parents who did not receive the services would have found them helpful. This allows for some analyses of missed opportunities to provide needed preventive care. The NSECH is a one-time endeavor, but it may serve as a model for incorporation of preventive care questions into ongoing national surveys.

CONCLUSION AND FUTURE CONSIDERATIONS

When considered together, this collection of national surveys covers a very large number of domains of children's health and many family, community, and medical influences on their health and development. When considered individually (because information from across surveys can rarely be combined), there remain substantial gaps in what is measured for children, particularly regarding positive functioning or health potential for children, family, or parenting processes, neighborhood and community influences, and aspects of health care quality. Moreover, with the exception of preventive care, there is almost no attempt to tailor measures to appropriate age groups or make them age-specific.

While recurrent surveys such as NHIS are well established and structured to routinely collect standard information about child health, their established nature makes them somewhat resistant to change other than through special supplements. The NHANES is, perhaps, one exception because it already collects biological samples from children, and these could be used to easily screen for additional biomarkers. Despite these gaps in measurement, a number of one-time surveys have successfully collected data on measures at the forefront of children's health issues. Collection of these data not only demonstrates that these issues can be successfully measured, but also serves as a testing ground for the validity and reliability of the measures, easing their transition into other ongoing national surveys.

TABLES B-1 THROUGH B-4 FOLLOW

TABLE B-1 Descriptive Characteristics of 12 National Surveys of Children's Health

Descriptive Characteristics	NHIS	NHANES	MEPS[a]	YRBS	NLSY[b]	Add Health
Year	2002	1994–2004	2002	2003	1997	2001–2002
Origination	1957	1971	1996	1991	1997	1994–1995
Sponsor(s)	NCHS/CDC	NCHS/CDC	AHRQ	NCHS/CDC	DOL	NICHD
Frequency	Annual	Annual since 1999	Annual	2 years	Various	3 waves, 1 and 6 years
Design	CS	CS	CS panels	CS	L	L
Sample size	N = 12,524; 26,191 children in person file	N = 5085 <20 years, 4,880 adults	N = 11,500 children/year	N = 13,000 adolescents	N = 8,984 adolescents	N = 20,745 adolescents
Age group	All ages	All ages	<18 years	14–17 years	12–16 years	<18 years
Respondent	Adult	Adult	Household respondent	Adolescent	Adolescent and adult	Adolescent and adult

NHIS = National Health Interview Survey; NHANES = National Health and Nutrition Examination Survey; MEPS = Medical Expenditure Panel Survey; YRBS = Youth Risk Behavior Survey; NLSY = National Longitudinal Survey of Youth; Add Health = National Longitudinal Survey of Adolescent Health; NSFH = National Survey of Families and Households; ECLS-K = Early Childhood Longitudinal Study Kindergarten Class; ECLS-B = Early Childhood Longitudinal Study-Birth Cohort; NHES = National Household Education Surveys; NSECH = National Survey of Early Childhood Health; NS-CSHCN = National Survey of Children with Special Health Care Needs

NSFH	ECLS-K	ECLS-B	NHES	NSECH	NS-CSHCN
2001–2002	2002	2001	2003	2000	2000–2002
1987–1988	1998–1999	2001	1991	2000	2000–2002
NICHD/ NIA	NCES	NCES	NCES	CDC/AAP	MCHB
3 waves: 5 and 8 years	Fall and Spring K and 1st. Spring 3rd and 5th.	5 waves: 9 months to 6 years	Approx. every 2 years	One time	One time
L	L	L	CS	CS	CS
N = 2,500 children	N = 22,000 children	N = 10,700 children	Varies: N = 7,000– 22,000	N = 2,068 children	N = 37,500 children
<18 years	5–10 years	9 months to 6 years	Varies: but always includes <18 years	4–35 months	<18 years
Child and adult	Adult, child, school records	Adult, child, child care provider, observation, and birth certificate	Adult and adolescent	Adult	Adult

CS = Cross-sectional study design
L = Longitudinal study design

[a]Prior to 1996, the MEPS was conducted in 1977 and 1987.
[b]The NSLY was started in 1979 with an original cohort of 12,686 children ages 14–22 that was interviewed annually until 1994. In this review, we focus only on a more recent and separate NSLY cohort study that began in 1997.

TABLE B-2 Child Health Condition Categories (by ICD9 Code) with Selected Highlights

ICD9 Code	Health Conditions, Disorders, or Diseases	NHIS	NHANES	MEPS
001–139	Infectious and parasitic diseases	●	○●●	●
	042: AIDS		○	
	079: Syphilis		○●	
	055: Measles		○	
140–239	Neoplasms		●●	●
240–279	Endocrine, nutritional, metabolic			●
	250: Diabetes mellitus	●	○●●	●
280–289	Blood and blood-forming organs	●	●	●
	280: Iron-deficiency anemia	●	○●	
	984: Lead poisoning		○●	
290–319	Mental disorders	●●	●●	●●
	300: Depression		●●	●
	314: ADD/ADHD	●	●●	●
	315: Mental retardation	●		●
320–389	Nervous system & sense organs	●●		●
390–459	Circulatory system	●		●
460–519	Respiratory system	●●	●●	●
	493: Asthma	●●	●●	●
520–579	Digestive system	●	●	●
	521: Oral health (cavities, etc)		○	●
580–629	Genitourinary system			
630–676	Pregnancy, childbirth, puerperium		○●	●
	635: Abortion			
680–709	Skin and subcutaneous tissue	●	○●●	●
710–739	Musculoskeletal/connective tissue	●		●
740–759	Congenital abnormalities	●		●
760–779	Conditions in perinatal period			
	765: Low birthweight	●	●	
	765: Very low birthweight	●	●	
780–799	Symptoms/ill-defined conditions	●		●
800–999	Injury and poisoning	●		●
	995: Child abuse			
V01–V82	Supplemental influences on health			
	V22: Pregnancy		●	
E800–E999	Supplemental injury, poisoning	●		
	E950–959: Suicide			
	Chronic condition (general measure)			

NHIS = National Health Interview Survey; NHANES = National Health and Nutrition Examination Survey; MEPS = Medical Expenditure Panel Survey; YRBS = Youth Risk Behavior Survey; NLSY = National Longitudinal Survey of Youth; Add Health = National Longitudinal Survey of Adolescent Health; NSFH = National Survey of Families and Households; ECLS-K = Early Childhood Longitudinal Study Kindergarten Class; ECLS-B = Early Childhood Longitudinal Study-Birth Cohort; NHES = National Household Education Surveys; NSECH = National Survey of Early Childhood Health; NS-CSHCN = National Survey of Children with Special Health Care Needs

YRBS	NLSY	Add Health	NSFH	ECLS-K	ECLS-B	NHES	NSECH	NS-CSHCN
		●					●	
		●○						
	●	●						
	●	●						
	●	●						
	●	●		●		●●		
	●	●						
	●			●●				
	●			●		●		
					●			
					●			
	●	●		●	●		●	
	●	●		●	●		●	
							●	
●	●	●●	●		bc			
	●	●						
		●					●	
	●							
					bc			
				●	bc		●	
	●	●		●	bc	●	●	
	●			●	bc	●	●	
		●			●●			
●	●							
		●						
●	●	●●	●					
	●							
	●	●						
		●			●		●	●●

●● Construct is measured "comprehensively" (i.e., at least 3–4 questions used to gather information on a topic).

● Construct is measured "adequately" (i.e., only 1–2 questions used to gather information on a topic).

○ Construct is measured through a biological or physical mechanism (e.g., withdrawal of a blood sample or physical exam).

bc Construct is measured using data from birth certificates.

TABLE B-3 Child Health Status, Functioning, and Health Potential Measures

Health Measures	NHIS	NHANES	MEPS
I. Functioning			
A. Physical functioning			
1. Diseases	●	○●	●
2. Injuries	●		●
3. Impairments			
Limitations in mobility	●	●	●
Impairments needing wheelchair, etc.	●	●	●
Gross and fine motor deficits		●	
Hearing difficulty, deafness	●		●●
Vision difficulty, blindness	●●	○●	●●
Speech difficulty	●		
Delays in growth or development			
Measurement of height	●	●	●
Measurement of weight	●	●●	●●
Restriction of usual activities	●●	●●	●●
Limitations due to oral health		●	
4. Symptoms			
B. Psychological functioning			
1. Cognitive functioning			
Alertness problems			
Confusion problems		●●	
Inattentiveness		●	
Concentration difficulty	●		
Problem-solving deficits			
Language use/comprehension deficits			
Reading difficulty			
Learning disability	●	●●	
2. Emotional functioning			
Limitations in usual activities		●	●
Attachment problems			
Negative affect, mood, or depression	●		●●
Consideration of suicide			
Infant temperament			
Temperament problems	●		●
Anxious, nervous, or worrisome	●		●
Trouble with self-regulation			
Poor self-esteem and self-perception			
Negative body image			
Self-sufficiency problems			
Difficulty getting to sleep	●		
C. Social functioning			
Relational capacity deficits	●		●
Cooperation problems	●		
Poor integration or connection			
Conduct/delinquency problems		●●	●
Poor academic performance			
School days missed	●	●	

Key on page 271

YRBS	NLSY	Add Health	NSFH	ECLS-K	ECLS-B	NHES	NSECH	NS-CSHCN
	●	●		●	●	●	●	
●	●	●			●			
		●	●		●	●		
	●	●●		●				
	●	●		●	●	●		
	●	●		●	●	●		
	●	●		●		●		
		●		●		●		
●		●	●	○	○			
●		●	●	○	○			
	●	●						●
		●						
				●●				
				●		●		
	●	●	●					
		●●						
		●			●●			
	●	●●		●		●		
	●							●
					●			
●	●	●●		●		●		
●●		●●	●●					
					●			
	●●	●●	●●	●	●●	●		
	●●	●	●●	●				
		●●		●●		●		
●	●●	●●						
	●	●			●			
	●	●●		●		●		
				●		●		
		●●						
	●●	●●	●●	●		●●		
	●●	●●	●	●●		●●		
	●●	●●	●	●		●		●

continued

TABLE B-3 Continued

Health Measures	NHIS	NHANES	MEPS
School drop out	●		
II. Health potential			
A. Physical well-being			
Self-assessed physical health		●	●
Self-assessed oral health		●	
Changes in physical health status	●	●	●
Gross and fine motor coordination			
Positive growth or development			
Participation in usual activities			●
Developmental milestones			
B. Psychological well-being			
1. Cognitive well-being			
Intelligence (IQ)			
Alertness			
Attentiveness			
Problem-solving ability			
Language use/comprehension ability			
Reading level or frequency			
Task persistence	●		
Curiosity			
Creativity			
2. Emotional well-being			
Obedience/compliance	●		
Self-assessed mental health status			●
Independence			
Positive personal affect or mood			●
Positive temperament			●
Impulse control			
Self-esteem and self-perception			
Positive body image			
Self-sufficiency			
C. Social well-being			
Relational capacity (parents, peers)			●
Cooperativeness			
Integration/connection (e.g. sports)			●
School readiness			
Academic performance			●
High school completion		●	
College plans/admission			
D. Resilience (e.g., seldom gets sick)			●●

NHIS = National Health Interview Survey; NHANES = National Health and Nutrition Examination Survey; MEPS = Medical Expenditure Panel Survey; YRBS = Youth Risk Behavior Survey; NLSY = National Longitudinal Survey of Youth; Add Health = National Longitudinal Survey of Adolescent Health; NSFH = National Survey of Families and Households; ECLS-K = Early Childhood Longitudinal Study Kindergarten Class; ECLS-B = Early Childhood Longitudinal Study-Birth Cohort; NHES = National Household Education Surveys; NSECH = National Survey of Early Childhood Health; NS-CSHCN = National Survey of Children with Special Health Care Needs

YRBS	NLSY	Add Health	NSFH	ECLS-K	ECLS-B	NHES	NSECH	NS-CSHCN
	●●	●	●					
	●	●		●	●		●	
	●	●			●			
	●●			●				
		●●		●				
					●●			
						●		
				●	●	●		
	●●	●●		●	●●			
	●●			●		●		
	●●			●				
				●				
				●				
				●				
	●	●	●					
			●	●				
	●●	●●	●	●				
	●●	●●	●	●	●			
		●		●	●			
		●		●				
	●●	●●				●		
		●						
	●●	●●	●●	●		●		
		●●		●				
●		●●	●●	●●		●●		
				●●		●●		
●	●●	●●	●●	●●		●●		
	●●	●●	●●					
	●●	●●	●●			●●		
		●●						

●●   Construct is measured "comprehensively" (i.e., at least 3–4 questions used to gather information on a topic).

●   Construct is measured "adequately" (i.e., only 1–2 questions used to gather information on a topic).

○   Construct is measured through a biological or physical mechanism (e.g., withdrawal of a blood sample or physical exam).

bc   Construct is measured using data from birth certificates.

TABLE B-4 Influences on Children's Health

Health Measures	NHIS	NHANES	MEPS
I. Children's biology			
1. Genetics			
2. Body burdens			
3. Biomarkers		○	
4. Body composition		○●	
5. Body anthropometry		○	
6. Cardiovascular fitness		○	
7. Blood pressure		○●	
II. Children's behavior			
1. Child social behaviors			
Peer contacts and support networks			
Romantic relationships			
Peer pressures/influences			
Employment/volunteering			●
Civic involvement			
2. Child health risk behaviors			
Smoking/chewing tobacco		○●●	
Alcohol use/riding drunk		●●	
Drug use		●●	
Overeating/undereating/dieting		●●	
Excessive television watching		●●	
High-risk sexual activity		●●	
Carrying a weapon to school			
Perceptions of risk			
3. Child health promotion behaviors			
Seat belt use			●
Exercise frequency/intensity		●●	
Nutrition adequacy		●●○	
Getting adequate sleep			
Sunscreen use		●●	
Use of bicycle/motorcycle helmets			
Eye protection during sports	●(periodic)		
4. Illness management behaviors			
Belief in medical care			
Compliance with treatments			
Attendance of scheduled visits			
Parent receipt of health education			
Child receipt of health education			
III. Social environment			
A. Family			
1. Family composition and size			
Single vs. two-parent families	●		●
Family disruption (e.g., divorce)	●	●	
Maternal age (e.g., teen birth)	●		
Foster care/guardian	●		●
Number/spacing of children			
Relocation and mobility		●	

Key on page 283

YRBS	NLSY	Add Health	NSFH	ECLS-K	ECLS-B	NHES	NSECH	NS-CSHCN
		○			●			
		○						
		○		○				
	●●	●●	●●	●				
	●●	●●	●●					
	●●	●●		●		●●		
	●●	●●	●●			●●		
		●●				●●		
●●	●●	●●	●					
●●	●●	●●	●					
●●	●●	●●						
●●	●	●●						
●	●●	●●		●●	●●	●	●	
●●	●●	●●	●					
●●	●●	●						
	●●	●●						
●	●	●						
●●	●●	●		●●				
●●	●	●		●	●			
	●	●●						
		●●						
●		●						
		●					●	
		●						
●		●●					●●	
●●	●	●●	●●	●●	●●	●	●	●
●●	●	●●	●●	●●	●●	●	●	
●●	●●	●●	●●	●	●	●	●	
●●	●	●●	●●	●●		●	●	●
●●	●	●●	●●	●●	bc ●	●	●	●
●●	●	●●	●●	●●	●	●	●	

continued

TABLE B-4 Continued

Health Measures	NHIS	NHANES	MEPS
2. Socioeconomic status			
Family income	●●	●●	●●
Difficulty paying for basic needs			●
Receipt of TANF	●●	●●	
Receipt of SSI		●●	●
Receipt of WIC	●	●	
Rental assistance/public housing			
Food insecurity	●●	●●	
Receipt of food stamps	●	●	
Participation in early intervention	●	●●	
Special education	●●	●	
Individualized education program			
Free or reduced price lunch		●●	
Maternal/paternal education	●●	●	●●
Maternal/paternal employment	●●	●●	●●
4. Parent health, mental health, substance use			
Parent health	●●		●●
Parent/partner support or arguing			
Maternal depression	●		●
Maternal frustration			
Maternal stress			
Parent social support			
Parent concerns about child health			
Parent exercise behaviors	●●		●
Parent smoking	●●	●●	●
Parent alcohol and drug use	●●	●●	
5. Pregnancy issues			
Whether the pregnancy was wanted			
Receipt of prenatal care			
Prepregnancy weight			
Supplement use during pregnancy			
Use of fertility treatments			
6. Parenting			
Paternal involvement/closeness			
Breastfeeding		●●	
Routines for sleeping, feeding			
Childrearing belief (age to toilet train)			
Parenting style (authoritarian, etc.)			
Time spent with children			
Monitoring and supervision			
Supportive nature			
Discipline			
Use of child care		●	
7. Family learning environments			
Home schooling	●		
Reading to children			

YRBS	NLSY	Add Health	NSFH	ECLS-K	ECLS-B	NHES	NSECH	NS-CSHCN
●●	●		●●	●●	●●	●	●●	●
	●			●●	●●		●●	●
●●	●			●	●	●		
●●	●				●			●
●●	●			●	●●	●	●	
●●								
	●			●●	●●	●		
●●	●			●	●	●		
					●	●		
	●			●●		●		●
				●●		●		●
				●●		●●		
●●	●		●●	●●	●●	●	●	●
●●	●		●●	●●	●●	●●	●	
●●	●		●●	●	●●			
●●				●	●●			
●			●●	●●	●●		●●	
			●●				●	
			●●				●	
			●●	●●	●●		●	
							●●	
		●	●		●●			
			●		●●			
		●			●			
		●			bc ●●			
					●			
		●			●			
					●			
●●	●				●●			
	●				●●		●●	
	●		●●	●●	●●	●	●●	
					●●			
●●	●		●●	●●	●●	●●	●●	
●●	●●		●●	●●	●●	●	●	
●	●		●●	●●	●●			
●	●●		●●	●●	●●	●		
●	●		●●	●●	●●	●	●●	
●●			●●	●●	●●	●●	●●	
						●●		
			●●	●●	●●	●	●	

continued

TABLE B-4 Continued

Health Measures	NHIS	NHANES	MEPS
Socialization and play			
Participation in school activities			
Providing learning opportunities			
Assisting with homework/projects			
Use of after school programs			
Availability of a computer at home			
8. Family provision of safe environments	●(periodic)		
Car seats and seat belts			
Use of smoke detectors			
Reduce hot water temperature			
Cabinet locks or safety latches			
Covering electrical sockets			
Baby gates and other barriers			
Water safety supervision			
Have syrup of Ipecac			
Safe storage of firearms			
B. Community			
1. Neighborhood demographics and SES			
Geographic setting (e.g., rural)			
Community socioeconomic level			
Unemployment rates			
Relative income distribution			
Affordable housing			
2. Neighborhood institutions			
Preschool availability and use		●	
Head Start availability and use		●	
Schools and class size			
Social (e.g., library/community centers)			
Child care programs			
Police protection			
3. Social organization of neighborhood			
Social cohesion (trust and values)			
Social control (monitoring)			
Social connection (e.g., to school)			
Social interaction and networks			
C. Culture			
Race/ethnicity	●●	●	●●
English-language proficiency		●●	●
Culture, beliefs, practices			
Citizenship or immigration status	●	●	●
Acculturation	●	●●	●
D. Discrimination			
Diversity and segregation			
Racism, classicism, etc.			

YRBS	NLSY	Add Health	NSFH	ECLS-K	ECLS-B	NHES	NSECH	NS-CSHCN
		●	●●	●●	●●	●●	●●	
	●	●	●●	●●	●	●●		
		●	●●	●●	●●	●●	●●	
		●	●	●●		●●		
				●●		●●		
	●	●		●●	●	●		
					●			
					●			
							●	
							●	
							●	
							●	
							●	
					●			
	●●					●		
	●	●●		●		●		
	●	●●			●	●		
	●	●●						
		●						
		●						
	●		●			●●		
				●●	●	●●		
	●	●		●●		●		
					●	●●		
						●		
		●●			●			
		●						
		●●	●●		●●	●●		
		●●		●●	●			
●	●●	●●	●	●	●●	●	●●	●
	●●	●		●	●●	●	●	
	●●			●		●		
	●●	●		●	●	●		
	●	●			●			
		●		●				

continued

TABLE B-4 Continued

Health Measures	NHIS	NHANES	MEPS
IV. Physical environment			
A. Micro-environment			
1. Prenatal exposures			
Nonconcurrent exposures			
Concurrent exposures (e.g., smoking)		●	
2. Postnatal exposures			
Air pollutants		●●	
Water pollutants			
Food contaminants			
Infectious agents		○	
Chemicals (e.g., lead) and pesticides		○●●	
Noise			
Radiation (UV and Ionizing)			
B. Macro-environment			
1. Physical exposures			
Noise and unwanted sound			
Environmental air pollution/ozone			
2. Physical safety and security			
Housing adequacy		●●	
Housing safety (e.g., lead paint)	●(periodic)	●●	
School safety (e.g., playground)			
Recreational safety (e.g., parks)			
Pedestrian safety (e.g., crosswalks)			
Vehicle accidents (e.g., car, bike)			
Community/school safety (violence)			
V. Services (health services)			
A. Structure			
1. Health insurance coverage and type	●●	●●	●●
Public vs. private sponsorship	●●	●●	●●
Comprehensiveness of benefits		●	
Cost-sharing requirements		●●	●●
Gaps in coverage	●	●	●●
2. Managed care plan restrictions			
Gatekeeping restrictions	●●	●●	●●
Network restrictions	●●	●●	●●
Provider incentives			
3. Regular source/provider of care	●	●	●
Specialty and training	●		●
Demographics (gender, race, or age)			●●
Language			●
4. Setting of care			
Clinic vs. private office	●	●	●
Health center (e.g., CHC)			●
Staffing and resources			
Geographic location			
Service capacity			

YRBS	NLSY	Add Health	NSFH	ECLS-K	ECLS-B	NHES	NSECH	NS-CSHCN
					••			
		••			••			
		••		•				
		••		••		••		
				•				
				•				
					•			
••	••	••		•	•	•		
	•	•		•	••	•	••	••
	•	•		•	•	•	••	••
								•
					•		••	••
					•		•	
							•	
					•		•	•
							•	•
							•	
		•			•		•	•
		•			•		•	
							•	

continued

TABLE B-4 Continued

Health Measures	NHIS	NHANES	MEPS
B. Process of care			
1. Accessibility	●		●●
Waiting time for/at appointment			●
Distance/transportation to office			●
Phone contact with provider	●		●
Delayed or missed care/prescriptions	●	●	●
Difficulty obtaining referrals			●
2. Continuity of care			
Same provider for sick and well care	●		●
Same provider seen regularly	●		
Length of time with same provider			
3. Interpersonal manner			
Duration of medical visit			
Enough time to ask questions			●
Provider listens/answers questions			●
Support and partnership in care			●●
4. Comprehensiveness of services			
Developmental assessment			
Use of reminders for immunizations			
Anticipatory guidance			●●
Injury prevention guidance			●●
Psychosocial counseling			
Lead poisoning screening			
Reproductive counseling/screening			
5. Coordination of care			
Need for coordination			
Type of care coordinator			
Actions of the provider/coordinator			●
Communication among providers			
Communication with school/teacher			
Receipt of Title V services			
6. Family-centered care			
7. Cultural competence			●
C. Utilization/receipt of care			
1. Primary care			
Well-child/routine checkup visits	●		●
Physician visits	●	●	●
Vision visits	●		●
Dental visits	●	●●	●
Prescription medication (use)	●	●	●
2. Up-to-date immunization schedule	●		
Hepatitis A	●	○●	
Hepatitis B	●	○●	
DTP (diphtheria, tetanus, pertussis)	●		
MMR (measles, mumps, rubella)	●	○	
IPV (inactivated polio)	●		

YRBS	NLSY	Add Health	NSFH	ECLS-K	ECLS-B	NHES	NSECH	NS-CSHCN
							●	●
		●						●
		●						●
							●	●
		●			●		●●	●
								●
								●
							●	●
							●	●
								●
								●
								●
							●	
							●●	
							●●	
							●●	
								●
								●
								●
								●
								●
						●		●
							●●	
		●		●	●	●	●	●
	●	●		●	●		●	●
		●		●	●			●
		●		●	●	●		●
●	●	●					●	●

continued

TABLE B-4 Continued

Health Measures	NHIS	NHANES	MEPS
Hib (Haemophilus influenzae)	●		
Varicella	●	○	
Influenza	●		
Pneumococcal	●	●	
3. Specialty and tertiary care			
Specialist visits	●		●
Mental health visits	●	●	●
Receipt of special therapy			●●
Hospitalization admission	●	●	●
Emergency department visit	●	●	●
Surgical procedures	●		●
Home care from professional	●		●

NHIS = National Health Interview Survey; NHANES = National Health and Nutrition Examination Survey; MEPS = Medical Expenditure Panel Survey; YRBS = Youth Risk Behavior Survey; NLSY = National Longitudinal Survey of Youth; Add Health = National Longitudinal Survey of Adolescent Health; NSFH = National Survey of Families and Households; ECLS-K = Early Childhood Longitudinal Study Kindergarten Class; ECLS-B = Early Childhood Longitudinal Study-Birth Cohort; NHES = National Household Education Surveys; NSECH = National Survey of Early Childhood Health; NS-CSHCN = National Survey of Children with Special Health Care Needs

YRBS	NLSY	Add Health	NSFH	ECLS-K	ECLS-B	NHES	NSECH	NS-CSHCN

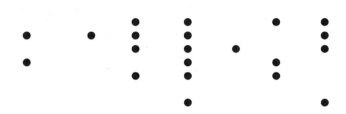

●● Construct is measured "comprehensively" (i.e., at least 3–4 questions used to gather information on a topic).

● Construct is measured "adequately" (i.e., only 1–2 questions used to gather information on a topic).

○ Construct is measured through a biological or physical mechanism (e.g., withdrawal of a blood sample or physical exam).

bc Construct is measured using data from birth certificates.

Appendix C

Selected Indicators from National Children's Data Syntheses

T his appendix highlights the types of measures used in national initiatives that present indicators on various aspects of children's health and may provide a useful reference for states and localities interested in developing state or local indicators. Details regarding specific data used to produce indicators are typically available on the web site of the data collection agency.

America's Children and the Environment

http://www.epa.gov/envirohealth/children/

A report by the U.S. Environmental Protection Agency, produced for the first time in 2000 and updated in 2003. It presents key information on the environmental exposures, biomonitoring, and environmentally related diseases that affect children's health and well-being. The measures in the report are based on data collected from state and federal agencies.

Measure/Indicator	Age	Frequency Measured	Level
Common air pollutants (1): percentage of children living in a county in which at least one air quality standard was exceeded during the year	Children ≤ 18 yrs	Annually: 1990–1998	County
Common air pollutants (2): percentage of children's days that were designated as having "unhealthy" air quality	Children ≤ 18 yrs	Annually: 1990–1998	County

Measure/Indicator	Age	Frequency Measured	Level
Hazardous air pollutants: percentage of children living in counties where at least one hazardous air pollutant concentration was greater than a health benchmark	Children ≤ 18 yrs	1990	County
Environmental tobacco smoke: percentage of homes with children under 7 in which someone smokes on a regular basis	Children < 7 yrs	1994, 1996, 1999 (total of 10 target years)	National— based on national survey
Drinking water standards: percentage of children served by public water systems that exceeded a maximum contaminant level or violated a treatment standard	Children ≤ 18 yrs	Annually: 1993–1998	National[a]
Nitrates and nitrites: percentage of children living in areas served by public water systems in which the nitrate/nitrite standard was exceeded	Children ≤ 18 yrs	Annually: 1993–1998	National[a]
Monitoring and reporting: percentage of children living in areas with major violations of drinking water monitoring and reporting requirements	Children ≤ 18 yrs	Annually: 1993–1998	National[a]
Pesticide residues in foods: percentage of fruits, vegetables, grains, dairy, and processed foods with detectable pesticide residues		Annually: 1993–1998	National[a]
Hazardous waste sites (1): percentage of children living in counties with Superfund sites	Children ≤ 18 yrs	Every 2 years: 1990–2000	County
Hazardous waste sites (2): percentage of children living in counties that had Superfund sites in 1990	Children ≤ 18 yrs	Every 2 years: 1990–2000	County
Concentrations of lead in blood (1): average concentrations of lead in blood for children 5 and under	Children ≤ 5 yrs	1976–1980, 1988–1991, 1992–1994	National[a]
Concentrations of lead in blood (2): percentage of children ages 1–5 with concentrations of lead in blood greater than 10 micrograms per deciliter	Children 1–5 yrs	1992–1994	National[a]

Measure/Indicator	Age	Frequency Measured	Level
Respiratory diseases (1): percentage of children under 18 with asthma and chronic bronchitis	Children ≤ 18 yrs	Annually: 1990–1996	National[a]
Respiratory diseases (2): percentage of children under 18 with asthma	Children ≤ 18 yrs	1997–1998	National[a]
Respiratory diseases (3): asthma hospitalization rate for children 0–14	Children 0–14 yrs	Annually: 1987–1998	National[a]
Childhood cancer (1): cancer incidence and mortality for children under 20	Children ≤ 20 yrs	Annually: 1975–1995	National[a]
Childhood cancer (2): cancer incidence for children under 20 by type	Children ≤ 20 yrs	Annually: 1973–1996	National[a]

[a]Based on data reported to rather than collected by the federal government.

America's Children: Key National Indicators of Well-Being

http://www.childstats.gov/americaschildren/

A report by the Federal Interagency Forum on Child and Family Statistics that includes federal and state statistics on the health and well-being of children and their families. The report includes indicators of well-being within the parameters of economic security, health, behavior, and social environment and education in addition to key contextual measures.

Measure/Indicator	Age	Frequency Measured	Level
Child poverty and family income: percentage of related children under age 18 in poverty by family structure	Children ≤ 18 yrs	Annually: 1980–2000	National
Child poverty and family income: percentage of related children under age 18 relative to the poverty line	Children ≤ 18 yrs	Annually: 1980–2000	National
Secure parental employment: percentage of children under age 18 living parents with at least one parent employed full time all year	Children ≤ 18 yrs	Annually: 1980–2000	National
Housing problems: percentage of households with children under age 18 that report housing problems	Children ≤ 18 yrs	1978, 1983, 1989, 1993, 1995, 1997, 1999	National

Measure/Indicator	Age	Frequency Measured	Level
Food security and diet quality (1): percentage of children under age 18 in households experiencing food insecurity reporting child hunger	Children ≤ 18 yrs	Annual: 1995–2000, however 1996 and 1997 omitted because not relevant for comparison	National
Food security and diet quality (2): percentage of children ages 2 to 5 and 6 to 9 with a good diet	Children 2–5 yrs 6–9 yrs	1994–1996, 1998	National
Access to health care: percentage of children under age 18 covered by health insurance	Children ≤ 18 yrs	Annual: 1987–2000, 1999 and 2000 not comparable with earlier years	National
Access to health care: percentage of children under age 18 with no usual source of health care by type of health insurance	Children ≤ 18 yrs	Annual: 1993–2000, 1997–2000 not comparable with earlier years	National
General health status: percentage of children under age 18 in very good or excellent health	Children ≤ 18 yrs	Annual: 1984–2000, 1997–2000 not comparable with earlier years	National
Activity limitation: percentage of children ages 5 to 17 with any limitation in activity resulting from chronic conditions	Children 5–17 yrs	2000	National
Childhood immunization: percentage of children ages 19 to 35 months who received combined series immunization coverage	Children 19–35 mos	Annual: 1994–2000	National
Low birthweight: percentage of infants weighing less than 5.5 pounds at birth	Children < 5.5 lbs	Annual: 1980–2000	National
Infant mortality: deaths before the first birthday per 1,000 live births	Children < 1 yr	Annual: 1983–1991, 1995–1999	National

Measure/Indicator	Age	Frequency Measured	Level
Child mortality (1): deaths per 100,000 children ages 1 to 4	Children 1–4 yrs	Annual: 1980–1999	National
Child mortality (2): deaths per 100,000 children ages 5 to 14 by race and by cause of death	Children 5–14 yrs	Annual: 1980–1999	National
Adolescent mortality: deaths per 100,000 adolescents 15 to 19 by cause of death	Children 5–19 yrs	Annual: 1980–1999	National
Adolescent mortality: injury deaths per 100,000 adolescents 15 to 19 by gender, race, and type of injury	Children 5–19 yrs	1999	National
Adolescent births: births per 1,000 females ages 15 to 17	Females 15–17 yrs	Annual: 1980–2000	National
Regular cigarette smoking: percentage of 8th grade students who reported smoking daily in the previous 30 days	Children 8th, 10th, and 12th grades	Annual: 1980–2001	National
Alcohol use: percentage of 8th grade students who reported having five or more alcoholic beverages in a row in the last 2 weeks	Children 8th, 10th, and 12th grades	Annual: 1980–2001	National
Illicit drug use: percentage of 8th grade students who have used illicit drugs in the previous 30 days	Children 8th, 10th, and 12th grades	Annual: 1980–2001	National
Youth victims and perpetrators of serious violent crimes: rate of serious violent crime victimization per 1,000 youth ages 12 to 17	Children 12–17 yrs	Annual: 1980–2000	National
Youth victims and perpetrators of serious violent crimes: serious violent crime offending rate by youth ages 12 to 17	Children 12–17 yrs	Annual: 1980–2000	National
Family reading to young children: percentage of children ages 3 to 5 who are read to every day by a family member	Children 3–5 yrs	1993, 1995, 1996, 1999, 2001	National
Early childhood care and education: percentage of children ages 3 to 5 who are enrolled in early childhood centers	Children 3–5 yrs	1991, 1993 not comparable for later years 1995, 1996, 1999, 2001	National

Measure/Indicator	Age	Frequency Measured	Level
Mathematics achievement (0–500 scale): average mathematics scale score of 9-, 13- and 17-year-olds	Children 9, 13, 17 yrs	1982, 1986, 1990, 1992, 1994, 1996, 1999	National
Reading achievement (0–500 scale): average reading scale score of 9-, 13- and 17-year-olds	Children 9, 13, 17 yrs	1980, 1984, 1988, 1990, 1992, 1994, 1996, 1999	National
High school academic course-taking: percentage of high school graduates who completed high-level coursework in mathematics, science, English, or foreign language	High school graduates	1982, 1987, 1990, 1992, 1994, 1998	National
High school completion: percentage of young adults ages 18 to 24 who have completed high school	Young adults 18–24 yrs	Annual: 1980–2000	National
Youth neither enrolled in school nor working: percentage of youth ages 16 to 19 who are neither in school nor working	Children 16–19 yrs	Annual: 1984–2001	National
Higher education: percentage of high school graduates ages 25 to 29 who have completed a bachelor's degree or higher	Young adults 25–29 yrs	Annual: 1980–2001	National
Children of at least one foreign-born parent: percentage of children under age 18 by nativity of child and parents	Children ≤ 18 yrs	Annual: 1994–2001	National

Child Health USA

http://www.mchirc.net/CH-USA.htm

An annual report by the Health Resources and Service Administration of the U.S. Department of Health and Human Services composed of secondary data for 59 health status indicators summarized both graphically and textually, including long-term trends.

Measure/Indicator	Age	Frequency Measured	Level
Related children under 18 years of age living in families below 100% of poverty level by race/ethnicity	Children ≤ 18 yrs	1970, 1980, 1990, 1998, 1999	National

Measure/Indicator	Age	Frequency Measured	Level
Related children under 18 years of age living in families below 100% of poverty level, by household status	Children ≤ 18 yrs	1999	National
Status school dropout rates for ages 16–24 by race/ethnicity	Children 16–24 yrs	Annual: 1988–1999	National
Mothers in the workforce	Children 6–17 yrs	Every 5 years— 1980–2000	National
Hours per week spent in child care by children under 5 with working mothers	Children < 5 yrs	1997	National
Percentage distribution of births by maternal age, by race	N/A	1999	National
Breastfeeding by race	N/A	Annual: 1990–1999	National
Percentage of infants born at low birthweight by race	N/A	Annual: 1984–1999	National
Percentage of infants born at very low birthweight by race	N/A	Annual: 1984–1999	National
Comparison of national infant mortality rates	N/A	1997	International, National
U.S. infant mortality rates by race of mother	N/A	Annual: 1980–1999	National
Preliminary neonatal mortality rates by race of mother	N/A	1999	National
Preliminary postneonatal mortality rates by race of mother	N/A	1999	National
Maternal mortality rates by race of mother	N/A	Annual: 1975–1998	National
Number of cases of reportable vaccine-preventable diseases among children under 5	Children < 5 yrs	1999	National
Percentage of child abuse and neglect victims by type of maltreatment	N/A	1999	National
Sources of maltreatment reports	N/A	1999	National

Measure/Indicator	Age	Frequency Measured	Level
Pediatric aids by race/ethnicity and exposure category	N/A	1981–2000	National
Major causes of hospitalization by age	Children 1–21 yrs	1999	National
Discharge rate of patients 1–14 years old for selected diagnosis	Children 1–14 yrs	Annual: 1985–1999	National
Leading causes of death in children ages 1–14	Children 1–14 yrs	1999	National
Childhood deaths due to external cause, by cause and age	Children 1–14 yrs	1999	National
Adolescent birth rates, by age and race of mother	N/A	1999	National
Percentage of high school students who have ever had sexual intercourse, by grade and gender	Children 9th, 10th, 11th, and 12th grades	1999	National
Sexual activity and condom use in high school students	Children 9th, 10th, 11th, and 12th grades	1999	National
Rates of sexually transmitted disease per 100,000 adolescents by age and race	Young adults 15–24 yrs	1999	National
Adolescent AIDS cases, by race/ethnicity and exposure category for ages 13–19	Children 13–19 yrs	1981–1999	National
Adolescent AIDS cases by gender and exposure category for ages 13–19	Children 13–19 yrs	1981–1999	National
Young adult AIDS cases by gender and exposure category for ages 20–24	Young adults 20–24 yrs	1981–1999	National
Percentage of high school students who carried a gun in the past 30 days, by sex and race	N/A	Annual: 1993–1999	National
Percentage of high school students who participated in vigorous, moderate, or strengthening physical activity, by race	N/A	1999	National

Measure/Indicator	Age	Frequency Measured	Level
Percentage of high school students who participated in moderate physical activity, by grade	Children 9th, 10th, and 11th grades	1999	National
Long-term trend in 30-days prevalence of cigarette smoking for 8th, 10th, and 12th graders	Children 8th, 10th, and 12th grades	Annual: 1975–2000	National
30-day prevalence of drug use among adolescent ages 12–17	Children 12–17 yrs	Annual: 1988–1999	National
Leading causes of death in adolescent ages 15–19	Children 15–19 yrs	1999	National
Motor vehicles crashes and firearms mortality among adolescents ages 15–19	Children 15–19 yrs	1998	National
Health insurance coverage of children under 18 yrs	Children ≤ 18 yrs	1999	National
Health insurance coverage of children under 18 yrs in poverty	Children ≤ 18 yrs	1999	National
Estimated vaccination coverage among children ages 19–35 months by race/ethnicity	Children 19–45 mos	2000	National
Recommended childhood immunization schedule, United States, January–December 2001	Children ≤ 18 yrs	2001	National
Percentage of children receiving an EPSDT preventive dental service	Children > 2 yrs	Annual: 1988–1998	National
Percentage of children with dental care needs and those receiving dental care in the last 12 months by income	Children > 2 yrs	1997	National
Percentage of children with no physician visits in the past year, by age and race/ethnicity	Children ≤ 19 yrs	1998	National
Usual source of acute care	Children ≤ 19 yrs	1998	National
Physician utilization by children with chronic activity limitation, by age	Children under 5 yrs, over 5 yrs	1998	National
Hospital utilization by income and race	N/A	1998	National

Measure/Indicator	Age	Frequency Measured	Level
Percentage of mothers beginning prenatal care in the first trimester, by age and race	N/A	1999	National
Percentage of mothers receiving late or no prenatal care, by age and race of mother	N/A	1999	National
Percentage of infants born at low birthweight, women receiving first trimester prenatal care, and births to women under 18, by race of mother and state	N/A	1999	State, national
Medicaid enrollees, expenditures, and reported EPSDT utilization for children under age 21	N/A	FY 1998 FY 1999	State, national
State Children's Health Insurance Program (SCHIP) aggregate enrollment statistics	N/A	FY 2000	State, national
Health insurance status for children under age 19	N/A	1999	County
Percentage of children under 19 who are uninsured	N/A	1999	State, national
Infant and neonatal mortality rates, by race of mother and state	N/A	1998	State, national
Percentage of infants born at very low birthweight in U.S. cities with populations over 100,000	N/A	Annual: 1989–1999	National
Percentage of infants born at very low birthweight in U.S. cities with populations over 100,000	N/A	Annual: 1989–1999	National
Infant mortality in U.S. cities with population over 100,000	N/A	Annual: 1989–1998	National
Percentage of pregnant women receiving first trimester prenatal care in U.S. cities with populations over 100,000	N/A	Annual: 1989–1999	National
Percentage of pregnant women receiving late or no prenatal care in U.S. cities with populations over 100,000	N/A	Annual: 1989–1999	National

KIDS COUNT Data Book

http://www.aecf.org/kidscount/kc2002/

A data book produced by the Annie E. Casey Foundation that tracks national and state-level indicators of the educational, social, economic, and physical well-being of children in the United States, with a focus on 10 core indicators.

Measure/Indicator	Age	Frequency Measured	Level
Number of children under age 18	N/A	2000	State, national
Race and Hispanic origin of children	N/A	2000	State, national
4th grade students who scored below basic reading level	Children 4th grade	1998	State, national
8th grade students who scored below basic reading level	Children 8th grade	1998	State, national
8th grade students who scored below basic writing level	Children 8th grade	1998	State, national
Median income of families with children	N/A	1998	State, national
Female-headed families receiving child support or alimony	N/A	1998	State, national
Children in working-poor families without a telephone at home	N/A	1998	State, national
Children in extreme poverty (income 50% below of poverty level)		1998	State, national
Children without health insurance		1998	State, national
Children in working-poor families who lack health insurance		1998	State, national
2-year-olds who were immunized	Children 2 yrs	1999	State, national
Juvenile violent crime arrest rate	Children 10–17 yrs	1998	State, national

Measure/Indicator	Age	Frequency Measured	Level
Juvenile property crime arrest rate	Children 10–17 yrs	1998	State, national
Number of children under 18 in working poor families	Children < 18 yrs	1998	State, national
Percentage of children under age 18 in working poor families	Children < 18 yrs	1998	State, national
Percentage change of low-birthweight babies		1990–1998	State, national
Percentage change of infant mortality rates		1990–1998	State, national
Percentage change of child death rates ages 1–14	Children 1–14 yrs	1990–1998	State, national
Percentage change of rate of teen deaths by accident, homicide, and suicide ages 15–19	Young adults 15–19 yrs	1990–1998	State, national
Percentage change of teen birth rate of females ages 15–17	Females 15–17 yrs	1990–1998	State, national
Percentage change of teens who are high school dropouts ages 16–19	Young adults 16–19 yrs	1990–1998	State, national
Percentage change of teens not attending school and not working ages 16–19	Young adults 16–19 yrs	1990–1998	State, national
Percentage change of children living with parents who do not have full-time, year-round employment		1990–1998	State, national
Percentage change of children in poverty		1990–1998	State, national
Percentage change of families with children headed by a single parent		1990–1998	State, national

Child Trends Databank

http://www.childtrendsdatabank.org/

Child Trends produces this continuously updated web-based bank of data of the latest estimates for indicators relating to child and family health and well-being. The data identifies and tracks trends and population subgroup disparities.

Measure/Indicator	Age	Frequency Measured	Level
Overweight children and youth	Children 6–19 yrs	1999	National
Disordered eating: symptoms of bulimia	Children 9th–12th grades	2001	National
Children with limitations	Children 5–17 yrs	1998–2000	National
Learning disabilities	Children 3–17 yrs	1997–2000	National
Asthma	Children < 18 yrs	1988–1998	National
Children with AIDS	Children < 13 yrs	1985–2001	National
Low- and very-low-birthweight infants		1970–2001	National
Suicidal teens	Children 9th–12th grades	2001	National
Adolescents who feel sad or hopeless	Children 9th–12th grades	1999, 2001	National
Parental symptoms of depression	Children < 18 yrs	2000	National
Vigorous physical activity by youth	Children 9th–12th grades	1993–2001	National
Mothers who smoke while pregnant	N/A	1989–2000	National

Measure/Indicator	Age	Frequency Measured	Level
Condom use	Children 9th–12th grades	1993–1999	National
Participation in school athletics	Children 8th–12th grades	1991–2000	National
Seat belt use	Children 5–15 yrs	1994–2000	National
Drunk driving	Children 9th–12th grades	1995–2001	National
Physical fighting by youth	Children 9th–12th grades	1993–2001	National
Students carrying weapons	Children 9th–12th grades	1991–2001	National
Adolescents who have ever been raped	Females 9th–12th grades	2001	National
Dating violence	Children 9th–12th grades	1999–2001	National
Child maltreatment	Children < 18 yrs	1990–2000	National
Youth who felt unsafe at school	Children 12–18 yrs	1999	National

In addition, the U.S. Department of Health and Human Services has identified in *Healthy People 2010* a set of health objectives intended to improve the health of the country. *Healthy People 2010* specifies 10 leading health indicators and 467 objectives within the overall goals of improving quality and years of healthy life and eliminating health disparities. Several of the objectives relate to children. The objectives are listed and can be searched at http://www.healthy people.gov/.

Appendix D

Glossary

Administrative Data   Data collected as part of the administration of a specific program (e.g., Medicaid, Temporary Assistance for Needy Families).

Children's Health   The extent to which individual children or groups of children are able or enabled to (a) develop and realize their potential; (b) satisfy their needs; and (c) develop the capacities that allow them to interact successfully with their biological, physical, and social environments.

Critical Periods   Refers to a time during which certain experiences or influences have a deterministic (positive or negative) affect. Although the terms "critical periods" and "sensitive periods" are often used interchangeably in the literature, there are relatively few, if any, critical periods outside of the biological arena. From a biological or molecular perspective, there can be several critical periods such as during gestational periods or with exposure to mutagens and other carcinogenic agents (see sensitive periods below).

Data Element   A specific data component (e.g., height, weight).

Data Linkage   The combination of data on specific individuals from two or more datasets.

Data System   A collection of two or more datasets integrated into one system. Multiple administrative or other datasets might be linked using unique identifiers or might be aggregated and then combined into a single system.

Dataset   Two or more data elements collected through a single mechanism, effort, or type of scientific investigation.

Development   The processes by which humans proceed through life in individual ways that lead to new and more complex forms and progressive growth in capacities and functions.

Dimensions   The multiple factors within a subdomain that are measurable; for example, within the physical functioning subdomain, dimensions might include mobility, growth, and age-specific activities.

Domains   The broad categories of health. For this report, we divide health into three domains: health conditions, functioning, and health potential.

Environments   The set of factors external to a child. For purposes of this report, these factors are organization as the social environment (including family, community, culture, and discrimination) and the physical environment (including air, food, and water as well as aspects of the larger environment such as the built environment).

Influences   The range of factors that can pose a risk to children's health or serve in a health-protecting or -promoting capacity. Influences, therefore, refer to risk, protective, and promotional factors.

Measures   Indicators of health or health influences that can assess the aspects of each dimension in order to quantify the quality of health. Measures may be single items or composites of items. For example within the growth dimension, a child's height and weight are periodically measured.

Population Health   Population health refers to the aggregate measures of health for individuals within a population as well as the distribution of these measures across the major subpopulations in the population. That is, population health is reflected both as average levels of health as well as the variability in those levels across the population.

Safety   Aspects of the environment that contribute to health, including the physical environment (i.e., absence of lead levels in paint, pesticides or pollutants in the ground water, etc.), social environment (i.e., low neighborhood crime rates, rates of risky behaviors either by the children or adults), and psychological environment (i.e., the perception of being in personal danger).

Sensitive Periods   Refers to a time when the child is especially receptive to certain kinds of environmental influences or experiences and the ideal time to provide or to avoid them. Though the term "critical and sensitive periods" is used in this report, there are relatively few critical periods (see critical periods above).

Subdomains   Based on a hierarchy, the subcategories that domains are divided into that contain various dimensions and indicators within them. For example, within the domain of functioning, subdomains include physical functioning, psychological functioning, and social functioning.

Well-being   Well-being is the sense of health and safety as appraised by the individual. Factors such as quality of life, fulfillment, and ability to contribute constructively to society and one's own family are also important aspects of well-being. Aspects of well-being are incorporated in the domain of health termed "health potential" by the committee.

Appendix E

Acronyms

AAP	American Academy of Pediatrics
ACS	American Community Survey
ACYF	Administration for Children, Youth and Families
Add Health	National Longitudinal Study of Adolescent Health
AHRQ	Agency for Health Care Research and Quality
AIDS	Acquired immune deficiency syndrome
ASPE	Assistant Secretary for Planning and Evaluation
BESSC	Built Environment Site Survey Checklist
CAHPS	Consumer Assessment of Health Plans Survey
CDC	Centers for Disease Control and Prevention
CHRIS	Children's Registry and Information System
CMS	Center for Medicare and Medicaid Services
CMV	Cytomegaliovirus
CPS	Current Population Survey
CSHCN	Children with Special Health Care Needs
CSPR	Child Services and Policy Research
DHHS	Department of Health and Human Services
DUF	Drug Use Forecasting
ECLS-K	Early Childhood Longitudinal Survey, Kindergarten Class
ECSL-B	Early Childhood Longitudinal Survey, Birth Cohort

EPA	Environmental Protection Agency
EPSDT	Medicaid Early Periodic Screening, Diagnosis and Treatment
FACCT	Foundation for Accountability
FDLRS	Florida Diagnostic and Learning Resources System
FERPA	Federal Education Right to Privacy Act
FIFCFS	Federal Interagency Forum on Child and Family Statistics
GYTS	Global Youth Tobacco Survey
HBSC	Health Behavior in School-Aged Children
HEDIS	Health Employer Data Information System
HHANES	Hispanic Health and Nutrition Examination Survey
HIPAA	Health Insurance Portability and Accountability Act
HIV	Human immunodeficiency virus
HP2010	*Healthy People 2010*
HRSA	Health Resources and Services Administration
IAP	Immunization Action Plan
ICD-10	International Classification of Diseases and Related Health Problems-10
ICF	International Classification of Functioning
ICPC	International Classification of Primary Care
IHDP	International Human Dimensions Program on Global Environmental Change
IOM	Institute of Medicine
MCHB	Maternal and Child Health Bureau
MEPS	Medical Expenditure Panel Surveys
MMWR	Morbidity and Mortality Weekly Report
MTO	Moving to Opportunity
NCANDS	National Child Abuse and Neglect Data System
NCES	National Center for Education Statistics
NCHS	National Center for Health Statistics
NCQA	National Committee for Quality Assurance
NCVHS	National Committee on Vital and Health Statistics
NEDSS	National Electronic Disease Surveillance System
NEGP	National Education Goals Panel
NHANES	National Health and Nutrition Examination Survey
NHES	National Household Education Survey
NHII	National Health Information Infrastructure
NHIS	National Health Interview Survey

NHTS	National Household Travel Survey
NHTSA	National Highway Traffic Safety Administration
NICHD	National Institute of Child Health and Human Development
NIH	National Institutes of Health
NIMH	National Institute of Mental Health
NIS	National Immunization Survey
NLSY	National Longitudinal Survey of Youth
NPTS	National Personal Transportation Survey
NRC	National Research Council
NSCSHCN	National Survey of Children with Special Health Care Needs
NSECH	National Survey of Early Childhood Health
NSFG	National Survey of Family Growth
NSFH	National Survey of Families and Households
ODPP	Office of Disease Prevention and Health Promotion
OECD	Organisation for Economic Co-operation and Development
PCB	Polychlorinated biphenyl
PM	Particulate matter
RCD	Research Data Centers
SAMHSA	Substance Abuse and Mental Health Services Administration
SARS	Severe acute respiratory syndrome respiratory syndrome
SCHIP	State Child Health Insurance Program
SES	Socioeconomic status
SIDS	Sudden infant death syndrome
SIPP	Survey of Income and Program Participation
SLAITS	State and Local Area Integrated Telephone Survey
SRC	Social Research Council
TANF	Temporary Assistance for Needy Families
TIPP	The Injury Prevention Program
UNICEF	United Nations Children's Fund
USCB	U.S. Census Bureau
USDA	U.S. Department of Agriculture
WHO	World Health Organization
WIC	Women, Infants and Children
YRBS	Youth Risk Behavior Survey

Appendix F

Biographical Sketches
of Committee Members and Staff

Greg J. Duncan (*Cochair*) is the Edwina S. Tarry chair in the Human Development and Social Policy Program at Northwestern University. An economist, Duncan has compiled a long history of research on poverty and welfare dynamics and their linkages to children's development outcomes. Much of Duncan's career was spent at the University of Michigan working on and ultimately directing the Panel Study of Income Dynamics data collection project. He is coeditor of *Consequences of Growing Up Poor* (with Brooks-Gunn) and the two-volume *Neighborhood Poverty* (with Brooks-Gunn and Aber). At the National Research Council, he was a member of the Committee on Integrating the Science of Early Childhood Development, which produced *From Neurons to Neighborhoods: The Science of Early Child Development* in 2000. He has been a member of the Child and Family Well-Being Research Network of the National Institute of Child Health and Human Development since its inception in 1993. He has a Ph.D. in economics from the University of Michigan.

Ruth E.K. Stein (*Cochair*) is professor of pediatrics at the Albert Einstein College of Medicine and former vice chairman in the Department of Pediatrics at the Albert Einstein College of Medicine and Children's Hospital at Montefiore. Her research on children's health and children with chronic conditions has been supported by a number of federal agencies and private foundations. For over a decade she was director and principal investigator of the National Institute of Mental Health–supported Preventive Intervention Research Center for Child Health at Albert Einstein College of Medicine/Montefiore Medical Center. She has published extensively on children with chronic conditions and measurement of outcomes for child health. She was a charter member of the Board of Directors and its Executive Committee of the Center for Child Health of the American Academy of Pediatrics. She is the editor of *Caring for Children with Chronic Illness: Issues and Strategies* and *Health Care for Children: What's Right What's Wrong What's Next.* She is chair of the New York Forum on Child Health. At the National Academies, she served on the Committee on Pediatric Emergency Medical Services and is a member of the Board on Children, Youth, and Families. She has a B.A. from Barnard College and an M.D. from the Albert Einstein College of Medicine.

Yolie Flores Aguilar is executive director of the Los Angeles County Children's Planning Council, the nation's largest partnership network bringing together the public and private sectors in Los Angeles to improve conditions for children through data, planning, and coordination, and by developing and supporting partnerships and collaboratives. She has directed efforts to develop a children's scorecard for the county with five outcome areas and indicators of child well-being, and works to help communities translate data into action. She has served as a senior consultant to the Annie E. Casey Foundation and its Making Connections initiative. She is the former director of child care policy and planning for the City of Los Angeles and the former work/family director of the Los Angeles Department of Water and Power, a nationally acclaimed employer-supported child care and work/family program. Between 1995 and 2000, she served as president and member of the Los Angeles County Board of Education, and vice president of the Pediatric and Family Medical Center. She is a former Coro fellow, a Casey fellow, and is an active member of the Annie E. Casey Foundation Children and Families Fellowship Network. She is a graduate of the University of Redlands and has an M.S.W. from the University of California, Los Angeles.

Cynthia Bearer is associate professor of pediatrics and neurosciences in the Department of Pediatrics at Case Western Reserve University. She is board certified in both pediatrics and neonatal-perinatal medicine and is currently the director of the Neonatology Fellowship Training Program at Rainbow Babies and Children's Hospital and director of medical education of the Mary Ann Swetland Center for Environmental Health. Her primary research interests are the mechanisms of developmental neurotoxicity, cell adhesion molecules, and the development of biomarkers of prenatal exposures. She has served on the U.S. Environmental Protection Agency's scientific advisory board, the American Academy of Pediatrics' Committee on Environmental Health, and the advisory group to the director of the National Center on Environmental Health at the Centers for Disease Control and Prevention. She is currently on the editorial boards of *Neurotoxicology* and *Alcohol Research & Health*, serves as a member of the neurotoxicology and alcohol study section, is chair of the science committee of the Children's Environmental Health Network, and is president of the Fetal

Alcohol Syndrome Study Group. She has a Ph.D. in biochemistry from Case Western Reserve University and an M.D. from Johns Hopkins University.

Cynthia García Coll (*Consultant*) is the Charles Pitts Robinson and John Palmer Barstow Professor; Professor of Education, Psychology and Pediatrics at Brown University. She has published numerous articles on the sociocultural and biological influences on child development with particular emphasis on at-risk and minority populations. She has also been on the editorial boards of many academic journals. She was a member of the MacArthur Foundation Network called Successful Pathways Through Middle Childhood. At the Society for Research on Child Development, she served as both chair and member of the Committee on Racial and Ethnic Issues; on the Governing Council from 1996–2002; and as its representative to the National Head Start Research Conference Committee from 1994 to 2001. García Coll has co-edited several books, including *Mothering Against the Odds: Diverse Voices of Contemporary Mothers* and *Nature and Nurture: The Complex Interplay of Genetic and Environmental Influences on Human Behavior and Development.* A fellow of the American Psychological Association, she also was a coeditor of the special issue for the journal Child Development entitled "Children and Poverty." She is the incoming editor of Developmental Psychology and has a Ph.D. in developmental psychology from Harvard University (1982).

Neal Halfon is professor of pediatrics in the School of Medicine of Community Health Sciences in the School of Public Health, and Policy Studies in the School of Public Policy and Social Research at the University of California, Los Angeles (UCLA). He is currently director of the UCLA Center for Healthier Children, Families, and Communities and directs the Child and Family Health Program in the School of Public Health. He also directs the Maternal and Child Health Bureau's National Center for Infancy and Early Childhood Health Policy Research. His primary research interests include the provision of developmental services to young children, access to care for poor children, and delivery of health services to children with special health care needs, with particular interest in children who have been abused and neglected and are being cared for by the foster care system. He has published investigations of immunizations for inner-city children, the health care needs of children in foster care, trends in chronic illnesses for children, the delivery of health care services for children with asthma, as well as investigations of new models of health service delivery for high-risk children. His recent work has focused on life-course models of health development. At the National Academies, he is a member of the Board on Children, Youth, and Families. He has an M.D. from the University of California, Davis, and an M.P.H. from the University of California, Berkeley and completed his residency in Pediatrics at the University of California, San Diego, and the University of California, San Francisco.

Peter Jensen is the director of the Center for the Advancement of Children's Mental Health—Putting Science to Work, and Ruane professor of child psychiatry at the Columbia University College of Physicians and Surgeons. Previously he was the associate director of child and adolescent research at the National Institute of Mental Health (NIMH). While at NIMH, he served as the lead investigator on the six-site study of Multimodal Treatment of ADHD (the MTA Study) and also as an investigator on other NIMH multisite studies. Dr. Jensen's current major areas of research include the integration of research findings into clinical settings, effectiveness and dissemination research, and studies of optimal approaches to facilitate the adoption of evidence-based mental health approaches by practitioners and parents on behalf of children with mental disorders. The author of over 200 scientific articles, book chapters, and editor or co-editor of a dozen books, Dr. Jensen has received many national awards for his research, writing, and teaching, including awards from the American Academy of Child and Adolescent Psychiatry, the American Psychiatric Association, the American Psychological Association, and family advocacy organizations including the National Alliance for the Mentally Ill and Children and Adults with Attention-Deficit/Hyperactivity Disorder. He has a bachelor's degree (cum laude) from Brigham Young University and an M.D. from George Washington University Medical School. He did his postgraduate training at the Letterman Army Medical Center and the University of California, San Francisco.

Donald Mattison is senior advisor to the director of the National Institute of Child Health and Human Development (NICHD) and Acting Chief of the Obstetrics and Pediatrics Pharmacology Research Branch in the Center for Research for Mothers and Children. In this role he chairs the advisory committee for the National Children's Study and provides oversight to the obstetrical and pediatric pharmacology programs of NICHD. Previously, he was medical director of the March of Dimes, and prior to that dean of the Graduate School of Public Health at the University of Pittsburgh, where he was professor of environmental and occupational health. He serves on various national committees related to environmental health, public health, and disease prevention, including the Children's Environmental Health Advisory Committee of the U.S. Environmental Protection Agency and the Collegiate Commission on Nursing Education, and was chair of the Board on Health Promotion and Disease Prevention of the Institute of Medicine. He is a fellow of the American Association for the Advancement of Science and the New York Academy of Medicine and a member of the Institute of Medicine. He is the author of numerous scientific journal articles, and coedited the seminal contribution on *Male Mediated Developmental Toxicology*. He has a B.A. from Augsburg College in Minnesota, an M.S. from the Massachusetts Institute of Technology, and an M.D. from the College of Physicians and Surgeons, Columbia University. He is a diplomat of the American Board of Toxicology and a fellow of the Academy of Toxicological Sciences.

Mary Ellen O'Connell (*Study Director*) is a senior program officer with the Board on Children, Youth, and Families. Her work with the board includes development of two standalone workshops, on welfare reform and children and gun violence. She was also the study director for the Committee on Developing a Strategy to Reduce and Prevent Underage Drinking and currently serves as study director for the Committee on Housing-Related Health Hazard Research Involving Children, Youth, and Families. Previously she worked at the U.S. Department of Health and Human Services (HHS), where she spent eight years in the Office of the Assistant Secretary for Planning and Evaluation (ASPE), most recently as director of state and local initiatives. During her tenure in ASPE, Mary Ellen focused on data, research, and policy related to homelessness and community-based health decision making. Prior to HHS, she worked at the U.S. Department of Housing and Urban Development on homeless policy and program design issues. She has a B.A. (with distinction) from Cornell University and an M.A. in the management of human services from the Heller School at Brandeis University.

Peter Simon is assistant medical director, Rhode Island Department of Health. He also is the deputy medical director of the Division of Family Health and the medical director of the Childhood Lead Poisoning Prevention Program and the Newborn Screening Programs. His programmatic responsibilities range across the spectrum of core public health functions for the traditional maternal and child health populations. He is certified by the American Board of Preventive Medicine and the American Board of Pediatrics. He has had multiple roles with the Title V program at the state, regional, and national level as well as serving the American Academy of Pediatrics at the state and national levels. He served as the chairman of the local chapter of the American Academy of Pediatrics and presently coedits the chapter newsletter and serves as the CATCH (Community Access to Child Health) coordinator. Since giving up his private practice in 1985, he continues to see pediatric patients at the Providence Community Health Centers and volunteers at the Hospital Albert Schweitzer in rural Haiti. He has an undergraduate degree from Cornell University, an M.P.H. from Johns Hopkins University (1976), and an M.D. from the State University of New York, Upstate Medical School.

Bonita Stanton is professor and Schotanus family chairperson of the Department of Pediatrics at Wayne State University. Previously she was professor and chairperson at West Virginia University and had been professor of pediatrics at the University of Maryland School of Medicine. She has published extensively in the fields of risk prevention, behavioral change, vaccine development, diarrheal diseases, and maternal child health care. She serves on the editorial board of *Youth and Society* and has served on advisory boards and study sections to numerous organizations, including the Child Health Foundation and the National

Institutes of Health. She has consulted with numerous national and international groups on issues related to urban health, HIV/AIDS transmission in youth, and health services research. Her special interests are pediatric infectious diseases, AIDS, HIV prevention in adolescents, and adolescent risk reduction low-income adolescents and community health. She has a B.A. (magna cum laude) from Wellesley College and an M.D. (cum laude) from Yale University; she completed her pediatric residency at the University Hospitals of Cleveland.

Barbara Starfield, a physician and health services researcher, is university distinguished professor and professor of health policy and pediatrics at Johns Hopkins University. Internationally known for her work in primary care, her books *Primary Care: Concept, Evaluation, and Policy* and *Primary Care: Balancing Health Needs, Services, and Technology* are widely recognized as the seminal works in the field. She has been instrumental in leading projects to develop important methodological tools, including the Primary Care Assessment Tool, the CHIP tools (to assess adolescent and child health status), and the Johns Hopkins Adjusted Clinical Groups for assessment of diagnosed morbidity burdens reflecting degrees of comorbidity. She was the codeveloper and first president of the International Society for Equity in Health, a scientific organization devoted to furthering knowledge about the determinants of inequity in health and ways to eliminate them. Her work thus focuses on quality of care, health status assessment, primary care evaluation, and equity in health. She is a member of the Institute of Medicine and has been on its governing council, as well as on the National Committee on Vital and Health Statistics, and many other government and professional committees and groups. She has a B.A. from Swarthmore College, an M.D. from the State University of New York, Downstate Medical Center, and an M.P.H. from Johns Hopkins University School of Public Health.

Fredia Stovall Wadley is medical director for the Delmarva Foundation for Medical Care, a not-for-profit organization with a mission to improve health care and human services. Previously she served as commissioner of the Tennessee Department of Health and the director of the Nashville/Davidson County Metropolitan Health Department. Her academic affiliations include the University of Tennessee Center for Health Sciences (Pediatric Department), Meharry Medical College (Pediatrics and Preventive Medicine), East Tennessee State University (Preventive Medicine), the University of Tennessee, and Vanderbilt Schools of Nursing; she is a board member of the Vanderbilt Children's Hospital. Her areas of interest include early intervention services for children, health services for foster children, and integrating children's health data across multiple departments of state government. She is currently a board member of the Public Health Foundation, has served on various committees of the Association of State and Territorial Health Officials and the National Association for State Health Policy, has been on the board of directors for a hospital managing corporation, and received recognition for accomplishments in public health and improving the health for children in Tennessee. She has an M.D. from the University of Tennessee Center for Health Sciences and an M.A. in health planning and administration from the University of Cincinnati.

Michelle Williams is professor of epidemiology at the University of Washington, School of Public Health and Community Medicine. Her areas of expertise are reproductive and perinatal epidemiology. Her current research involves identifying genetic and nongenetic biological markers of placental pathology and relating those markers to potentially modifiable exogenous risk factors of adverse pregnancy outcomes, including preterm delivery, abruptio placentae, pregnancy-induced hypertension (preeclampsia), and gestational diabetes. As codirector of the Center for Perinatal Studies at Swedish Medical Center, her current research includes both clinical epidemiological studies, such as assessment of prenatal screening protocols for diagnosing birth defects and infant chromosomal abnormalities. She is director of the university's Multidisciplinary International Research Training Program, which provides research training opportunities to undergraduate and graduate students. She has a B.A. from Princeton University, an M.S. from Tufts University and S.M. and Sc.D. degrees from Harvard University.

Index

Academic performance
  health outcomes and, 76
  parental educational attainment, 133–134
  parental influences, 72
  television/video viewing and, 80–81
Access to care, 84, 88–89, 152, 153
Accidents and injuries, 2
  built environment design and, 66–67
  childhood risk, 64–65
  health care utilization related to, 65
  mortality, 15, 64–65
  prevention, 65, 87
  trends, 65
  workplace, 64
Adherence to treatment, 55–57
Administration for Children and Families, 66, 100, 197
Agency for Healthcare Research and Quality, 6, 93–94, 99, 156–157, 197, 205
Age-related subpopulations, 113
  biomarkers of susceptibility, 120
Aggregated data systems, 167–170, 205, 207–208
Aggressive behavior
  electronic entertainments and, 79
  parenting style and, 71
  See also Violence
Air pollutants, 59, 64, 67
  recommendations for research, 9, 203

Alcohol use and abuse
  during pregnancy, 58
  genetic factors, 48, 49
  parental, 73
All Kids Count, 101, 173–174
Allergies, 50
American Community Survey, 9, 137, 203
Annie E. Casey Foundation, 98
Antibiotic resistance, 62
Arboviruses, 62
Asbestos, 64
Asthma, 2
  hygiene theory, 50
Attachment formation and development, 54–55, 71
Attention deficit disorder, 2
Attitudes and beliefs, 126–127
  assessing perceptions of built environment, 132
  in chronic illness, 56
  influence on health, 54, 55–56, 126–127
  interventions targeting, 56
  measurement, 126
Automobile accidents, 65, 66–67, 132

Back to Sleep campaign, 158
Bacteria, 59

Behavioral factors in children's health, 45
    adaptation in development, 54–55
    behavior as health outcome and, 57, 128–
        129
    cognitive factors, 54, 55–56, 126–127
    conceptual model of health, 3–4, 38–49,
        40–43
    current data sources, 125–127
    early programming concept, 53
    education and, 76
    emotion-related factors, 54
    environmental influences and, 56–57, 132
    genetic influences and, 31, 48
    importance of, 57, 128
    measurement, 124–129
    scope of, 53
    See also Influences on children's health
Behavioral Risk Factor Surveillance Survey,
    208
Biological influences on children's health, 45
    body stores, 51–52
    conceptual model of health, 3–4, 38–49,
        40–43
    early programming concept, 52–53
    future prospects for noninvasive
        assessment, 124
    genetic factors, 47–51
    interaction with external environment, 47,
        48–51
    measurement, 118–124
    See also Influences on children's health
Biomarkers, 7, 118–124, 158, 209
Body burden, 51–52
    biomonitoring programs, 120–121
Built environment, 66–67, 77–78, 131–133

Canada, 159–160, 183
Cat scratch disease, 62–63
Census Bureau, 9, 137, 180, 181, 203
Centers for Disease Control and Prevention,
    5–6, 92, 120, 121, 187, 197, 205
Chemical exposures, 129–130, 209
Child abuse and neglect, 73, 134–135
Child and Adolescent Health Measurement
    Initiative, 151
Child Health USA, 97–98
Child Trends, Inc., 98
Child Well-Being and Welfare, 134
Children, defined, 2, 18
Children's ScoreCard, 169–170, 171

Chronic health conditions
    current health measurement system, 92
    prevalence, 14
    treatment compliance in, 56
CityMatCH, 100–101
Cognitive functioning, 36
    attitudes and beliefs as health
        determinants, 54, 55–56
    electronic entertainments and, 80–81
    influence on child's health, 53
    toxin exposures affecting, 51
Coining, 82
Committee on Evaluation of Children's
    Health: Measures of Risk, Protective,
    and Promotional Factors for Assessing
    Child Health in the Community,
    17–18
Community environment
    data collection and management, 100–101,
        137–142, 169–170, 185–186, 189
    demographic factors, 74–75, 137
    health care service delivery system, 152–153
    health measurement considerations, 25
    influences on health, 74
    neighborhood design, 77–78, 131–133
    process factors, 75
    recommendations for research, 8–9, 203–
        204
    report cards, 170, 171
    schools, 76
    scope of, 74
    social organization, 77–78, 137–138
    violence in, 77, 138–139, 141
    See also State and local data collection
Comorbidity, 102
Computer and video games, 78–81
Confidentiality, 109, 176–178
    in aggregated data systems, 167
    in assessment and monitoring of health
        influences, 117
    of geocoded data, 9, 203, 204
    informed consent for sharing of data, 178–
        179
    in linked data systems, 172–173
    recommendations for research, 9–10, 204
    security of data systems, 179–180
Consumer Assessment of Health Plans Survey,
    151, 187
Cost of care, 149
Crime, 203, 204
    law enforcement data, 169–170

Critical periods, 39, 50–51
    early programming, 52–53
    in fetal development, 58
Culture, 24–25
    acculturation effects, 143, 145, 202
    concepts of children and children's health,
        28–29
    definition, 81, 143
    family beliefs, 68
    family learning environment, 72
    health measurement considerations, 43,
        81–83, 108, 118, 142–146, 200, 202
    parenting style, 71
    research needs, 209
    treatment compliance and, 57
Cupping, 82
Current Population Survey, 133, 135, 143
Cystic fibrosis, 49, 85
Cytomegalovirus, 62

Data collection
    on access to care, 152, 153
    access to data, 9–10, 168–169, 178–180,
        189–191, 203, 204, 205
    assessing effectiveness of health services,
        150, 151–152, 153
    on behavioral influences on health, 124–129
    on biological influences on health, 118–124
    biological samples, 121–123, 124, 180–182
    on built environment, 131–133
    on child functioning, 103, 113, 199
    clinical data, inadequacies in, 98–100, 102–
        103, 136
    on community influences on health, 100–
        101, 137–142
    competing stakeholder interests in, 185
    confidentiality in, 9–10, 109, 176–178
    creating profiles and integrative measures of
        health, 104–106, 154–155, 158–159, 165
    on cultural factors, 43, 81–83, 108, 118,
        142–146, 200, 202
    current system, 1, 12, 21, 26–27, 91–101,
        193, 199
    discrimination effects, 146–149
    environmental factors, 8–9, 199–200, 203–
        204
    family factors, 133–137
    future prospects, 124, 209
    geographic variation, 8–9, 203–204
    on health conditions, 102–103
    on health potential, 103–104, 199

    health-related quality of life, 105
    informed consent issues, 178–179
    infrastructure for, 183–185
    investigator-initiated surveys, 95–96, 126
    to monitor health policy outcomes, 25,
        149–150, 155–162
    national data syntheses, 97–98
    newborn screen testing, 120, 180–181
    as ongoing effort, 159–160
    on positive factors, 114, 118
    proxy respondents, 107
    rationale, 165–166, 192–193
    recommendations for, 5–9, 196–204
    on referrals from primary care to
        specialists, 154
    reliability and validity, 107–109
    security concerns, 179–180
    standardization, 10–11, 182–183, 204–205,
        206, 207–208
    state and local government role in, 206–208
    on subgroup disparities, 8, 118, 201–202
    survey methodology, inadequacies in, 95,
        96–97, 102–103, 109, 110, 117–118
    terminology, 165
    toxin exposure, 120–121, 129–130
    See also Measurement system for children's
        health; State and local data collection
Data element, defined, 165
Data system, defined, 165
Dataset, defined, 165
David and Lucile Packard Foundation, 100
Definition and framework for children's
        health, 12, 13–14, 17, 18, 19–20, 26
    conceptual model of health, 37–38, 41–43
    cultural variation, 24–25
    current conceptualizations, 32–33
    domains of health, 4, 6, 33–37, 195, 199
    historical and conceptual development,
        28–32
    implications for measurement, 13–14, 197–
        198
    policy development and, 160–161
    recommendations, 3–5, 194–196
Department of Health and Human Services, 5–
        6, 9, 10, 196–197, 203, 204–205
Depression, 69
    parental, 72–73
Developing a Daddy Survey, 96
Development, 12
    assessing discrimination effects, 146–147
    behavioral adaptation in, 54–55, 127

body stores and, 51–52
childhood precursors of adult health, 24,
    40, 114, 192
conceptual model of health, 3–5, 38–40,
    41–43, 45–46, 192, 194–196
considerations in measurement of
    children's health, 6, 12, 39, 107, 108–
    109, 110–112, 113, 192, 199, 208–209
dependency of children, 23
early programming concept, 52–53
family influence and, 69
gene expression patterns, 50–51
parenting and, 71
peer influences, 78
rationale for children's health research, 22–
    24
sensitive and critical periods, 39, 49–50
sociocultural context, 29
transition stages, 40, 112
Diabetes, 2
Diagnostic classification, 30
inadequacies in children's health data
    collection, 98–100, 102–103
Diet and nutrition
    biomonitoring program, 121
    during pregnancy, 52–53
    early programming concept, 52–53
    family factors in, 72
    fetal exposure to toxins, 59
    food contaminants, 61–62
    television viewing and, 80
Dioxin exposure, 121
Disability-adjusted life years, 105–106
Disadvantaged groups
    assessing effectiveness of health policies,
        157–158
    current disparities in health care delivery, 15
    opportunities for improving health
        measurement, 112
    poverty and health, 69–70
    recommendations for children's health
        measurement, 7, 8, 201
    See also Minority populations
Discrimination, 82–83
    measuring health effects of, 146–149
    research challenges, 146, 147–148
    research needs, 148–149
    stress of worrying about, 148
Divorce, 70
Domains of children's health, 4, 6, 33–37, 43,
    101–104, 195, 199

Drinking water, 58–61, 87, 88
Drug use and abuse
    current data collection efforts, 126
    during pregnancy, 58
    parental, 73
    See also Alcohol use and abuse

Early Childhood Comprehensive Systems
    Initiative, 155
Early Childhood Longitudinal Studies,
    8, 199
Early Childhood Longitudinal Study, 96, 127
    Birth Cohort, 96, 127
    Kindergarten Class, 96, 127
Early intervention, 84, 155
Early warning, 3, 16–17, 194, 198
Economic analysis, 105–106
Electronic media, 78–81
Emotional functioning, 36
    behavioral adaptation in development, 55
    inadequacies in children's health data
        collection, 102–103
    influence on child's health, 53, 54
    treatment compliance and, 56
Empacho, 82
Environmental factors, 3–4, 14
    assessing effects of environmental policy, 158
    behavioral influences on health and, 56–57,
        132
    built environment, 66–67, 77–78, 131–133
    community environment, 74–78, 137–142
    concept of safety, 19
    in conceptual model of health, 3–4, 195
    culture, 81–83, 142–146
    emotional response to, as health influence,
        54
    family factors, 68–73
    health influence of, 14, 57
    home exposures, 64
    injury risk, 64–65
    interaction with biological factors, 47, 48–
        51
    measurement of health influence of, 6–7,
        129–133, 199–200
    noise exposure, 63
    radiation exposure, 63
    recommendations for children's health
        measurement, 8–9, 203–204
    recommendations for research, 11–12, 208,
        209
    school exposures, 64

scope of, 45, 57
shortcomings of current measurement
   system, 7, 158, 162
workplace exposures, 58, 64, 130
See also Toxin exposure
Environmental Protection Agency, 9, 98, 203,
   208

Families
   composition, 70
   data collection and analysis, 133–137
   demographic factors, 68, 69–70
   influence on children's health, 68–69
   learning environment, 72
   parental mental health, 72–73
   parental substance abuse, 73
   process factors, 68, 71–73
   See also Parent–child interaction
Federal Education Right to Privacy Act, 177–
   178
Federal government
   data collection efforts, 92–100, 184, 186–
      189
   historical evolution of child protection
      policies, 29–30
   recommendations for agencies and
      departments, 5–6, 9, 10, 11–12, 196–
      197, 203, 204–205, 208–210
   spending on children, 149
   standardization of health data, 182
   support for state and local data collection,
      10, 204–206
Federal Interagency Forum in Child and
   Family Statistics, 98, 197
Fetal alcohol syndrome, 58
Fetal development. *See* Prenatal health
Florida Children's Registry and Information
   System, 173, 174
Fluoridation of drinking water, 87, 88
Folate, 51
Folic acid, 85
Forecasting, 3
Foster care, 153, 173
Foundation for Accountability, 151
Fragile Families and Child Well-Being Study,
   95–96
Functioning domain of health, 4, 35–37
   inadequacies in children's health data
      collection, 103, 199
   measurement, 7, 8, 11–12, 113–114, 199, 201
Furan exposure, 121

Galactosemia, 120
Genetics, 45
   behavior and, 48
   disorders of, 47–48
   ethics issues regarding genetic data, 181–
      182
   gene expression biology, 50–51
   influence on health, 20
   interaction with environmental exposures,
      48–51
   screening, 121
   susceptibility genes, 49, 120
Geographical variation
   current data collection, 17, 169–170, 185–
      186
   recommendations for data collection, 8–9,
      203–204
   shortcomings of behavioral data collection,
      129
Growth curve analysis, 210

Health care system
   assessing effectiveness of service delivery, 3,
      25, 149–155, 194
   community service system, 152–153
   effectiveness of health services, 83–85, 87
   evolution of children's health services, 29–
      32
   goals for monitoring, 3, 151, 193–194
   inappropriate interventions, 150
   rationale for children's health research, 21–
      25, 192–193, 210
   referrals from primary care to specialist, 154
   research needs, 154–155
   services for special populations, 153
   shortcomings and accomplishments, 1–2,
      13–16
   types of health services for children,
      85–87
Health conditions, 4, 34–35, 102–103
Health Employer Data Information System,
   151–152
Health Insurance Portability and
   Accountability Act, 178
Health Interview Survey, 149
Health potential, 4, 35, 37
   inadequacies in children's health data
      collection, 103–104, 199
   measurement, 7, 8, 12, 199, 201
Health-related behaviors, 53–54
   access to care, 84

attitudes and beliefs as determinant of, 54, 55–56
cultural influences, 81–82
data collection and security, 179
Health Resources and Services Administration, 5, 94, 197
Healthy People 2010 initiative, 4, 37, 41, 98, 158–159, 170, 196
Hearing, 49
childhood noise exposure, 63
Hemoglobinopathies, 120
Huntington's disease, 48
Hyperphenylalaninemia, 120
Hypothyroidism, 120

Immigrant paradox, 82
Immune function, hygiene theory of, 50
Immunization, 14, 29, 84–85
Infectious disease, 1–2
childhood risk, 62–63
current health measurement system, 92
food contaminants, 61–62
vector-borne, 62–63
water-borne disease, 59
Influences on children's health, 20–21, 26
behavioral, 3–4, 45, 53–57
biological, 3–4, 45, 47–53
challenges in assessment and monitoring of, 116–118, 121–124, 127–128, 133, 135–136, 139–140, 143–144, 152–153, 160–161
conceptual model of health, 3–5, 37–38, 41–43, 45–47, 192, 195–196
cultural environment, 81–83, 142–146
definition of health and, 32
developmental, 23, 38–40, 41–43, 45–46
discrimination experience, 83, 146–149
electronic media, 78–81
family factors, 67–73, 133–137
health services delivery, 83–87, 149–155
interactions among, 4, 30–31, 40–41, 46, 47, 117, 147, 161, 195, 196, 200
limitations of research on, 46–47, 198–199
measurement system goals, 6, 16–17, 196
policy environment, 87–90
research needs, 90, 162–163, 200–201, 210
scope of, 45
See also Environmental factors
Informed consent, 178–179
Insecticides. *See* Pesticides and insecticides

Insurance, 88–89, 157
datasets, 98–99
Integrated measurement system, 104–106, 154–155, 165, 205–206
aggregated data systems, 167–170
confidentiality issues, 167, 172–173, 176–178
defined, 165
future prospects, 166–167, 188–189
Internet access, 168–169
linked data systems, 170–175
rationale, 165–166
recommendations for, 11, 207–208
resource needs, 184
strategies, 167
International Classification of Diseases of Related Health Problems, 30, 35
International Classification of Functioning, Disability and Health, 103
International Classification of Primary Care, 103
International comparisons
children's health, 14, 15–16
health measurement, 159
Internet, 168–169, 189–191, 205
Intervention in children's health
access, 84
assessing effectiveness of service delivery, 149–155
compliance, 56
conceptual and clinical evolution, 30–31
early intervention services, 84, 155
effectiveness of health services, 83–85, 87
injury prevention, 65, 66–67
to prevent adult morbidity, 24
sociocultural differences, 25
spending, 149
types of, 85–87
Investigator-initiated surveys, 95–96, 126
Iron, 51–52

KIDS COUNT, 98, 170
KIDSNET, 173–174, 175

Language skills, 72
Law enforcement data, 169–170
Lead, 14, 51, 60–61
Life-style-related health conditions, 127
Linked data systems, 170–175, 176–178, 184
geocoding, 9, 203, 204

Low birthweight babies, 15–16
  current health measurement system, 91
Lyme disease, 62

Maine Marks, 190
Mandated reporting, 92, 176
Mass media, 78–81
MassCHIP, 170, 172
Maternal and Child Health Bureau, 5, 94, 97–
  98, 100, 113, 155, 156–157, 186–187,
  197, 205
Measurement system for children's health
  assessing effectiveness of service delivery,
    149–155
  challenges in assessment and monitoring of
    health influences, 116–118, 121–124,
    127–128, 133, 135–136, 139–140, 143–
    144, 146–148, 152–153, 160–161
  conceptualization gaps, 106–107
  coordination and linkage among studies,
    96, 97
  criteria for, 43–44
  current system, 6–7, 26–27, 91–101, 193
  definition of health in, 13–14, 19–20, 197–
    198
  developmental considerations, 39, 107,
    108–109, 110–112, 113, 192, 199
  domains of health, 33–37, 43
  goals, 2–3, 114–115, 193–194, 198
  historical development, 30, 31–32
  international comparison, 159
  methodological gaps, 107–110, 209, 210
  opportunities for improving, 101–114,
    162–163
  rationale, 1, 2, 16–17, 21, 192–193, 210
  recommendations, 9–12, 204–210
  See also Data collection; Integrated
    measurement system
Medicaid, 89, 149, 151, 157, 178, 182
Medical Expenditure Panel Surveys, 94, 157
Melanoma, 63
Meningitis, 85
Mental health, 2, 36
  behavioral assessment, 128–129
  discrimination experience and, 83
  parental, 72–73
  prevalence of disorders, 14
  service delivery, 153
  socioeconomic status and, 69
Mercury, 51

Minority populations
  current disparities in health care delivery, 15
  data collection, 134, 142–146
  discrimination, 82–83, 146–149
  recommendations for children's health
    measurement, 8, 200
  See also Disadvantaged groups
Monitoring the Future, 126
Monoamine oxidase, 49
Mortality
  automobile accident-related, 65
  childhood, 64–65
  community violence, 77
  current health measurement system, 91
  current patterns, 15
  health care system performance to date, 1–
    2, 14–15
  infant, 158
  infectious disease, 62
  injury-related, 15, 64–65
  international comparisons, 15–16
  socioeconomic status and, 69
  workplace, 64

National Action Alliance, 184–185
National Center for Educational Statistics, 96
National Center for Environmental Health, 95
National Center for Health Statistics, 5–6, 92–
  94, 156–157, 166, 197, 205
National Child Abuse and Neglect Data
  System, 134–135
National Children's Study, 8, 96, 199, 201
National Committee on Quality Assurance,
  151–152
National Committee on Vital and Health
  Statistics, 187, 207
National Electronic Disease Surveillance
  System, 187, 207
National Health and Nutrition Examination
  Survey, 8, 93, 110, 113, 120, 121, 124,
  125, 149, 199
National Health Information Infrastructure,
  187–188
National Health Interview Survey, 8, 92, 93,
  113, 125, 157, 199, 200
National Hospital Discharge Data Set, 99
National Household Education Surveys, 96
National Household Survey of Drug Use and
  Health, 94, 126
National Household Travel Survey, 132

National Immunization Survey, 93
National Institute for Child Health and
    Human Development, 6, 96, 197
National Institutes of Health, 6, 95, 197
National Labor Survey on Youth, 126
National Longitudinal Survey of Adolescent
    Health, 95, 126, 139
National Longitudinal Survey of Youth, 149
National Survey of Children with Special
    Health Care Needs, 134, 150
National Survey of Children's Health, 95, 150
National Survey of Early Childhood Health,
    94, 113, 134, 150
Nephron development, 52–53
No Child Left Behind Act, 182–183
Noise exposure, 63

Obesity, 2
    electronic entertainments and, 79–80
    prevalence, 14
Odor analysis, 124
Office of Disease Prevention and Health
    Promotion, 6, 197
Office of the Assistant Secretary for Planning
    and Evaluation, 6, 98, 197
Otitis media, 84–85
Ozone, 67

Parent–child interaction
    adaptations in development, 54–55
    attachment formation, 54–55, 71
    child development and, 71
    child health-related behaviors and, 54
    data collection, 134
    early programming concept, 53
    influence on child's health, 71
    maternal substance abuse and, 73
    parental depression and, 72–73
    parental monitoring, 69
    parenting styles, 71
    See also Families
Peer relations, 78, 139, 141–142
Perfect pitch, 49
Persistent organic pollutants, 121
Pesticides and insecticides, 59, 62, 121
Pets, 62–63
Phenylketonuria, 85
Phobias, 48
Phthalate metabolite, 121
Physical activity, 36
    built environment and, 67, 131, 132

electronic entertainments and, 79–80
    school physical education programs, 76
Phytoestrogens, 121
Playground injuries, 65
Policy development
    historical concepts of children and
        children's health, 29–30
    influence on children's health, 87–90
    integrated data systems for, 165–166, 167
    measurement system goals, 3, 198
    monitoring policy effects, 25, 155–162
    to promote health-related behaviors, 53–54
    risk assessment in, 161
    role of data collection and analysis, 1, 16–
        17, 25–26, 117, 149–150
Polyaromatic hydrocarbons, 121
Polychlorinated biphenyls, 51, 52, 121
Population subgroups
    age-related, 113
    current health disparities among, 15
    data collection and management, 167
    health services for special populations, 153
    opportunities for improving health
        measurement, 112–114, 144–146
    origins and development of health
        disparities among, 8
    profiles and integrative measures of health,
        104
    recommendations for children's health
        measurement, 8, 200, 201–202
    shortcomings of current health
        measurement system, 7, 46–47, 118,
        142–144
    sources of health disparities, 202, 209
    types of, 202
    vulnerable subpopulations, 112
    See also Disadvantaged groups; Minority
        populations
Pornography, 80
Pregnancy
    among unmarried women, 70
    teenage, 14, 15
    See also Prenatal health
Prenatal health, 18, 45
    early programming, 52–53
    recommendations for data collection, 201
    toxin exposures, 51–52, 58–59
Profiles of health, 104, 105–106
Project on Human Development in Chicago's
    Neighborhoods, 138
Promoting Healthy Development Survey, 151

Protective factors
  behavioral, 53–54
  environmental exposures, 51–52
  genetic, 49
  health potential conceptualization, 37
  measurement, 114, 118
  See also Influences on children's health;
    Resilience factors
Psychosocial functioning. *See* Mental health;
    Social functioning
Public health departments, 166, 167, 206

Quality of care, 150–152
Quality of life, 105

Racial and ethnic minorities. *See* Minority
    populations
Radiation exposure, 63
Radon, 63, 64, 130
Reading skills, 72
Referrals, from primary care to specialist, 154
Reliability of data collection methodology,
    107–109
Religion and spirituality, 71–72
Report cards, 169–170, 171
Research
  access to health data, 9–10, 168–169, 178–
    180, 189–191, 203, 204, 205
  rationale for children's health research, 21–
    25, 192–193, 210
  recommendations for, 3, 6, 11–12, 200–
    201, 208–210
  See also Data collection
Resilience factors, 37
  cultural, 82–83
  families as, 68–69
  measurement, 104, 114
  measurement system goals, 198
  See also Protective factors
Respiratory syncytial virus, 62
Risk factors
  behavioral, 53–54
  behavioral assessment, 128–129
  biomarkers of susceptibility, 120
  cultural, 82–83
  environmental exposures, 51–52
  evaluation in policy development, 161
  families as, 68–69
  genetic, 48–49
  health potential conceptualization, 37
  parenting style, 71

socioeconomic status, 69–70, 74–75
  See also Influences on children's health
Robert Wood Johnson Foundation, 101, 173–
    174
Rocky Mountain spotted fever, 62

Safety, defined, 19
Schools and schooling, 64, 76, 78
  child behavior data collection, 125–126, 127
  confidentiality of education data, 177–178,
    179
  school readiness measures, 205–206
  standardization of education data, 182–183
Score cards, 169–170, 171
Screening, newborn, 120
Sensitive periods, 39
  early programming, 52–53
Sexual behavior
  media portrayals, 80
  sexually transmitted disease, 92
  teen pregnancy, 14, 15
Sickle cell trait, 49
Single-parent families, 70
Sleep disorders, 48
Social functioning, 36
  behavioral adaptation in development, 55
  community interaction and organization,
    75, 77–78, 137–142
  family influences on health, 68–73, 133–137
  genetic factors in, 49
  peer relations, 78, 139, 141–142
Social Security Act, 178
Socioeconomic status, 45
  community characteristics, 74–75, 203
  current health disparities, 15, 69
  data collection, 133–134, 135–136, 137,
    202, 203
  influence on health, 69–70
  opportunities for improving health
    measurement, 112
  recommendations for children's health
    measurement, 8
  welfare policy, 90
  See also Disadvantaged groups
Special populations, 3
State and Local Area Integrated Telephone
    Survey, 94–95, 187, 188
State and local data collection
  access, 168–169
  administrative structure, 10–11, 191, 206–
    207